Essentials of Cancer Survivorship

Essentials of Cancer Survivorship

A Guide for Medical Professionals

Edited by Lidia Schapira, MD, FASCO

Professor of Medicine at Stanford University School of Medicine

Director of Cancer Survivorship at the Stanford Comprehensive
Cancer Center and Stanford Cancer Institute, Stanford, CA

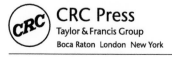

CRC Press
Taylor & Francis Group
Boca Raton London New York

CRC Press is an imprint of the
Taylor & Francis Group, an **informa** business

CRC Press
Boca Raton and London
First edition published 2022

by CRC Press
6000 Broken Sound Parkway NW, Suite 300, Boca Raton, FL 33487-2742
and by CRC Press

2 Park Square, Milton Park, Abingdon, Oxon, OX14 4RN

© 2022 Taylor & Francis Group, LLC

CRC Press is an imprint of Taylor & Francis Group, LLC

Library of Congress Cataloging-in-Publication Data

Names: Schapira, Lidia, editor.
Title: Essentials of cancer survivorship: a guide for medical professionals / edited by Lidia Schapira.
Description: First edition. | Boca Raton: CRC Press, 2021. | Includes bibliographical references and index. |
Summary: "This new concise guide is intended for cancer clinicians as well as generalists and specialists who meet cancer survivors in their practices for routine check-ups or specialized consultations"— Provided by publisher.
Identifiers: LCCN 2021031151 (print) | LCCN 2021031152 (ebook) | ISBN 9780367518509 (hardback) | ISBN 9780367518486 (paperback) | ISBN 9781003055426 (ebook)
Subjects: MESH: Cancer Survivors—psychology | Rehabilitation—methods | Needs Assessment
Classification: LCC RC271.M4 (print) | LCC RC271.M4 (ebook) | NLM QZ 260 | DDC 616.99/40651—dc23
LC record available at https://lccn.loc.gov/2021031151
LC ebook record available at https://lccn.loc.gov/2021031152

ISBN: 978-0-367-51850-9 (hbk)
ISBN: 978-0-367-51848-6 (pbk)
ISBN: 978-1-003-05542-6 (ebk)

DOI: 10.1201/9781003055426

Typeset in Times LT Std
by KnowledgeWorks Global Ltd.

Contents

Contributors

Catherine Benedict, PhD
Psychiatry and Behavioral Sciences
Stanford University School of Medicine
Stanford, CA

Roberto M. Benzo, PhD
Sylvester Comprehensive Cancer Center
Miller School of Medicine
University of Miami, FL

Phyllis Butow, PhD
Psycho-Oncology Co-operative Research Group
    (PoCoG) and School of Psychology
University of Sydney
Sydney, Australia

**Martin Chasen, MD, MBChB, FCP(SA), MPhil
(Pall Med)**
Survivorship and Palliative Medicine
William Osler Health System
Brampton
and Department of Family Medicine and
    Community Health
University of Toronto
Toronto, ON, Canada

Susan Dent, MD, FRCPC
Duke Cancer Center and Duke Cancer Center
    Breast Clinic
Duke University
Durham, NC

Kathleen Gali, PhD
Stanford Prevention Research Center
Stanford University
Stanford, CA

Madeline Graf, MS, CGC
Department of Pediatrics
Stanford University School of Medicine
Stanford, CA

Avirup Guha, MD, RPVI, FACC
Harrington Heart and Vascular Institute
Case Western Reserve University
Cleveland, OH

Rebecca A. Harrison, MD
Department of Neuro-Oncology
University of Texas MD Anderson Cancer
    Center
Houston, TX

Tara O. Henderson, MD, MPH
Department of Pediatrics and Childhood
    Cancer Survivor Center at The University
    of Chicago
Chicago, IL

Doris Howell, RN, PhD, FAAN
Princess Margaret Cancer Centre
ELLICSR Health, Wellness and Survivorship
    Centre
Lawrence Bloomberg Faculty of Nursing and
    Institute for Health Policy, Management and
    Evaluation
Dalla Lana School of Public Health
University of Toronto
Toronto, ON, Canada

Michael Jefford, PhD, FRACP
Department of Cancer Experiences Research
    and Australian Cancer Survivorship
    Centre
Peter MacCallum Cancer Centre, and Sir Peter
    MacCallum Department of Oncology
University of Melbourne
Victoria, Australia

Lauren Jimenez-Kurlander, MD
Pediatrics Long-Term Follow-Up
Memorial Sloan Kettering Cancer Center
New York, NY

Shelli R. Kesler, PhD
School of Nursing
Department of Diagnostic Medicine
Department of Oncology and Livestrong Cancer
    Institute
University of Texas at Austin
Austin, TX

Jennifer Kim, MD
Department of Medicine, Primary Care and
    Population Health
Stanford University, CA

Cristina Kline-Quiroz, DO
Department of Physical Medicine &
    Rehabilitation
Vanderbilt University Medical Center
Nashville, TN

Allison W. Kurian, MD, MSc
Departments of Medicine and Epidemiology and
    Population Health
Stanford University School of Medicine
Stanford, CA

Karolina Lisy, PhD, BSc
Department of Cancer Experiences
    Research and Australian Cancer
    Survivorship Centre
Peter MacCallum Cancer Centre,
    and Sir Peter MacCallum Department
    of Oncology
University of Melbourne
Victoria, Australia

Ioannis Milioglou, MD
University Hospitals Cleveland Medical Center
Case Western Reserve University
Cleveland, OH

Ana Patricia Navarrete-Reyes, MD
Department of Geriatrics
Instituto Nacional de Ciencias Medicas y
    Nutricion Salvador Zubiran
Mexico City, Mexico

Juan Pablo Negrete-Najar, MD
Department of Geriatrics
Instituto Nacional de Ciencias Medicas y
    Nutricion Salvador Zubiran
Mexico City, Mexico

Blanca Noriega Esquivels, MD
Sylvester Comprehensive Cancer Center
Miller School of Medicine
University of Miami, FL

Danielle Novetsky Friedman, MD, MS
Pediatrics
Memorial Sloan-Kettering Cancer Center
New York, NY

Harsh Patolia, MD
Internal Medicine
Duke University Hospital Program
Durham, NC

Brandy Patterson, MD
Cardiovascular Disease
University of Virginia Medical Center
Charlottesville, VA

Frank J. Penedo, PhD
Sylvester Comprehensive Cancer Center
Miller School of Medicine
University of Miami, FL

Andrea Perez-de-Acha, MD
Department of Geriatrics
Instituto Nacional de Ciencias Medicas y
    Nutricion Salvador Zubiran
Mexico City, Mexico

Judith J. Prochaska, PhD, MPH
Stanford Prevention Research Center
Stanford University
Stanford, CA

Jennifer B. Reese, PhD
Cancer Prevention and Control
Fox Chase Cancer Center
Philadelphia, PA

Lindsay Schwartz, MD
Department of Pediatrics
The University of Chicago
Comer Children's Hospital
Chicago, IL

Raman Sharma, MD
Cancer Rehabilitation
Oncology Hematology Associates
Edison, NJ

Louise Sharpe, PhD
School of Psychology
University of Sydney
Sydney, Australia

Anish Singh Jammu, HBSc, MSc (C)
William Osler Health System
Brampton, ON
and McMaster University Global Health Program
Hamilton, ON, Canada

Stephanie M. Smith, MD MPH
Division of Hematology/Oncology
Department of Pediatrics
Stanford University School of Medicine
Stanford, CA

Enrique Soto-Perez-de-Celis, MD
Department of Geriatrics
Instituto Nacional de Ciencias Medicas y
    Nutricion Salvador Zubiran
Mexico City, Mexico

Michael D. Stubblefield, MD
Cancer Rehabilitation
Kessler Institute for Rehabilitation
ReVital Cancer Rehabilitation, and Department of
    Physical Medicine and Rehabilitation
Rutgers New Jersey Medical School
West Orange, NJ

Ilana Yurkiewicz, MD
Stanford University
Department of Medicine
Division of Oncology
Stanford, CA

Lauren A. Zimmaro, PhD
Cancer Prevention and Control
Fox Chase Cancer Center
Philadelphia, PA

After Cancer
A Vision of Integrated Care

1

Lidia Schapira

In a moving essay published a few months before her death from lung cancer, Dr. Gene Bishop spoke of feeling grateful for having survived Hodgkin lymphoma in 1965; at the age of 18 (1), I had the privilege of speaking with Dr. Bishop a few weeks before her death in March of 2020. She shared that she did not think of herself as a cancer survivor for the first 20 years, as she never lost her hair or vomited or missed a day of college at Radcliffe during the weeks of her radiation therapy. But after three more bouts with cancer and surgery for radiation-induced cardiac disease, she understood her story was a warning for medicine, reminding us that today's cures may be tomorrow's illnesses.

Herself an accomplished internist, Dr. Bishop wrote and spoke of having her symptoms dismissed by doctors when they did not fit into recognizable categories. She found more useful information in an online group of Hodgkin survivors, a community that understood the difficulties of facing uncertainty and shared the experience of living with treatment-related toxicities and symptom clusters. For years, she felt doctors celebrated the cure and dismissed new symptoms as psychologic, without being open to consider the association between a current problem and prior exposures. Her essay serves as a call to action for all clinicians who encounter cancer survivors in their medical practice.

Pediatric oncologists have led the way in the emerging field of cancer survivorship, by organizing dedicated survivorship clinics and gathering long-term outcomes data that inform customized survivorship care plans. Still, the fate of the young adults who attend survivorship clinics is far from certain, as they may require access to expert consultation for the rest of their lives. Primary care physicians (PCPs) and general practitioners (GPs) face significant challenges as they assume the central role in caring for cancer survivors of all ages and backgrounds. As Dr. Bishop put it to me, "there is no way a primary care doctor can know all about this." She is right. There are well-documented gaps in medical education about cancer survivorship and many clinicians feel ill prepared to handle the complexities of the many physical and emotional sequelae of cancer and cancer therapies.

With growing numbers of cancer survivors across the world, it is urgent that we enlist all clinicians into the workforce and integrate cancer survivorship in the curricula of healthcare professionals and postgraduate medical education. If "cancer" is on the medical problem list, we want clinicians to feel prepared to bring it into the conversation, and to at least consider if it could affect the problem that is being discussed in the moment. We need attentive listeners who can empathize with patients who seem anxious waiting for test results or shy about sharing the extent of their physical and emotional disabilities. As the science of cancer survivorship grows and provides more evidence-based effective and practical interventions to ameliorate the symptoms and suffering incurred during or after treatment, it is imperative that clinicians recognize these problems and refer patients who may benefit in a timely manner.

We are learning to recognize the variety of experiences, to move away from a "one size fits all" approach to cancer survivorship and to honor the lived experience of individual patients and caregivers.

DOI: 10.1201/9781003055426-1

While there is a general consensus that cancer survivorship begins at diagnosis and persists for the remainder of a person's life, there are some who do not and will not identify as survivors, whereas others who embrace the status find relief in that designation. The purpose of cancer survivorship education is to increase awareness and share evidence-based knowledge and best practices among all who live with, and care for individuals seeking medical attention after cancer. Generalists and specialists alike need to engage with cancer survivors on a daily basis, but it is the GPs and PCPs who ultimately have the responsibility for organizing and coordinating their care, and it is with them in mind that we have written and organized the content of this textbook.

Cancer survivorship is not only about recognizing long-term and late effects of cancer therapies, but fundamentally about integrating preventive health into longitudinal care. Cancer survivors need to understand their genetic risk and be guided to understand how to mitigate inherited risk through lifestyle, pharmacologic and non-pharmacologic interventions. PCPs and GPs need to recognize the fear that lies behind the requests for more and more testing, as cancer survivors seek reassurance where none can be found (2). Generalists and specialists need to recognize the symptom burden that can be disabling and work to resolve them using a personalized framework to guide symptom management in survivorship. Incorporating the patient's voice, through patient-reported outcome measures in clinical encounters, can facilitate engagement and communication and forms the basis for supportive self-management in chronic illness, a model that is well suited and easily adapted to inform the care of cancer survivors. With the goal of building confidence in patients and caregivers, self-management shifts the role from passive recipients of care to active partners, and this will be clear to the reader in subsequent chapters.

While there is much excitement about discoveries that impact health outcomes for adult survivors of childhood cancer, there is an urgent need to define best practices and efficient strategies for customizing cancer care for older individuals and those with extensive comorbidities. Prehabilitation and rehabilitation, as well as integrated care between specialists and generalists, come into sharp focus when the patient has a life-threatening cancer and compromised organ function or inadequate social supports. We have addressed these common scenarios through vignettes embedded in chapters that focus on older survivors. Special attention is given to cardiovascular complications of cancer therapy with a rigorous review of existing guidelines and a new practical synthesis that can inform decisions regarding cardiac monitoring and the need for specialized referrals and testing. With an eye on future health and the teachable moment offered by survivorship-focused consultations, we present an update on novel techniques for quitting tobacco that can be easily integrated in the scope of primary care. Oncologists have listened to cancer survivors who relate losses in cognitive capacity and for years have struggled to find the proper way to report these troubling symptoms that may lead to disability. Readers will find an outstanding summary of the state of the field in the chapter addressing the effects of cancer therapy on cognition, and feel better prepared to converse with their patients who describe losses in verbal, spatial, and numerical skills and the ability to multitask and maintain their focus and attention.

Early on in my medical oncology practice and long before cancer survivorship was recognized as a distinct phase of the continuum of cancer care, I realized that my patients needed a pep talk or exit chat at the end of active cancer therapy. The transition to "after cancer" did not appear smooth and so I made it my practice to take my time and have the "life after cancer" conversation. I learned from listening to patients talk about their parenting concerns, the impact of treatment on intimacy and sexual health, career interruptions and shifts in relationships. I am grateful to them and to my colleagues who are content experts in the many dimensions of the science and art of cancer survivorship, and who have collaborated with me to present this book to you in the hope that it will guide you in the care of future cancer survivors.

REFERENCES

1. Bishop G. The Arc of Therapy: From Cure to Humbling Legacy. J Clin Oncol. 2019;37(34):3320–2.
2. McCoy R. Searching for Evidence-Based Reassurance Where None Can Be Found. J Clin Oncol. 2018;36(12):1266–7.

From Learning to Survive to Learning to Live

Meeting a Cancer Survivor's Needs

2

Ilana Yurkiewicz

When Rob Wong (named changed) came to establish care with me, I did not yet have the language of cancer survivorship. Rob and I were both in our late twenties and imagining a life ahead of us. But that is where our similarities ended.

When Rob was a college student, his life was put on a multi-year hold by acute lymphoblastic leukemia (ALL). He left school for treatment and never went back. He was pulled from his friends, his goals, and his life. For nearly 4 years, the entirety of his existence focused on survival.

He underwent multiple rounds of chemotherapy and too many lumbar punctures to count. He endured neutropenic fevers and infections. He spent months tethered to an IV pole in fluorescent hospital rooms and knew every nurse in the leukemia ward by name. He received a bone marrow transplant from his brother, which kept him cloistered within the hospital's narrow radius for 3 months and afraid to venture outside without the protective gear he called his "Darth Vader mask." He developed graft-versus-host-disease (GvHD) that scarred his skin and damaged his gut.

The transplant put him into a lasting remission, but his transplant doctor was hesitant to declare victory until enough time had passed. When it finally did, even she was comfortable saying it. Rob was cured.

There were no fireworks or confetti, but a cold new reality: the work was just beginning.

I don't remember exactly what I expected the day I met Rob, but I believe it was some version of a grateful person. I was a new doctor in my primary care continuity clinic of residency. I read his chart and grasped the intensity of what he had been through. But now – according to the chart at least – Rob was doing well. The enemy that had been threatening his mortality and ravaging his life for years was gone.

Rob's leukemia may have been gone, but in its place was a host of new medical challenges, emotional trauma, and unrelenting uncertainties. The part missing from Rob's chart was the toll his cancer saga had taken on him. It was all-encompassing. As we got to know each other, he shared more details.

He was depressed, he told me one day.

"I never thought I would be the guy living in my parents' basement," he said. "No job. No friends. No girlfriend."

DOI: 10.1201/9781003055426-2

He thought a lot about the cancer coming back.

"If the leukemia does come back, I don't think I want to treat it. I can't deal with all that again," he said. There were many times he had wanted to give up, he told me, and it was mainly for his parents that he pushed through. But if his leukemia relapsed and the prognosis was that much more dire, he couldn't go through treatment just for his parents again. He would take stock of his savings, travel the world, and not look back.

He was angry, he admitted.

The GvHD still affected him, and it was likely it always would. Most bothersome were his eyes. They always felt gritty and dry, like sand had been thrown in them. He tried different medications and procedures, but he still couldn't drive when the sun beamed in his direction, and he had to take breaks from reading when the page got too blurry. He recalled his first eye doctor who had not suspected his symptoms were a manifestation of GvHD. It was this delay in initiating treatment, Rob believed, that led to permanent damage.

Finally, he was anxious.

Around the time I became Rob's doctor, our hospital launched an open notes initiative to give patients better access to their charts. Sharing my notes with Rob resulted in an inbox flood of frantic messages. Any careless word choice, abnormal vital sign, or blood test that came back in red signifying out of range provoked a slew of questions. The meaning behind these messages was not difficult to interpret. Rob feared the leukemia was coming back.

What he didn't know was that I was worried, too. Was I checking the right labs? Was I thinking about the differential diagnoses thoroughly? Behind the scenes, I was in frequent communication with his bone marrow transplant doctor. Even as we shared care for Rob, I saw how easily something important could slip through the cracks. I didn't want to fail him as yet another provider who didn't take him seriously.

I was Rob's doctor for 3 years. After much encouragement and the power of my signature on mountains of paperwork, he returned to the same college he had left 7 years earlier. Meanwhile, I embarked on a hematology and oncology fellowship. I couldn't have been more excited; becoming an oncologist felt like going behind the curtain. I imagined that my intensive oncology training would give me the extra expertise and focus to care for patients like Rob in a holistic way. I was eager to manage not only my patients' cancers but also everything else cancer left in its wake.

I had the privilege of caring for hundreds of cancer survivors, but I learned that being on the oncology "side" did not magically fix the gaps. For many oncologists, survivorship is framed as a story of unmitigated success. You *have* to see this patient, oncologists would tell me in clinic – no evidence of disease for 5 years! Outside the room, we would review in detail the cocktail of immunotherapy drugs that finally worked or the third-line chemotherapy that secured a lasting remission. How is the patient doing? I'd ask. Great, the oncologist would often say. And it was great. The cancer was gone.

And though each patient was unique, they shared what Rob had – a new world of problems. There was the woman with breast cancer whose endocrine therapy torpedoed her mood and her productivity, and she grappled with the tough choice of whether to continue. There was the elderly man with prostate cancer who shyly brought up intimacy problems with his wife after keeping it under wraps for nearly 2 years. There was the breast cancer survivor who developed a secondary angiosarcoma after the radiation therapy that was supposed to keep her cancer-free. There was the lymphoma survivor who blamed himself for the multiple rounds of treatment that nearly bankrupted him, cursing his failure to factor a potential devastating illness into his financial planning.

The breadth of my patients' experiences humbled me. They also made me wonder: what else was lurking beneath the surface? As oncologists, we are trained in the basic tenets of palliative care, our field recognizing the importance of providing thoughtful and compassionate care at the end of life. But we receive little guidance on how to care for patients at their new beginnings. As Suleika Jaouad, who survived acute myeloid leukemia (AML) in her twenties, wrote in her memoir, *Between Two Kingdoms*: "Now that I've survived, I'm realizing I don't know how to live."

In 1986, the advocacy organization National Coalition for Cancer Survivorship (NCCS) generated the language for survivorship we still use today. A cancer survivor, they said, is any individual who has experienced cancer from the day of diagnosis. Notably, they extended the definition to include family members, friends, and caregivers.[1] In 2006, the Institute of Medicine (IOM) published its seminal report, "From Cancer Patient to Cancer Survivor: Lost in Transition," which outlined ten recommendations aimed at improving care for cancer survivors.[2] The report broadened the recognition of cancer survivorship as a distinct phase along the cancer care spectrum, called for the development and dissemination of survivorship care plans (SCPs) to better inform patients of what to expect in the post-treatment period, and called to improve gaps in the education of health care providers and patients.

These calls boldly named what I saw in my patients. Cancer does not simply disappear without a trace. Rather, its ghosts embed themselves in a survivor's life, sometimes in unexpected places. As of 2019, there were an estimated 16.9 million cancer survivors in the United States;[3] that number is poised to reach 26.1 million by 2040.[4] Addressing cancer survivors meaningfully means addressing the persistent "brain fog" limiting career dreams, the anxiety over recurrence that turns everyday aches into panic attacks, and the strained relationships with loved ones who have developed compassion fatigue. It means delineating clear roles and cultivating communication between primary care and oncology and helping patients navigate what can feel like a strange limbo between the two. It means taking care not to send the spoken or unspoken message that issues of survivorship take short shrift compared to cancer.

In the 15 years since the IOM report was published, the movement has achieved large strides. We have listened to our patients and we have learned. We have organized. We have increased our educational efforts. The number of providers versed in tackling these issues head-on and championing a better way is growing.

But there is still much work to be done. The time is now to go deeper than glossy websites and checkboxes toward developing real infrastructure, supporting broad education, and changing the conversation to establish cancer survivorship as an urgent medical need – one that is valued, prioritized, and funded.

Today, Rob has completed a degree in criminal justice. He lives with two roommates, and recently he joined a martial arts group. His eyes continue to feel gritty, but he has gained a level of acceptance over this new normal. Though he does not know exactly what his future will hold, he is motivated that there is one to be had.

The population of cancer survivors is expanding. They have complex medical, psychosocial, and emotional needs that are demanding to be met. Are we ready?

REFERENCES

1. National Coalition for Cancer Survivorship (NCCS). https://canceradvocacy.org/.
2. Hewitt M, Greenfield S, Stovall E. From Cancer Patient to Cancer Survivor: Lost in Transition. Washington, DC: National Academies Press; 2006.
3. Miller KD, Nogueira L, Mariotto AB, et al. Cancer treatment and survivorship statistics, 2019. CA Cancer J Clin. 2019;69:363.
4. Bluethmann SM, Mariotto AB, Rowland JH. Anticipating the "silver tsunami": prevalence trajectories and comorbidity burden among older cancer survivors in the United States. Cancer Epidemiol Biomarkers Prev. 2016;25:1029–36.

Adult Survivors of Childhood Cancers

3

Stephanie M. Smith, Lauren Jimenez-Kurlander,
Lindsay Schwartz, Tara O. Henderson*, and
Danielle Novetsky Friedman*

INTRODUCTION

The population of adult survivors of childhood cancer continues to grow due to improvements in treatment and supportive care. Five-year survival rates for children and adolescents with cancer have increased steadily since the 1970s and exceed 85% for patients diagnosed during 2010–2016 (1). Accordingly, it is likely that all primary care physicians will encounter patients with a history of childhood cancer over the course of their careers. Moreover, adult survivors of childhood cancer are at increased risk of morbidity and mortality due to their prior cancer treatment. As recommended by the National Academy of Medicine in 2003, life-long risk-based medical care is essential to optimize survivors' overall health. The goal of this chapter is to provide a practical framework for a generalist to approach the care of an adult survivor of childhood cancer.

Historical Perspective

Following early successes treating childhood cancer in the 1960s and 1970s, pediatric oncologists discovered that long-term survivors were developing new health problems after completing cancer treatment (late effects; Table 3.1) at a greater frequency than would be expected in the general population. In the late 20th century, physicians and researchers collaborated to establish large prospective cohort studies of childhood cancer survivors, which have linked prior cancer treatment exposures with risk of late effects and subsequent cancers (2, 3). Researchers found that nearly three-quarters of childhood cancer survivors treated during 1970–1986 developed a chronic health condition by 30 years after diagnosis, with 42% having a severe, disabling, life-threatening, or fatal condition (4).

Building from the extensive literature linking therapeutic exposures with late effects, contemporary childhood cancer treatment protocols aim to minimize late effects while maintaining cure rates.

Framework for Childhood Cancer Survivorship Care

Care of the childhood cancer survivor requires an individualized approach due to the wide variety of cancers and treatment regimens. Patient's age and developmental stage at diagnosis are important

---

* Indicates co-senior authors.

DOI: 10.1201/9781003055426-3

TABLE 3.1   Definitions

Long-term effects	Health problems arising *during* cancer treatment and persisting after completion of treatment
Late effects	Health problems arising at any time *after* completion of cancer treatment
Risk-based care	Tailored approach that accounts for cancer treatment exposures and associated risk of late effects

considerations and add to the complexity. At first glance, this task may seem daunting for non-oncologists. However, there are several key underlying principles that simplify the approach and can be applied regardless of prior experience:

1. Therapeutic exposures are linked with risk of late effects
2. Risk of late effects tends to increase with increasing age and time since treatment
3. Cancer treatment during childhood is associated with accelerated aging
4. Clinical practice guidelines for childhood cancer survivorship care are readily available (5)

Individualized care that is tailored according to cancer treatment exposures and risk of late effects is referred to as "risk-based survivorship care" (Table 3.1). This draws from the principle that specific cancer treatment exposures are associated with specific late health effects.

Therapeutic Exposures Are Linked with Risk of Late Effects

For adult survivors of childhood cancer, risk of late effects is determined by a number of factors, including those that are unmodifiable, such as past treatment exposures and underlying genetics, and those that are modifiable, such as health behaviors and management of comorbidities (Figure 3.1). Recognizing that some risk factors are *not* modifiable emphasizes the importance of optimizing the *modifiable* risk factors in order to reduce the overall risk of late effects. Additionally, specific surveillance based on prior cancer treatment exposures is recommended to enable early detection and treatment of late effects, when possible.

The most important information to identify from a patient's cancer treatment history includes the **type of treatment** received (chemotherapy, radiotherapy, immunotherapy, targeted biologic therapy) and **age at the time of treatment**, as some therapies have different effects depending on the patient's age and developmental stage. For some chemotherapies such as anthracyclines and alkylating agents, the **cumulative dose** is an important factor in determining risk of late effects. For radiotherapy, the **cumulative dose** and **body part(s) exposed** are the most important details. Newer therapies such as immunotherapy and targeted biologic therapy have not yet been incorporated into childhood cancer survivorship clinical practice guidelines due to lack of data but remain an active area of investigation.

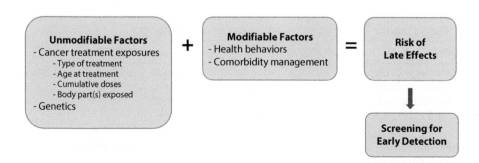

FIGURE 3.1   Factors contributing to risk of late effects in childhood cancer survivors.

Risk of Late Effects Tends to Increase with Increasing Age and Time since Treatment

It is important to understand the trajectory of late effects risks over a patient's lifetime. In general, the risk of late effects in adult survivors of childhood cancer increases with aging and longer time since treatment. For example, the risk of subsequent solid tumors arising in prior radiotherapy fields increases steadily over time and does not plateau (6, 7). Similarly, the incidence of cardiovascular disease increases with age, especially among those who received cardiotoxic therapies at a young age (8, 9). By age 50 years, childhood cancer survivors had developed an average of 4.7 severe, disabling, life-threatening, or fatal chronic health conditions, which were twice as many as similarly aged controls in the general population (10). This risk trajectory emphasizes why adult survivors of childhood cancer require ongoing medical care even many years after completing cancer treatment (see "Models of Survivorship Care" section on the following text for additional details regarding approaches for provision of survivorship care).

Cancer Treatment during Childhood Is Associated with Accelerated Aging

Many adult survivors of childhood cancer experience an earlier onset of chronic health conditions than would be predicted based on age-related, genetic, and behavioral risks alone, which has been called premature physiologic aging (11, 12). Frailty, typically associated with aging, is as prevalent among young adult childhood cancer survivors (mean age 33 years) as among older adults in the general population (age 65 and older) (11), and three times more prevalent in childhood cancer survivors than in their siblings (13).

Recognition of accelerated physiologic aging and frailty in adult survivors of childhood cancer presents opportunities for intervention and rehabilitation (see Chapter 13 for further detail).

Clinical Practice Guidelines for Childhood Cancer Survivorship Care Are Readily Available

In order to synthesize the research linking childhood cancer treatments and late effects into clinically actionable recommendations, experts have developed evidence-based clinical practice guidelines that are reviewed and updated on an ongoing basis (Table 3.2). The Children's Oncology Group (COG) Long-Term Follow-Up Guidelines, which are exposure-based screening guidelines, are widely implemented in childhood cancer survivorship programs in the United States (5, 14). Alternatively, the International Guideline Harmonization Group for Late Effects of Childhood Cancer (IGHG) provides systems-based screening recommendations and clinical practice guidelines for survivorship care in Europe and North America (15, 16).

TABLE 3.2 Clinical practice guidelines for childhood cancer survivorship care

ORGANIZATION	NOTES	WEBSITE
Children's Oncology Group Long-Term Follow-Up Guidelines for Survivors of Childhood, Adolescent, and Young Adult Cancers	• Organized by treatment exposure; searchable PDF available online • Includes patient education sheets ("Health Links") on specific late effects	www.survivorshipguidelines.org
International Guideline Harmonization Group for Late Effects of Childhood Cancer	• Organized by specific late effects; available online	www.ighg.org

Importantly, prospective cohort studies continue to collect data as childhood cancer survivors' age, and new data will emerge as upfront therapeutic approaches evolve. Thus, it is essential to know where to find updated, expert-vetted information to guide the care of childhood cancer survivors (Table 3.2). The COG guidelines, for example, are updated by experts every 5 years.

Survivorship Care Plans

In order to facilitate high-quality survivorship care that adheres to the aforementioned guidelines, all survivors should receive a copy of a survivorship care plan, or a written document that summarizes all prior therapeutic exposures and includes a surveillance schedule for recurrence and late effects (17–19). These individualized documents appear to increase survivors' personal risk awareness (20) while also providing clinicians with a critical roadmap for lifelong risk-based screening for each survivor (17, 19, 21). Pediatric oncology teams should provide patients and clinicians with a cancer treatment summary or survivorship care plan after completion of therapy. If a patient does not have a cancer treatment summary, it is reasonable for the primary care clinician to contact the patient's pediatric oncologist or survivorship team from the primary cancer center and request an updated copy.

In the following sections, we will review two clinical cases to illustrate how to apply these principles in practice. While Case 1 uses an **exposure-based** approach, Case 2 combines an **exposure-based** and **systems-based** approach. Both algorithms represent a sound approach when considering an individual survivor's risk of developing late effects.

CASE 1

Tyrone B. is a 25-year-old biological male who has history of childhood high risk pre-B cell acute lymphoblastic leukemia (ALL). He presents to your office to establish care 7 years post-completion of prior cytotoxic therapies. He has not seen a clinician since he graduated from high school 6 years ago. After probing further, Tyrone reveals that he had recent development of difficulty achieving and maintaining an erection, so he thought it was time to "get checked out." He works as a computer engineer and reports that it takes him much longer than his coworkers to complete tasks.

As noted above, in order to anticipate the potential effects of Tyrone's specific therapies, there are a number of factors to consider to best conceptualize and communicate his risks, including:

- Treatment exposures
- Biological sex
- Race/ethnicity
- Age at diagnosis and age at time of treatment
- Diagnosis
- Time since end of treatment of all cytotoxic therapies
- Attained age

Using the risk-based care framework, you learn that Tyrone was first diagnosed when he was 15 years old. His age at diagnosis identifies him as an **adolescent and young adult (AYA)** survivor, a group that includes patients diagnosed between 15 and 39 years old as defined by the Adolescent and Young Adult Oncology Progress Review Group (AYAO PRG) and the National Cancer Institute (NCI). This population has been recognized to have distinctive tumor biology, difficulties accessing medical care, and unique psychosocial needs (22). Tyrone's treatment likely impacted his education, sexual health, financial health, and his routine vaccination schedule. Considering Tyrone is 7 years post-completion of cytotoxic therapies for leukemia, you recognize that some risks will continue to increase over time (e.g., endocrinopathies,

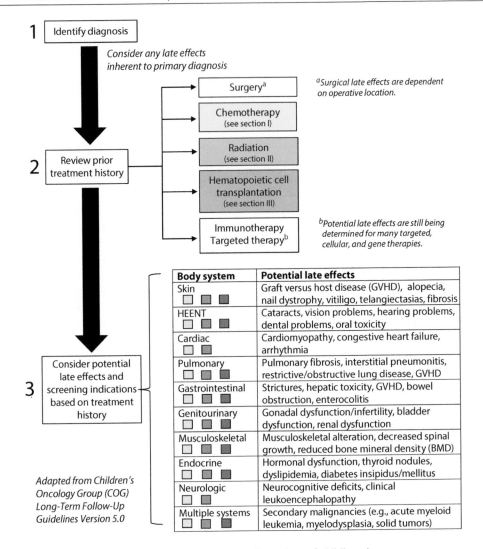

FIGURE 3.2 Sample algorithm for approaching the adult survivor of childhood cancer.

cardiovascular disease, secondary malignancies), while others would have more likely occurred closer to the time of treatment with low risk of later-onset development (23). After consideration of these factors, you take an algorithmic approach to assess Tyrone's specific risks as depicted in Figure 3.2.

Chemotherapy

You ask Tyrone for records of his prior treatment. He shows you a list of chemotherapies as follows: Vincristine, dexamethasone, prednisone, methotrexate, pegaspargase, daunorubicin, cyclophospha-mide, cytarabine, mercaptopurine, thioguanine, etoposide. He asks you the relevance of these che-motherapies at this time since he received them over 8 years prior.

Patients treated as children, adolescents, or young adults often have a limited understanding of their treatment history (24). It is critical to review treatment history and potential late effects for patients with a history of childhood cancer treatment, in addition to periodically reviewing relevant potential and/or devel-oping late effects as the patient ages. You explain Tyrone's exposure-based risks, as shown in Table 3.3.

TABLE 3.3 Common exposure-based late effects and recommended screening for males

CHEMOTHERAPY	DRUG CLASS	DOSE CONSIDERATIONS	POTENTIAL LATE EFFECTS	INDICATED SCREENING
Vincristine	Plant alkaloid	N/A	Peripheral neuropathy	Annual neurologic history and exam (until 2–3 years after therapy)
Dexamethasone	Corticosteroid	N/A (25)	Cataracts, reduced BMD, osteonecrosis	Annual ophthalmology exam
Annual musculoskeletal exam
Baseline bone density evaluation (DXA) at entry to LTFU; repeat as clinically indicated
Prednisone	Corticosteroid	Higher risk for BMD deficits if >9000 mg/m² (26)	Cataracts, reduced BMD, osteonecrosis	Annual ophthalmology exam
Annual musculoskeletal exam
Baseline DXA at entry to LTFU
Methotrexate	Anti-metabolite	Higher risk for BMD deficits if >40,000 mg/m² (26)	Reduced BMD, hepatic dysfunction, neurocognitive deficits, clinical leukoencephalopathy	Baseline DXA at entry to LTFU
LFTs at entry to LTFU
Annual gastrointestinal exam
Refer for formal neuropsychological testing
Annual neurologic exam
Pegaspargase	Enzyme	N/A	N/A	N/A
Daunorubicin	Anthracycline antibiotic	Higher risk for cardiac dysfunction if doxorubicin equivalent dose ≥250 mg/m² (27)	Cardiac toxicity	EKG at entry to LTFU
Echo every 2–5 years
(Refer to Chapter 12 for detailed cardiac screening guidelines)
Cyclophosphamide	Classical alkylating agent	Higher risk for Sertoli cell dysfunction if ≥4 g/m², Leydig cell dysfunction if ≥20 g/m², urinary tract toxicity if ≥3 g/m² (28)	Testicular hormone dysfunction, impaired spermatogenesis, urinary tract toxicity, acute myeloid leukemia, bladder toxicity	Urinalysis, urine culture, spot urine calcium/creatinine ratio for patients with positive history of renal dysfunction (assess for risk annually)
Yearly dermatologic exam (pallor, petechiae, bruising) up to 10 years after exposure
(Refer to Chapter 4 for detailed fertility guidelines)
Cytarabine	Anti-metabolite	Risk for neurocognitive deficits exists only if dose ≥1000 mg/m²	Neurocognitive deficits	Refer for formal neuropsychological testing
Mercaptopurine and Thioguanine	Anti-metabolite	N/A	Hepatic dysfunction, sinusoidal obstructive syndrome (SOS)	LFTs at entry to LTFU
Annual gastrointestinal exam
Etoposide	Epipodophyllotoxin	N/A	Acute myeloid leukemia	Yearly dermatologic exam (pallor, petechiae, bruising) up to 10 years after exposure

Source: Adapted from Children's Oncology Group (COG) Long-Term Follow-Up (LTFU) Guidelines Version 5.0 (5).

Radiation

On further history, Tyrone reports that he had a central nervous system relapse with bone marrow infiltration when he was 16 years old. As a result, in addition to the systemic chemotherapies he had already shown you, he also received total body irradiation (TBI) with a cranial boost prior to hematopoietic stem cell transplantation (hSCT).

With this new information, you review the various late effects that can result from TBI and/or cranial irradiation. You reference Figure 3.3 to remind yourself which organs were impacted by the radiation that Tyrone received.

With an understanding of Tyrone's potential impacted organs, you then review with him potential late effects related to his prior TBI exposure, as shown in Table 3.4.

Endocrinopathies refer to any hormone dysregulation(s) and are common late effects in patients who received cranial radiation, TBI, or have a history of a central nervous system tumor. In a study of 310 adult survivors, Brignardello et al. reported at least one endocrine disorder in more than half of survivors 16 years after their childhood cancer diagnosis (30).

Endocrinopathies result from either direct injury to the organ responsible for hormone production or disruption of secondary signaling organs, the most common of which include the hypothalamus and pituitary. The anterior pituitary is particularly susceptible to injury by irradiation, and therefore all anterior pituitary hormones can be affected (i.e., growth hormone [GH], adrenocorticotropic hormone [ACTH], luteinizing hormone [LH], follicle-stimulating hormone [FSH], and thyroid-stimulating hormone [TSH]) in a dose-dependent manner (Figure 3.4) (31).

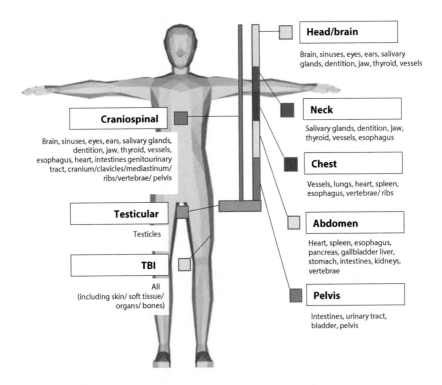

Head/brain

Brain, sinuses, eyes, ears, salivary glands, dentition, jaw, thyroid, vessels

Craniospinal

Brain, sinuses, eyes, ears, salivary glands, dentition, jaw, thyroid, vessels, esophagus, heart, intestines genitourinary tract, cranium/clavicles/mediastinum/ribs/vertebrae/ pelvis

Neck

Salivary glands, dentition, jaw, thyroid, vessels, esophagus

Chest

Vessels, lungs, heart, spleen, esophagus, vertebrae/ ribs

Testicular

Testicles

Abdomen

Heart, spleen, esophagus, pancreas, gallbladder liver, stomach, intestines, kidneys, vertebrae

TBI

All
(including skin/ soft tissue/ organs/ bones)

Pelvis

Intestines, urinary tract, bladder, pelvis

FIGURE 3.3 Impacted organs by radiation field (males). (Adapted from Children's Oncology Group Long-Term Follow-Up Guidelines for Survivors of Childhood, Adolescent, and Young Adult Cancers, Version 5.0. Available from: http://survivorshipguidelines.org.)

TABLE 3.4 Potential late effects after TBI for males

AFFECTED ORGAN(S)	LATE EFFECT(S)[a]	OTHER CONSIDERATIONS
Central nervous system	• Neurocognitive deficits • Leukoencephalopathy	Younger children (particularly if treated at age <3) and girls have highest risk. *Refer to Chapter 8 regarding effects of cancer therapy on cognition.*
Eyes	• Cataracts	
Dentition	• Dental abnormalities	
Endocrine	• Growth hormone (GH) deficiency • Primary hypothyroidism • Primary hyperthyroidism • Thyroid nodules • Metabolic syndrome • Sertoli cell dysfunction and impaired spermatogenesis • Leydig cell dysfunction and testosterone deficiency	There may be benefit to adulthood GH replacement in cases of GH deficiency even after achieving final adult height (29). Fertility preservation techniques are constantly evolving. *Refer to Chapter 4 regarding sexual function and infertility.*
Pulmonary	• Pulmonary toxicity	
Cardiac	• Cardiac toxicity	Physical activity is generally safe and should be encouraged in survivors with normal LV function. Consider cardiology consultation to define limits of physical activity for high-risk survivors who plan to participate in intensive exercise. *Refer to Chapter 12 regarding late effects on cardiac function.*
Renal	• Renal toxicity	
Gastrointestinal	• Diabetes mellitus • Central adiposity	
Musculoskeletal	• Growth problems • Decreased BMD • Osteonecrosis	
Multiple	• Second cancers (skin, bone, soft tissue, hematologic)	

Source: Adapted from Children's Oncology Group Long-Term Follow-Up Guidelines for Survivors of Childhood, Adolescent, and Young Adult Cancers, Version 5.0. Available from: http://survivorshipguidelines.org.

[a] For females, additional potential late effects include breast cancer, breast tissue hypoplasia, and ovarian dysfunction.

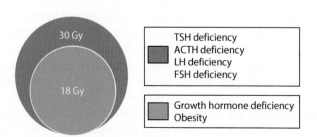

FIGURE 3.4 Endocrinopathy risks based on hypothalamic-pituitary axis radiation doses.

TABLE 3.5   Hematopoietic stem cell transplantation (hSCT) potential late effects

POTENTIAL EFFECTS OF THE HSCT EXPERIENCE	ADDITIONAL POTENTIAL EFFECTS IN PATIENTS WITH CHRONIC GVHD
Graft versus host disease (acute or chronic)	Xerophthalmia
Dental abnormalities	Xerostomia or dental abnormalities
Renal toxicity	Genitourinary strictures
Hepatic toxicity	Gastrointestinal strictures
Low BMD	Pulmonary toxicity
Avascular necrosis	Skin and joint changes
Psychosocial disability/impaired quality of life	Psychosocial disability/impaired quality of life
Mental health disorders	Immune deficiency
Secondary malignancies	Secondary malignancies

Source: Adapted from Chow EJ, Anderson L, Baker KS, Bhatia S, Guilcher GM, Huang JT, et al. Late effects surveillance recommendations among survivors of childhood hematopoietic cell transplantation: a Children's Oncology Group Report. Biol Blood Marrow Transplant. 2016;22(5):782–95.

With this knowledge, you ask Tyrone for records of his radiation treatment. He has records showing prior TBI (15 Gy) but the dose of his cranial boost is unknown. You cannot appropriately stratify his risk without this dose (as radiation dose thresholds to the hypothalamic-pituitary axis are cumulative); given this uncertainty, you conservatively opt to screen for all potential endocrinopathies.

Hematopoietic Stem Cell Transplantation (hSCT)

The majority of late effects from hematopoietic stem cell transplantation (hSCT) are secondary to the conditioning regimen, which often includes high-dose chemotherapies and/or irradiation. hSCT itself is also associated with a variety of possible effects, as shown in Table 3.5.

Following myeloablation prior to hSCT, a temporary state of combined immunodeficiency occurs in all patients. Functional recovery of humoral and cell-mediated immunity often takes a year or longer (33). This effectively eliminates prior antibody responses from childhood vaccinations (33). While universal consensus regarding specific revaccination practices is lacking, most clinicians promote revaccination after completion of therapy (34).

Case Wrap-Up

Given Tyrone's chief complaint of erectile dysfunction, you explain that this common condition may be a result of nerves but could alternatively reflect low testosterone levels, particularly in the context of his treatment-related risks. You explain that you will order gonadotropins and morning testosterone levels and also use this as an opportunity to discuss Tyrone's risk of future infertility as well as alternative methods of family-building (see Chapter 4 on sexual and reproductive health for additional detail). You also order other baseline screening labs, including a comprehensive metabolic panel, ferritin, lipid panel, HbA1c, TSH, morning cortisol, echocardiogram, and EKG. You refer him to an endocrinologist for consideration of GH stimulation testing. You begin his revaccinations as per the Infectious Diseases Society of American (IDSA) catch-up schedule. You also make referrals to ophthalmology for cataract screening, dermatology for secondary malignancy screening after radiation exposure, and dental for regular cleanings every 6 months. Finally, you recommend that Tyrone meet with a genetic counselor to explore his pedigree and potentially schedule genetic testing, if clinically indicated. This may impact cancer screening guidelines for Tyrone as well as other members of his family. Finally, given concerns about adverse academic/vocational, cognitive, and psychosocial outcomes among childhood and AYA cancer survivors (35–37), you do a psychosocial assessment with attention to depression, anxiety, and post-traumatic stress, and refer Tyrone to neuropsychology for formal neurocognitive testing (see Chapters 5 and 7 for additional details).

CASE 2

Jessica L. is a 33-year-old biological female, who is a new patient to your primary care clinic. During your initial history taking, she mentions she was diagnosed with Hodgkin Lymphoma when she was 12 years old and was told she was "cured" after completing treatment at age 13.

Hodgkin lymphoma accounts for approximately 3% of childhood and 13% of AYA cancer diagnoses in the United States (38, 39). It is the most common childhood cancer in the 15- to 19-year-old age group (38, 39). It also represents one of the great success stories in modern oncology: currently, children and AYAs with Hodgkin lymphoma have a 5-year survival of 90–95% compared to an 80% survival in the 1970s (39, 40). With improved survival rates, however, clinicians began to recognize that far too many Hodgkin lymphoma survivors were dying from late complications of their treatment (41–43). Therefore, standard treatment of Hodgkin lymphoma has evolved over the last several decades to utilize lower doses and smaller fields of radiation and less toxic chemotherapy while maintaining survival rates (44–47). This has resulted in significantly lower all-cause mortality (i.e., deaths from Hodgkin lymphoma plus deaths from late complications of therapy) and decreased long-term morbidity in patients treated in more recent eras (47, 48).

Currently, treatment of Hodgkin lymphoma may include chemotherapy and radiation, as well as hSCT in the relapsed and refractory setting. Targeted therapy (i.e., antibody-drug conjugate therapy) and immunotherapy are being studied for upfront therapy but are currently used only in the relapsed and refractory setting. Treatment is based on initial staging as well as disease response throughout therapy (49). Like any childhood cancer, late effects from treatment depend on the type and dose of the therapy received. As mentioned above, all cancer survivors should have a copy of their cancer treatment summary, a record of their cancer diagnosis, therapy, and any complications that occurred during active treatment (14). Templates of these summaries are available to download at http://www.survivorshipguidelines.org/, but should be requested directly from the patient's primary pediatric oncologist if unavailable at the time of transition to primary care.

You request a copy of Jessica's "Summary of Cancer Treatment" and discover that she was diagnosed with "stage IVA Hodgkin lymphoma, nodular sclerosis subtype," with disease in her bilateral cervical and axillary lymph nodes as well as lung nodules. Treatment included chemotherapy (including 145 mg/m² of anthracyclines, 3.6 g/m² of alkylating agents, and steroids) and mantle radiation (21 Gy).

Cardiac Dysfunction

This patient has two risk factors for developing late cardiotoxicity: anthracycline exposure and chest radiation.

Anthracycline-related cardiovascular toxicity is progressive and can take decades to fully develop (41, 50). While this can initially present as subclinical disease, this can progress to serious and life-threatening cardiac conditions, including congestive heart failure, stroke, and myocardial infarction (51–54). Higher cumulative doses of anthracyclines carry the highest risk (55). However, cardiac

TABLE 3.6   Recommended frequency of cardiac screening after cardiotoxic therapy

ANTHRACYCLINE DOSE[a]	CHEST RADIATION DOSE[b]	RECOMMENDED CARDIAC SCREENING INTERVAL
None	<15 Gy (including no exposure)	None
	≥15 to <35 Gy	Every 5 years
	≥35 Gy	Every 2 years
<250 mg/m²	<15 Gy (including no exposure)	Every 5 years
	≥15 Gy	Every 2 years
≥250 mg/m²	Any (including no exposure)	Every 2 years

Source: Children's Oncology Group Long-Term Follow-Up Guidelines for Survivors of Childhood, Adolescent, and Young Adult Cancers, Version 5.0. Available from: http://survivorshipguidelines.org.
[a] Based on Doxorubicin equivalent doses; dose equivalency ratios are located in COG Long-Term Follow-Up Guidelines Version 5.0.
[b] Radiation to chest, abdomen, spine (thoracic or whole), and/or TBI.

abnormalities have been noted in patients with lower dose exposures, suggesting there are no "safe" doses of anthracyclines (56).

"Mantle" field radiation involves exposure of the neck, chest, mediastinum, and axillae to radiation (57). Chest and mediastinal radiotherapy have been associated with a variety of cardiovascular complications, including pericarditis, myocardial fibrosis, coronary artery disease, valvular abnormalities, and arrhythmias leading, over time, to myocardial infarction and stroke (53, 58–60). Other potential sites for radiotherapy in childhood cancer treatment include abdominal radiation and TBI, a common therapy given to patients prior to hSCT (see Case 1). Both of these types of radiotherapy carry increased risk for dyslipidemia (61). Exposure to both anthracyclines and radiotherapy in the presence of modifiable risk factors such as hypertension confer risks for major cardiovascular events that extend beyond an additive expectation (62, 63).

The current COG recommendations for cardiac screening for patients exposed to anthracyclines and/or chest radiation are based on cumulative anthracycline dose in doxorubicin equivalents and chest radiation dose (5), as shown in Table 3.6.

If an echocardiogram is suboptimal, cardiac MRI is recommended adjunctly (5). Additional evaluation, including referrals to cardiology and high-risk obstetrics, is warranted in female survivors who are pregnant or planning to become pregnant and received ≥250 mg/m² of anthracyclines alone, ≥35 Gy of chest radiation alone, or any dose of anthracyclines combined with chest radiation of ≥15 Gy due to increased risk for cardiac failure (5). A fasting lipid panel is recommended every 2 years for patients exposed to abdominal radiation or TBI (64, 65). Abnormal results warrant a referral to a cardiologist, preferably a physician with experience treating childhood cancer survivors.

Jessica mentions that she saw an ophthalmologist "a few years after [she] completed treatment" and currently does not wear glasses or contacts. She asks whether she should resume care with an ophthalmologist.

Ocular Toxicity

Childhood cancer survivors are at increased risk for several ocular late effects, including cataracts, glaucoma, legal blindness, retinal damage, optic nerve damage, diplopia, and dry eye (66, 67). Treatments that pose the greatest risk of early or accelerated cataract formation are high-dose steroids, busulfan, and radiation to the head/brain or TBI (25, 68–70). Regardless of current symptoms, survivors with a history of exposure to any of these therapies require an annual visit with an ophthalmologist for visual acuity and fundoscopic exams.

You finish taking her history and begin the physical exam, which includes a breast exam. You palpate a hard lump, approximately 1.5 cm × 1.5 cm in size, in the lateral upper quadrant of her left breast.

Radiation-Associated Subsequent Malignant Neoplasms

Research has shown that childhood cancer survivors have increased risk for developing subsequent malignant neoplasms (SMNs) and non-melanoma skin cancers compared to unaffected peers, and this risk increases as patients age (71). Incidence is highest for survivors treated with radiation and those whose primary cancer was Hodgkin lymphoma – the patient in our case meets both these criteria (71).

Non-melanoma skin cancer

Currently, it is recommended that any childhood cancer survivor with a history of radiation receive an annual evaluation by a dermatologist for surveillance of skin findings ranging from atypical nevi to melanoma (5).

Breast cancer

Breast cancer is one of the most common subsequent malignancies occurring in adult survivors of childhood cancer (71), especially among female survivors treated with chest radiation during childhood (72, 73). Childhood cancer survivors are also more likely to die from their breast cancers compared to women with de novo breast cancer (74).

Research has shown that female survivors of childhood cancer treated with chest radiation benefit from early and lifelong breast cancer surveillance (75). Current recommendations are for female survivors with a history of chest radiation (including TBI) to undergo yearly screening with mammograms and breast MRI (76) beginning at age 25 or 8 years after radiation therapy, whichever occurs later (5). Women with a genetic predisposition to breast cancer should undergo early breast cancer screening as well.

Colorectal cancer

Childhood cancer survivors exposed to radiation fields that include the colon and rectum have an elevated risk of developing colorectal cancer and developing it at an early age compared to their healthy counterparts (77, 78). High doses of alkylating agents have also been associated with risk of developing colorectal cancer (78). Currently, COG recommends that survivors with a history of any radiation to the abdomen, pelvis, thoracolumbar or whole spine undergo colonoscopy every 5 years beginning 5 years after radiation therapy or at age 30 years, whichever occurs last (5). Though colonoscopy is considered the gold standard for colorectal cancer screening, an acceptable alternative is to undergo "multitarget stool DNA testing" every 3 years, provided that any positive result is followed up with a timely colonoscopy. Earlier and more intense screening may be recommended for those with a genetic predisposition to developing colorectal cancer as well (79).

Unfortunately, colorectal cancer screening compliance has historically been poor – greater than 70% of childhood cancer survivors deemed high-risk for developing early-onset colorectal cancer remain unscreened (77). Therefore, it is extremely important for clinicians to partner with their patients to determine the best screening option to fit the personal health values of each at-risk survivor.

Case Wrap-Up

After reviewing the appropriate risk-based screening tests mentioned above, as well as the recommended intervals for testing, you schedule Jessica for screening labs, including thyroid function tests, as well as a mammogram, echocardiogram, and colonoscopy. You explain that you will schedule Jessica's breast MRI in 6 months to ensure that she receives recommended breast cancer surveillance with both mammogram and breast MRI annually (80). You also take a menstrual history, discuss Jessica's risk for premature ovarian insufficiency (81), and review the options available for post-treatment fertility preservation if she is interested (see Chapter 4 for additional detail). You also recognize that she may be experiencing vocational, neurocognitive, and/or psychosocial difficulties related to her prior cancer therapy (82) and thus perform a thorough psychosocial assessment as well (see Chapters 5 and 7 for additional details).

MODELS OF SURVIVORSHIP CARE

As highlighted by these two cases, survivors of childhood, adolescent, and young adult cancer have unique long-term risks and require proactive medical follow-up. Importantly, as childhood cancer survivors age and become more likely to develop chronic health conditions, they are less likely to receive specialized care at a cancer center (83) and more likely to be followed by a primary care clinician. However, research has found that survivorship care is often heterogenous across institutions and practice settings (84). It is unclear how best to overcome these barriers and ensure that survivors receive appropriate, evidence-based risk-based care.

In a landmark consensus report from 2006, the National Academy of Medicine outlined the central components of survivorship care, which included the need for comprehensive coordination between specialists and primary care clinicians to meet the medical and psychosocial needs of survivors (85). One approach that has been suggested to address these concerns is the **shared-care model**, which involves two or more clinicians with different training who work together to provide high-quality survivorship care in a risk-stratified fashion (86). Using this approach, survivors are transitioned to (1) oncology-based, (2) primary care-based, or (3) shared-care survivorship models based on the survivor's risk for development of treatment-related late effects. For example, a "low-risk patient," or an individual treated with low-intensity therapy who has a low risk for cancer recurrence, might be followed exclusively by a primary care clinician. In contrast, a "high-risk survivor," previously treated with high-intensity therapy and at substantial risk for recurrence and/or subsequent cancers, might be followed by an oncologist and a primary care clinician in a shared-care program (87). Others have suggested that an **oncogeneralist**, or a primary care clinician with formal training in survivorship, may be helpful to define and integrate the multilayered needs and concerns of the higher risk cancer survivor, and can also be available within this shared-care model (88, 89).

In order for these models to be successful, primary care–focused clinicians should have access to a personalized treatment summary as well as patient-specific surveillance guidelines for late effects (90). Primary care clinicians have also highlighted the importance of having expedited routes of referral and/or access to evaluations for suspected recurrence as critical modalities for providing comprehensive survivorship care (91).

Even with these modalities in place, previous surveys of adult primary care clinicians have identified significant knowledge gaps in clinician knowledge of late effects and appropriate risk-based screening guidelines (89, 92). These data underscore the need for continued education about cancer survivorship in the primary care setting.

Education and Training

Given that 85% of adult survivors of childhood cancer receive their care in the community (83, 93), and that the number of adult survivors of childhood cancer continues to grow (38), it is likely that an increased number of community-based primary care clinicians will encounter and provide longitudinal care for adult survivors of childhood cancer. As such, it is critical to maximize educational opportunities for primary care clinicians in a variety of forums. Select medical schools and cancer centers have begun to introduce survivorship-focused educational curricula for medical students and formal training programs for physicians and advanced practice providers (94–96). These platforms will allow non-oncologists to become familiar with the epidemiology of cancer survivorship and proficient in the screening and management of late effects. Efforts should be made to expand educational opportunities through continuing medical education programs, both in-person and online, and through print materials targeted at the primary care community, such as the current volume.

CONCLUSION

Adult survivors of childhood cancer are a growing population with complex medical and psychosocial needs. Risk-based survivorship care may allow for early detection and treatment of late effects. Clinical practice guidelines are available to ensure that survivors are appropriately screened for treatment-related health conditions as they age. Educational opportunities should be made available to the primary care community to ensure that survivors receive lifelong, high-quality care across practice settings in the years to come.

REFERENCES

1. Howlader NNA, Krapcho M, Miller D, Brest A, Yu M, Ruhl J, et al. (eds). SEER Cancer Statistics Review, 1975–2016. Bethesda, MD: National Cancer Institute; 2019.
2. Bhatia S, Armenian SH, Armstrong GT, van Dulmen-den Broeder E, Hawkins MM, Kremer LC, et al. Collaborative research in childhood cancer survivorship: the current landscape. J Clin Oncol. 2015;33(27):3055–64.
3. Norsker FN, Pedersen C, Armstrong GT, Robison LL, McBride ML, Hawkins M, et al. Late effects in childhood cancer survivors: early studies, survivor cohorts, and significant contributions to the field of late effects. Pediatr Clin North Am. 2020;67(6):1033–49.
4. Oeffinger KC, Mertens AC, Sklar CA, Kawashima T, Hudson MM, Meadows AT, et al. Chronic health conditions in adult survivors of childhood cancer. N Engl J Med. 2006;355(15):1572–82.
5. Children's Oncology Group Long-Term Follow-Up Guidelines for Survivors of Childhood, Adolescent, and Young Adult Cancers, Version 5.0. Available from: http://survivorshipguidelines.org.
6. Turcotte LM, Liu Q, Yasui Y, Arnold MA, Hammond S, Howell RM, et al. Temporal trends in treatment and subsequent neoplasm risk among 5-year survivors of childhood cancer, 1970–2015. JAMA. 2017;317(8):814–24.
7. Turcotte LM, Whitton JA, Friedman DL, Hammond S, Armstrong GT, Leisenring W, et al. Risk of subsequent neoplasms during the fifth and sixth decades of life in the childhood cancer survivor study cohort. J Clin Oncol. 2015;33(31):3568–75.
8. Armstrong GT, Oeffinger KC, Chen Y, Kawashima T, Yasui Y, Leisenring W, et al. Modifiable risk factors and major cardiac events among adult survivors of childhood cancer. J Clin Oncol. 2013;31(29):3673–80.
9. van der Pal HJ, van Dalen EC, van Delden E, van Dijk IW, Kok WE, Geskus RB, et al. High risk of symptomatic cardiac events in childhood cancer survivors. J Clin Oncol. 2012;30(13):1429–37.
10. Bhakta N, Liu Q, Ness KK, Baassiri M, Eissa H, Yeo F, et al. The cumulative burden of surviving childhood cancer: an initial report from the St Jude Lifetime Cohort Study (SJLIFE). Lancet. 2017;390:2569–82.

11. Ness KK, Krull KR, Jones KE, Mulrooney DA, Armstrong GT, Green DM, et al. Physiologic frailty as a sign of accelerated aging among adult survivors of childhood cancer: a report from the St Jude Lifetime Cohort Study. J Clin Oncol. 2013;31(36):4496–503.
12. Ness KK, Wogksch MD. Frailty and aging in cancer survivors. Transl Res. 2020;221:65–82.
13. Hayek S, Gibson TM, Leisenring WM, Guida JL, Gramatges MM, Lupo PJ, et al. Prevalence and predictors of frailty in childhood cancer survivors and siblings: a report from the childhood cancer survivor study. J Clin Oncol. 2020;38(3):232–47.
14. Landier W, Bhatia S, Eshelman DA, Forte KJ, Sweeney T, Hester AL, et al. Development of risk-based guidelines for pediatric cancer survivors: the children's oncology group long-term follow-up guidelines from the children's oncology group late effects committee and nursing discipline. J Clin Oncol. 2004;22(24):4979–90.
15. International Guideline Harmonization Group for Late Effects of Childhood Cancer. Available from: http://ighg.org/guidelines.
16. Kremer LC, Mulder RL, Oeffinger KC, Bhatia S, Landier W, Levitt G, et al. A worldwide collaboration to harmonize guidelines for the long-term follow-up of childhood and young adult cancer survivors: a report from the international late effects of childhood cancer guideline harmonization group. Pediatr Blood Cancer. 2013;60(4):543–9.
17. Ganz PA, Casillas J, Hahn EE. Ensuring quality care for cancer survivors: implementing the survivorship care plan. Semin Oncol Nurs. 2008;24(3):208–17.
18. McCabe MS, Jacobs L. Survivorship care: models and programs. Semin Oncol Nurs. 2008;24(3):202–7.
19. Salz T, Oeffinger KC, McCabe MS, Layne TM, Bach PB. Survivorship care plans in research and practice. CA Cancer J Clin. 2012;62(2):101–17.
20. Landier W, Chen Y, Namdar G, Francisco L, Wilson K, Herrera C, et al. Impact of tailored education on awareness of personal risk for therapy-related complications among childhood cancer survivors. J Clin Oncol. 2015;33(33):3887–93.
21. Chow EJ, Baldwin LM, Hagen AM, Hudson MM, Gibson TM, Kochar K, et al. Communicating health information and improving coordination with primary care (CHIIP): rationale and design of a randomized cardiovascular health promotion trial for adult survivors of childhood cancer. Contemp Clin Trials. 2020;89:105915.
22. Burkart M, Sanford S, Dinner S, Sharp L, Kinahan K. Future health of AYA survivors. Pediatr Blood Cancer. 2019; 66(2):e27516.
23. Hudson MM, Ness KK, Gurney JG, Mulrooney DA, Chemaitilly W, Krull K, et al. Clinical ascertainment of health outcomes among adults treated for childhood cancer. JAMA 2013;309(22):2371–81.
24. Kadan-Lottick NS, Robison LL, Gurney JG, Neglia JP, Yasui Y, Hayashi R, et al. Childhood cancer survivors' knowledge about their past diagnosis and treatment: Childhood Cancer Survivor Study. JAMA. 2002;287(14):1832–9.
25. Alloin AL, Barlogis V, Auquier P, Contet A, Poiree M, Demeocq F, et al. Prevalence and risk factors of cataract after chemotherapy with or without central nervous system irradiation for childhood acute lymphoblastic leukaemia: an LEA study. Br J Haematol. 2014;164(1):94–100.
26. Mandel K, Atkinson S, Barr RD, Pencharz P. Skeletal morbidity in childhood acute lymphoblastic leukemia. J Clin Oncol. 2004;22(7):1215–21.
27. Armenian SH, Hudson MM, Mulder RL, Chen MH, Constine LS, Dwyer M, et al. Recommendations for cardiomyopathy surveillance for survivors of childhood cancer: a report from the International Late Effects of Childhood Cancer Guideline Harmonization Group. Lancet Oncol. 2015;16(3):e123–36.
28. Kenney LB, Cohen LE, Shnorhavorian M, Metzger ML, Lockart B, Hijiya N, et al. Male reproductive health after childhood, adolescent, and young adult cancers: a report from the Children's Oncology Group. J Clin Oncol. 2012;30(27):3408–16.
29. Felicetti F, Fortunati N, Arvat E, Brignardello E. GH deficiency in adult survivors of childhood cancer. Best Pract Res Clin Endocrinol Metab. 2016;30(6):795–804.
30. Brignardello E, Felicetti F, Castiglione A, Chiabotto P, Corrias A, Fagioli F, et al. Endocrine health conditions in adult survivors of childhood cancer: the need for specialized adult-focused follow-up clinics. Eur J Endocrinol. 2013;168(3):465–72.
31. Mostoufi-Moab S, Seidel K, Leisenring WM, Armstrong GT, Oeffinger KC, Stovall M, et al. Endocrine abnormalities in aging survivors of childhood cancer: a report from the Childhood Cancer Survivor Study. J Clin Oncol. 2016;34(27):3240–7.
32. Chow EJ, Anderson L, Baker KS, Bhatia S, Guilcher GM, Huang JT, et al. Late effects surveillance recommendations among survivors of childhood hematopoietic cell transplantation: a Children's Oncology Group Report. Biol Blood Marrow Transplant. 2016;22(5):782–95.
33. Johnston BL, Conly JM. Immunization for bone marrow transplant recipients. Can J Infect Dis. 2002;13(6):353–7.
34. Brodtman DH, Rosenthal DW, Redner A, Lanzkowsky P, Bonagura VR. Immunodeficiency in children with acute lymphoblastic leukemia after completion of modern aggressive chemotherapeutic regimens. J Pediatr. 2005;146(5):654–61.
35. Stefanski KJ, Anixt JS, Goodman P, Bowers K, Leisenring W, Baker KS, et al. Long-term neurocognitive and psychosocial outcomes after acute myeloid leukemia: a Childhood Cancer Survivor Study Report. J Natl Cancer Inst. 2020.
36. Crochet E, Tyc VL, Wang M, Srivastava DK, Van Sickle K, Nathan PC, et al. Posttraumatic stress as a contributor to behavioral health outcomes and healthcare utilization in adult survivors of childhood cancer: a report from the Childhood Cancer Survivor Study. J Cancer Surviv. 2019;13(6):981–92.
37. Phillips SM, Padgett LS, Leisenring WM, Stratton KK, Bishop K, Krull KR, et al. Survivors of childhood cancer in the United States: prevalence and burden of morbidity. Cancer Epidemiol Biomark Prev. 2015;24(4):653–63.
38. Siegel RL, Miller KD, Jemal A. Cancer statistics, 2020. CA Cancer J Clin. 2020;70(1):7–30.

39. Noone AM HN, Krapcho M, Miller D, Brest A, Yu M, Ruhl J, et al. (eds). SEER Cancer Statistics Review, 1975–2015. Bethesda, MD: National Cancer Institute; based on November 2017 SEER data submission, posted to the SEER website, April 2018. Available from: https://seer.cancer.gov/csr/1975_2015/.

40. DeVita Jr VT. A selective history of the therapy of Hodgkin's disease. Br J Haematol. 2003;122(5):718–27.

41. Castellino SM, Geiger AM, Mertens AC, Leisenring WM, Tooze JA, Goodman P, et al. Morbidity and mortality in long-term survivors of Hodgkin lymphoma: a report from the Childhood Cancer Survivor Study. Blood. 2011;117(6):1806–16.

42. Thomson AB, Wallace WHB. Treatment of paediatric Hodgkin's disease: a balance of risks. Eur J Cancer. 2002;38(4):468–77.

43. Kelly KM. Hodgkin lymphoma in children and adolescents: improving the therapeutic index. Blood. 2015;126(22):2452–8.

44. Friedman DL, Chen L, Wolden S, Buxton A, McCarten K, FitzGerald TJ, et al. Dose-intensive response-based chemotherapy and radiation therapy for children and adolescents with newly diagnosed intermediate-risk Hodgkin lymphoma: a report from the Children's Oncology Group Study AHOD0031. J Clin Oncol. 2014;32(32):3651–8.

45. Schwartz CL, Constine LS, Villaluna D, London WB, Hutchison RE, Sposto R, et al. A risk-adapted, response-based approach using ABVE-PC for children and adolescents with intermediate- and high-risk Hodgkin lymphoma: the results of P9425. Blood. 2009;114(10):2051–9.

46. Tebbi CK, Mendenhall NP, London WB, Williams JL, Hutchison RE, Fitzgerald TJ, et al. Response-dependent and reduced treatment in lower risk Hodgkin lymphoma in children and adolescents, results of P9426: a report from the Children's Oncology Group. Pediatr Blood Cancer. 2012;59(7):1259–65.

47. Oeffinger KC, Stratton K, Hudson MM, Leisenring W, Howell RM, Wolden SL, et al. Impact of risk-adapted therapy for pediatric Hodgkin lymphoma on risk of long-term morbidity: A report from the Childhood Cancer Surivovr Study. J Clin Oncol 2021. Epub ahead of print: doi 10.1200/JCO.20.01186, PMID 33630659.

48. Armstrong GT, Chen Y, Yasui Y, Leisenring W, Gibson TM, Mertens AC, et al. Reduction in late mortality among 5-year survivors of childhood cancer. N Engl J Med. 2016;374(9):833–42.

49. Board PDQPTE. Childhood Hodgkin Lymphoma Treatment (PDQ®): Health Professional Version. PDQ Cancer Information Summaries. Bethesda, MD: National Cancer Institute (US); 2020.

50. Franco VI, Lipshultz SE. Cardiac complications in childhood cancer survivors treated with anthracyclines. Cardiol Young. 2015;25 Suppl 2:107–16.

51. Lipshultz SE, Alvarez JA, Scully RE. Anthracycline associated cardiotoxicity in survivors of childhood cancer. Heart. 2008;94(4):525–33.

52. Mulrooney DA, Yeazel MW, Kawashima T, Mertens AC, Mitby P, Stovall M, et al. Cardiac outcomes in a cohort of adult survivors of childhood and adolescent cancer: retrospective analysis of the Childhood Cancer Survivor Study cohort. BMJ. 2009;339:b4606.

53. Bowers DC, McNeil DE, Liu Y, Yasui Y, Stovall M, Gurney JG, et al. Stroke as a late treatment effect of Hodgkin's disease: a report from the Childhood Cancer Survivor Study. J Clin Oncol. 2005;23(27):6508–15.

54. Bhakta N, Liu Q, Yeo F, Baassiri M, Ehrhardt MJ, Srivastava DK, et al. Cumulative burden of cardiovascular morbidity in paediatric, adolescent, and young adult survivors of Hodgkin's lymphoma: an analysis from the St Jude Lifetime Cohort Study. Lancet Oncol. 2016;17(9):1325–34.

55. Armenian S, Bhatia S. Predicting and preventing anthracycline-related cardiotoxicity. Am Soc Clin Oncol Educ Book. 2018(38):3–12.

56. Leger K, Slone T, Lemler M, Leonard D, Cochran C, Bowman WP, et al. Subclinical cardiotoxicity in childhood cancer survivors exposed to very low dose anthracycline therapy. Pediatr Blood Cancer. 2015;62(1):123–7.

57. U.S. National Institutes of Health NCI. SEER Training Modules, Radiation Therapy. Available from: https://training.seer.cancer.gov/lymphoma/treatment/radiation.html.

58. Armstrong GT, Oeffinger KC, Chen Y, Kawashima T, Yasui Y, Leisenring W, et al. Modifiable risk factors and major cardiac events among adult survivors of childhood cancer. J Clin Oncol. 2013;31(29):3673–80.

59. Adams MJ, Lipsitz SR, Colan SD, Tarbell NJ, Treves ST, Diller L, et al. Cardiovascular status in long-term survivors of Hodgkin's disease treated with chest radiotherapy. J Clin Oncol. 2004;22(15):3139–48.

60. Piovaccari G, Ferretti RM, Prati F, Traini AM, Gobbi M, Caravita L, et al. Cardiac disease after chest irradiation for Hodgkin's disease: incidence in 108 patients with long follow-up. Int J Cardiol. 1995;49(1):39–43.

61. Friedman DN, Tonorezos ES, Cohen P. Diabetes and metabolic syndrome in survivors of childhood cancer. Horm Res Paediatr. 2019;91(2):118–27.

62. Hancock SL, Tucker MA, Hoppe RT. Factors affecting late mortality from heart disease after treatment of Hodgkin's disease. JAMA. 1993;270(16):1949–55.

63. Pihkala J, Happonen J-M, Virtanen K, Sovijärvi A, Siimes MA, Pesonen E, et al. Cardiopulmonary evaluation of exercise tolerance after chest irradiation and anticancer chemotherapy in children and adolescents. Pediatrics. 1995;95(5):722–6.

64. Baker KS, Chow E, Steinberger J. Metabolic syndrome and cardiovascular risk in survivors after hematopoietic cell transplantation. Bone Marrow Transpl. 2012;47(5):619–25.

65. DeFilipp Z, Duarte RF, Snowden JA, Majhail NS, Greenfield DM, Miranda JL, et al. Metabolic syndrome and cardiovascular disease following hematopoietic cell transplantation: screening and preventive practice recommendations from CIBMTR and EBMT. Bone Marrow Transpl. 2017;52(2):173–82.

66. Whelan KF, Stratton K, Kawashima T, Waterbor JW, Castleberry RP, Stovall M, et al. Ocular late effects in childhood and adolescent cancer survivors: a report from the childhood cancer survivor study. Pediatr Blood Cancer. 2010;54(1):103–9.

67. Gurney JG, Ness KK, Rosenthal J, Forman SJ, Bhatia S, Baker KS. Visual, auditory, sensory, and motor impairments in long-term survivors of hematopoietic stem cell transplantation performed in childhood. Cancer. 2006;106(6):1402–8.

68. Benyunes MC, Sullivan KM, Deeg HJ, Mori M, Meyer W, Fisher L, et al. Cataracts after bone marrow transplantation: long-term follow-up of adults treated with fractionated total body irradiation. Int J Radiat Oncol Biol Phys. 1995;32(3):661–70.

69. Chodick G, Sigurdson AJ, Kleinerman RA, Sklar CA, Leisenring W, Mertens AC, et al. The risk of cataract among survivors of childhood and adolescent cancer: a report from the Childhood Cancer Survivor Study. Radiat Res. 2016;185(4):366–74.

70. Horwitz M, Auquier P, Barlogis V, Contet A, Poiree M, Kanold J, et al. Incidence and risk factors for cataract after haematopoietic stem cell transplantation for childhood leukaemia: an LEA study. Br J Haematol. 2015;168(4):518–25.

71. Friedman DL, Whitton J, Leisenring W, Mertens AC, Hammond S, Stovall M, et al. Subsequent neoplasms in 5-year survivors of childhood cancer: the Childhood Cancer Survivor Study. J Natl Cancer Inst. 2010;102(14):1083–95.

72. Henderson TO, Moskowitz CS, Chou JF, Bradbury AR, Neglia JP, Dang CT, et al. Breast cancer risk in childhood cancer survivors without a history of chest radiotherapy: a report from the Childhood Cancer Survivor Study. J Clin Oncol. 2016;34(9):910–8.

73. Moskowitz CS, Chou JF, Wolden SL, Bernstein JL, Malhotra J, Novetsky Friedman D, et al. Breast cancer after chest radiation therapy for childhood cancer. J Clin Oncol. 2014;32(21):2217–23.

74. Moskowitz CS, Chou JF, Neglia JP, Partridge AH, Howell RM, Diller LR, et al. Mortality after breast cancer among survivors of childhood cancer: a report from the Childhood Cancer Survivor Study. J Clin Oncol. 2019;37(24):2120–30.

75. Henderson TO, Amsterdam A, Bhatia S, Hudson MM, Meadows AT, Neglia JP, et al. Systematic review: surveillance for breast cancer in women treated with chest radiation for childhood, adolescent, or young adult cancer. Ann Intern Med. 2010;152(7):444–55; w144–54.

76. Ng AK, Garber JE, Diller LR, Birdwell RL, Feng Y, Neuberg DS, et al. Prospective study of the efficacy of breast magnetic resonance imaging and mammographic screening in survivors of Hodgkin lymphoma. J Clin Oncol. 2013;31(18):2282–8.

77. Daniel CL, Kohler CL, Stratton KL, Oeffinger KC, Leisenring WM, Waterbor JW, et al. Predictors of colorectal cancer surveillance among survivors of childhood cancer treated with radiation: a report from the Childhood Cancer Survivor Study. Cancer. 2015;121(11):1856–63.

78. Nottage K, McFarlane J, Krasin MJ, Li C, Srivastava D, Robison LL, et al. Secondary colorectal carcinoma after childhood cancer. J Clin Oncol. 2012;30(20):2552–8.

79. Lieberman DA, Rex DK, Winawer SJ, Giardiello FM, Johnson DA, Levin TR. Guidelines for colonoscopy surveillance after screening and polypectomy: a consensus update by the US Multi-Society Task Force on Colorectal Cancer. Gastroenterology. 2012;143(3):844–57.

80. Mulder RL, Hudson MM, Bhatia S, Landier W, Levitt G, Constine LS, et al. Updated breast cancer surveillance recommendations for female survivors of childhood, adolescent, and young adult cancer from the International Guideline Harmonization Group. J Clin Oncol. 2020;38(35):4194–207.

81. van Dorp W, Mulder RL, Kremer LC, Hudson MM, van den Heuvel-Eibrink MM, van den Berg MH, et al. Recommendations for premature ovarian insufficiency surveillance for female survivors of childhood, adolescent, and young adult cancer: a report From the International Late Effects of Childhood Cancer Guideline Harmonization Group in Collaboration with the PanCareSurFup Consortium. J Clin Oncol. 2016;34(28):3440–50.

82. Bitsko MJ, Cohen D, Dillon R, Harvey J, Krull K, Klosky JL. Psychosocial late effects in pediatric cancer survivors: a report from the Children's Oncology Group. Pediatr Blood Cancer. 2016;63(2):337–43.

83. Nathan PC, Greenberg ML, Ness KK, Hudson MM, Mertens AC, Mahoney MC, et al. Medical care in long-term survivors of childhood cancer: a report from the childhood cancer survivor study. J Clin Oncol. 2008;26(27):4401.

84. Halpern MT, Viswanathan M, Evans TS, Birken SA, Basch E, Mayer DK. Models of cancer survivorship care: overview and summary of current evidence. J Oncol Pract. 2015;11(1):e19–e27.

85. Hewitt M, Greenfield S, Stovall E. From Cancer Patient to Cancer Survivor: Lost in Transition. Washington, DC: National Academies Press; 2005.

86. Oeffinger KC, McCabe MS. Models for delivering survivorship care. J Clin Oncol. 2006;24(32):5117–24.

87. McCabe MS, Bhatia S, Oeffinger KC, Reaman GH, Tyne C, Wollins DS, et al. American Society of Clinical Oncology statement: achieving high-quality cancer survivorship care. J Clin Oncol. 2013;31(5):631.

88. Hong S, Nekhlyudov L, Didwania A, Olopade O, Ganschow P. Cancer survivorship care: exploring the role of the general internist. J General Intern Med. 2009;24(2):495–500.

89. Nekhlyudov L, Aziz NM, Lerro C, Virgo KS. Oncologists' and primary care physicians' awareness of late and long-term effects of chemotherapy: implications for care of the growing population of survivors. J Oncol Pract. 2014;10(2):e29–36.

90. Nathan PC, Daugherty CK, Wroblewski KE, Kigin ML, Stewart TV, Hlubocky FJ, et al. Family physician preferences and knowledge gaps regarding the care of adolescent and young adult survivors of childhood cancer. J Cancer Surviv. 2013;7(3):275–82.

91. Del Giudice ME, Grunfeld E, Harvey BJ, Piliotis E, Verma S. Primary care physicians' views of routine follow-up care of cancer survivors. J Clin Oncol. 2009;27(20):3338–45.

92. Suh E, Daugherty CK, Wroblewski K, Lee H, Kigin ML, Rasinski KA, et al. General internists' preferences and knowledge about the care of adult survivors of childhood cancer: a cross-sectional survey. Ann Intern Med. 2014;160(1):11–7.

93. Nathan PC, Ford JS, Henderson TO, Hudson MM, Emmons KM, Casillas JN, et al. Health behaviors, medical care, and interventions to promote healthy living in the Childhood Cancer Survivor Study cohort. J Clin Oncol. 2009;27(14):2363–73.
94. Nekhlyudov L, O'Malley DM, Hudson SV. Integrating primary care providers in the care of cancer survivors: gaps in evidence and future opportunities. Lancet Oncol. 2017;18(1):e30–e38.
95. Tonorezos ES, Barnea D, Sklar CA, Friedman DN. Training in long-term follow-up: fellowship in childhood cancer survivorship. J Cancer Educ. 2021;36(4):689–92.
96. Smith SM, Williams P, Kim J, Alberto J, Schapira L. Health after cancer: an innovative continuing medical education course integrating cancer survivorship into primary care. Acad Med. 2021;96(8):1164–67.

Genetic Risk and Cancer Susceptibility

4

Madeline Graf and Allison W. Kurian

INTRODUCTION

Over the past two decades, germline genetic testing for assessment of cancer risk has become increasingly integrated into cancer care. Detection of a hereditary pathogenic variant in a cancer susceptibility gene has implications throughout the cancer care continuum, from the previvor phase in which pathogenic variant carriers may undergo intensive cancer surveillance or risk-reducing procedures; to the treatment phase in which genetically targeted therapies are increasingly routine; to the survivorship period in which subsequent cancer risk reduction is an important consideration. For some patients, the survivorship period is an optimal time to pursue genetic counseling and testing, once the immediate demands of acute cancer treatment are lessened. Genetic counseling and testing can enable personalized cancer risk management for both the cancer survivor and their family members. In this chapter, we will summarize the principles of cancer genetic risk assessment, genetic counseling, and testing of cancer survivors and their relatives.

IDENTIFICATION OF PATIENTS FOR GENETICS EVALUATION

In general, suspicion for a hereditary cancer syndrome should be heightened when an individual has had:

- A cancer diagnosis at a younger age than expected for that cancer type (typically <50 years old), and/or
- A specific cancer type known to have relatively high heritability (i.e., ovarian, pancreatic, metastatic prostate), and/or
- Multiple primary cancers, and/or
- Rare cancers (i.e., adrenocortical carcinoma, male breast cancer), and/or
- Multiple affected family members in multiple generations (1–3).

When considering a patient for cancer genetics evaluation and/or testing, it is important to gather factors of a patient's personal and family history. Relevant personal history includes cancer type(s) and specific

DOI: 10.1201/9781003055426-4

pathology, age(s) of diagnosis, presence of suggestive physical features, ancestry, and whether any genetic testing (tumor or germline) has been previously performed. Other factors such as carcinogen exposure history (i.e., radiation, smoking tobacco), body mass index, reproductive history, and personal hormonal factors should be noted, but generally should not be used to exclude an individual from referral to genetics who would otherwise be an appropriate candidate (1, 3, 4).

Basic family history should be solicited for close family members (first-, second-, and third-degree relatives). For those who have had cancer, the type(s) and age(s) of diagnosis should be collected. It is also pertinent to know whether other family members have already undergone genetic testing for hereditary cancers. A genetic specialist such as a genetic counselor will collect a more detailed three-generation family history at the time of intake. If an individual has no knowledge or limited knowledge of their family medical history, such as those who were involved in closed adoptions, clinicians should operate conservatively and have a lower threshold for sending those patients for genetics evaluation (1, 3, 4).

There are some indications for cancer genetics evaluation that are satisfied by personal history alone and some which require a combination of personal and family history. The National Comprehensive Cancer Network and other groups deliver guidelines or statements periodically regarding which individuals should be offered genetic testing for hereditary cancers. There are many patients whose clinical scenarios are not covered in these guidelines, especially those with rarer hereditary cancer syndromes, that may still warrant genetics evaluation.

Below are reference tables for clinicians when considering a patient for genetics evaluation (Tables 4.1–4.3). Note that these tables are meant to be a guide and are not comprehensive. Additionally, indications for referral to a cancer genetics professional change and expand frequently. Clinicians are encouraged to consult updated resources and/or genetics professionals when determining patient candidates for genetics evaluation.

TABLE 4.1   Personal history indications for cancer genetics evaluation

BREAST CANCER
• Bilateral lobular breast cancer diagnosed <70 years old
• Breast cancer at any age with Ashkenazi Jewish ancestry
• Breast cancer diagnosed ≤45 years old
• Male breast cancer
• Multiple breast primaries, with the first diagnosed ≤50 years old
• Triple-negative breast cancer diagnosed ≤60 years old

GASTROINTESTINAL CANCERS
• ≥10 colonic adenomas
• ≥5 serrated colonic polyps

• Colorectal cancer **AND** ≥1 of the following:
  • Diagnosed <50 years old
  • Another synchronous or metachronous primary of specific type[1]

• Diffuse gastric cancer diagnosed <50 years old
• Pancreatic exocrine cancer

GYNECOLOGIC CANCERS

• Endometrial cancer **AND** ≥1 of the following:
  • Diagnosed <50 years old
  • Another synchronous or metachronous primary of specific type[1]

• Ovarian/fallopian tube/primary peritoneal epithelial cancer

(Continued)

TABLE 4.1 (*Continued*) Personal history indications for cancer genetics evaluation

GENITOURINARY CANCERS

- Bilateral or multifocal renal cancer
- Metastatic, intraductal/cribriform, or high-risk to very high-risk prostate cancer
- Renal cancer diagnosed at ≤46 years old

ENDOCRINE AND NEUROENDOCRINE CANCERS

- ≥2 of the following tumors: parathyroid, pituitary, well-differentiated endocrine tumors of the gastro-entero-pancreatic tract
- Adrenocortical carcinoma
- Cribriform-morular variant of papillary thyroid cancer
- Neuroendocrine tumors of the pancreas
- Pheochromocytoma or paraganglioma

SARCOMA

- Desmoid tumor
- Rhabdomyosarcoma (anaplastic embryonal subtype)

PATHOLOGY OR MOLECULAR FINDINGS

- Individuals with cancer who may benefit from germline testing to determine eligibility for targeted treatment (i.e., poly (ADP-ribose) polymerase inhibitor for ovarian, breast, pancreatic, or prostate cancer)
- Known pathogenic variant for hereditary cancer in any blood relative
- Pathogenic variant identified on tumor profiling which has clinical implications if identified to be germline
- Tumor with mismatch repair deficiency (tissue phenotype suggestive of Lynch syndrome)
- Uterine fibroid with loss of fumarate hydratase (FH) staining and positive cytoplasmic staining for S-(2-succino) cysteine

OTHER

- Endolymphatic sac tumor
- Multiple tumors in the following spectrum: soft tissue sarcoma, osteosarcoma, central nervous system tumor, breast cancer, adrenocortical carcinoma
- Retinal or central nervous system hemangioblastoma

Source: Refs. (4–10).

[1] Colorectal, endometrial, ovarian, gastric, pancreatic, urothelial, brain, biliary tract, small intestinal, sebaceous adenomas / carcinomas, or keratoacanthomas.

TABLE 4.2 Personal and family history indications for cancer genetics evaluation

PERSONAL CANCER HISTORY		FAMILY CANCER HISTORY
Breast cancer diagnosed at age 46–50	AND	• ≥1 close relative[1] with breast, ovarian, pancreatic, or prostate cancer OR • An unknown or limited family history (i.e., closed adoption or estranged)
Breast cancer at any age	AND	• ≥1 close relative[1] with breast cancer ≤50 years old or ovarian, male breast, pancreatic, or prostate[2] cancer OR • ≥2 additional diagnoses of breast cancer (in patient and/or close relatives[1])

TABLE 4.2 (*Continued*)   Personal and family history indications for cancer genetics evaluation

PERSONAL CANCER HISTORY		FAMILY CANCER HISTORY
Prostate cancer	AND	• ≥1 close relative[1] with breast cancer ≤50 years old or ovarian, pancreatic, or prostate[2] cancer *OR* • ≥2 close relatives[1] with breast or prostate cancer
Colorectal or endometrial cancer <50 years old	AND	• One first- or second-degree relative with specific cancer type[3] diagnosed <50 years old *OR* • ≥2 first- or second-degree relatives with specific cancer type[3]
Sarcoma diagnosed ≤46 years old	AND	• First- and/or second-degree relatives with cancer, especially when diagnosed <45 years old, or with tumors from specific spectrum[4], or with multiple primary cancers
Diffuse gastric cancer	AND	• One first- or second-degree relative with lobular breast cancer <70 years old *OR* • One first- or second-degree relative with diffuse gastric cancer

Source: Refs. (4–6).

[1] First-, second-, or third-degree relative.
[2] Must be metastatic, intraductal/cribriform, or high-risk to very high-risk.
[3] Colorectal, endometrial, ovarian, gastric, pancreatic, urothelial, brain, biliary tract, small intestinal, sebaceous adenomas or carcinomas, or keratoacanthomas.
[4] Soft tissue sarcoma, osteosarcoma, CNS tumor, breast cancer, or adrenocortical carcinoma.

There are rare cancer syndromes that can have pathognomonic or very suggestive features. It is recommended that whenever clinicians encounter a rare cancer or neoplasm, they investigate whether this could be related to a hereditary cancer syndrome. For a more exhaustive list of referral indications, consider consulting practice guidelines of the American College of Medical Genetics (2), the National Comprehensive Cancer Network (4), or similar guidelines in other countries (12, 13) with attention to updated guidelines and publications.

TABLE 4.3   Childhood cancer indications for cancer genetics evaluation

Personal history indication	• Choroid plexus carcinoma • Retinoblastoma • Pheochromocytoma • Hepatoblastoma
Personal history consideration, especially based on family history	• Acute leukemia • Burkitt lymphoma • Hodgkin lymphoma • Medulloblastoma • Neuroblastoma • Non-Hodgkin lymphoma • Optic glioma • Osteosarcoma • Wilms tumor

Source: Ref. (11).

THE GENETIC COUNSELING PROCESS

Genetic counseling is a relatively new profession, with just over 5,000 genetic counselors practicing in the United States and Canada and increasingly more globally (14, 15). Most genetic counselors work in a clinical setting with direct patient care and most specialize in areas including prenatal, cancer, and general/pediatric genetics. Genetic counselors achieve a master's degree and are trained in molecular biology in addition to advanced counseling skills. The traditional genetic counseling model includes pre- and post-test counseling.

The National Society of Genetic Counseling's definition of genetic counseling states that genetic counseling is the process of helping people understand and adapt to the medical, psychological, and familial implications of the genetic contributions to disease. This process integrates:

- Interpretation of family and medical histories to assess the chance of disease occurrence or recurrence.
- Education about inheritance, testing, management, prevention, resources, and research.
- Counseling to promote informed choices and adaptation to the risk or condition (3).

Pre-Test Counseling

The pre-test visit involves education, risk assessment, discussion of genetic testing options, and genetic test coordination.

Generally, patient education in cancer genetic counseling includes an explanation of different etiologies of cancer, typically emphasizing that hereditary cancers are a relatively small proportion of all cancers. Explanation of inheritance, hereditary cancer syndromes, and different cancer screening or prevention options for hereditary cancer are also discussed (Figure 4.1).

The genetic counselor will collect information about a patient's cancer history and risk factors including:

- Cancer type
- Pathology
- Age of diagnosis
- Stage
- Treatment

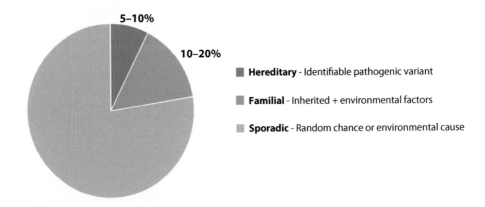

FIGURE 4.1   Proportion of cancers that are sporadic, familial, and hereditary.

- Exposure history such as radiation and smoking
- Surgical history such as hysterectomy or oophorectomy
- Prior germline (hereditary) or tumor genomic testing

Construction of Family History

A detailed three-generation family history, or pedigree, is prepared to identify cancer syndromes, determine the need for genetic testing, assist with management recommendations, and identify at-risk family members. The process of taking a family history also allows the counselor to assess relationships between family members and understand a patient's experience with cancer in their lifetime (Figure 4.2).

After gathering personal and family history, a genetic counselor will make an assessment, including building a differential diagnosis for potential causes of the cancers in the family. They may include information on whether the patient meets clinical testing criteria and the estimated yield in detecting a pathogenic variant on genetic testing.

In discussion with the patient, a genetic counselor will clarify the purpose of genetic testing, which can involve all or a portion of the following: (a) to provide an explanation for personal and/or family history of cancer, (b) to access targeted therapies, (c) to understand future cancer risks for the patient, and (d) to help family members understand their cancer risks.

Genetic counseling also provides the opportunity for a patient to explore their personal relationship to cancer and address any emotions surrounding genetic testing. In the survivorship phase, a patient may feel hesitancy to undergo genetic testing because they fear learning that they have a higher-than-average risk to develop a subsequent cancer. Genetic counselors can provide some reframing – helping the patient see that knowing about cancer risk can result in prevention or earlier diagnosis of cancer. Understanding that a patient's genetic test results can benefit family members, whether a pathogenic variant is identified or not, can also be motivating to patients.

Genetic counseling emphasizes patient autonomy; thus, the genetic counselor and patient will work together to determine the most appropriate test given both the clinical scenario and the patient's preferences. In most circumstances, genetic testing can be performed on a blood or saliva sample. Once an order has been placed, the genetic testing usually takes one to four weeks depending on the laboratory and test ordered.

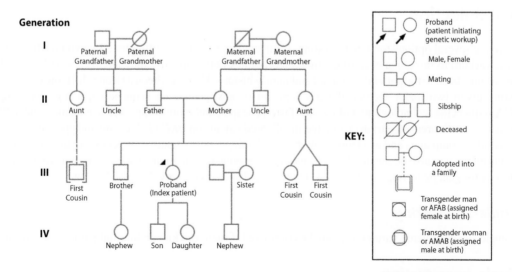

FIGURE 4.2 Three-generation pedigree as used in genetic counseling. (Image adapted from Bennett RL, French KS, Resta RG, Doyle DL. Standardized human pedigree nomenclature: update and assessment of the recommendations of the National Society of Genetic Counselors. J Genet Couns. 2008;17(5):424–33.

Post-Test Counseling

The role of a genetic counselor when a clinically significant finding is identified through genetic testing is to review the result with the patient including any risks associated with any pathogenic variants identified, typical management recommendations, reproductive risks, and which family members are also at risk. In some cases, results' reviews include a genetic counselor and a physician who can discuss the management recommendations and risk-reducing options more completely. This is particularly relevant in cancer genetics because the results of germline genetic testing increasingly inform cancer treatment selection (e.g., the use of poly(ADP-ribose) polymerase inhibitors for carriers of pathogenic variants in *BRCA1/2* or the use of immune checkpoint inhibitors for patients with tumor mismatch repair deficiency, frequently associated with Lynch Syndrome) (17, 18).

GENETIC TEST SELECTION

Laboratory Selection

The number of genetic testing laboratories has increased significantly over time, resulting in a competitive market; however, not all laboratories offer tests of equivalent quality. When choosing a laboratory for clinical genetic testing, important factors to consider are qualifications, test options, technical limitations, billing transparency and costs, turn-around time, and customer relations and communication. Qualified labs may be determined differently by country, but the United States requires clinical genetics laboratories to be certified by both the College of American Pathologists (CAP) and the Clinical Laboratory Improvement Amendments (CLIA) (19). Fortunately for many patients, the cost of genetic testing is no longer a significant barrier to undergoing testing. However, even with substantial decline in cost over the last decade, health disparities in access to genetic counseling, testing, and appropriate management recommendations remain and are key targets for quality improvement (20).

Test Selection

There are several options for genetic testing, from single-site analysis (often for a known familial pathogenic variant) to broad panel testing which incorporates both clinically indicated genes and genes that may be unrelated to the patient's personal and family history. There has been a strong shift toward broader testing given two major factors: the development of next-generation sequencing, a high-throughput DNA sequencing technology that allows for faster, cheaper, and more comprehensive testing, and a 2013 United States Supreme Court decision that invalidated patents on *BRCA1/2* testing and opened testing to many other companies and academic centers (21). Testing a larger number of genes can maximize clinical utility but can also be medically unnecessary or provide information a patient does not wish to know. Options for genetic testing and their advantages and disadvantages are discussed below.

Single-site testing

A single site or targeted variant test may be considered if there is a known familial pathogenic variant.

Single-gene testing

Testing a single gene may be considered when there is a clear clinical scenario that is likely attributable to a single gene. For example, one may test solely the *VHL* gene in an individual with multiple hemangioblastomas and bilateral renal cancer with high suspicion for Von Hippel Lindau syndrome.

Multi-gene panels

Most often, a multi-gene panel will be ordered in the hereditary cancer clinic. These panels vary greatly in size and can be focused to particular cancer types or broad to capture multiple cancer types. Some clinics will routinely offer multi-cancer panels that include all genes known to be related to hereditary cancers.

Limited-evidence genes

Increasingly, laboratories offer options to test genes with a paucity of evidence associating them to increased cancer risk. These are sometimes termed "limited-evidence" genes. Many of these genes are added to laboratory test menus because they operate in the same molecular pathway as other known hereditary cancer genes. A finding in a limited evidence gene may not be immediately relevant to an individual or their family but may be relevant over time as more is learned about that gene's associated cancer risks.

As shown in Figure 4.3, there are many options for genetic testing and choices are becoming increasingly complex. Advantages of single site, single gene, or panels tailored to personal and family history can include lower cost and fewer uncertain results. These targeted approaches can also be helpful for those currently undergoing cancer treatment who wish to limit exposure to information that may not be immediately useful to their cancer treatment or relevant to their cancer type. Cancer survivors may tend toward testing focused to their specific cancer type, or they may choose to obtain maximal cancer risk information to reduce the risks of a subsequent cancer.

Testing fewer genes has the chance to miss clinically relevant pathogenic variants. Data show that approximately 5% of patients tested on multigene panels have two pathogenic variants related to hereditary cancer, suggesting that larger gene panels should be discussed and considered even in the case of a

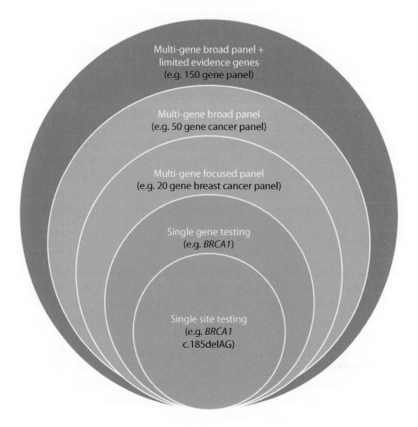

FIGURE 4.3 Genetic testing options in the hereditary cancer clinic.

known pathogenic variant in the family (22). Additionally, limiting the genes tested may fail to identify individuals who harbor pathogenic variants in unexpected genes. Studies show that when testing specific genes based on clinical testing criteria alone, up to 65% of individuals harboring a pathogenic variant in an important, medically actionable gene could be missed (23–25). Thus, performing broader genetic testing identifies a significant number of individuals and families with pathogenic variants that have important, sometimes life-saving implications for individuals and their families.

Genetic testing options offered can vary widely by institution, clinician, and the patient's clinical presentation. Clinicians should understand that selection of the appropriate genetic test is nuanced and requires exploration of personal and family history, patient preferences, and available data. It is important that a clinician navigate this decision-making process with the patient and discuss the benefits and limitations of each test option. Additionally, given the steady evolution of genetic data, genetic test results from even a few years prior to the current date, may be incomplete based on current practice. Thus, clinicians and their patients should consider periodic referral for updated genetic testing, especially in the event of an initially uninformative result.

INTERPRETATION OF GENETIC TEST RESULTS

Genetic testing can have three different types of results: positive (likely pathogenic or pathogenic variant), negative, and uncertain (variant of uncertain significance), each of which require special interpretation within the clinical context. A variant is anything identified on a genetic test that is different from the reference sequence to which it is compared. The reference used is the human genome, which was determined through the Human Genome Project (HGP). The publicly funded HGP was managed jointly by the National Institutes of Health and the United States Department of Energy and completed over a period of 13 years, with the first draft published in 2001. The goal of the project was to identify the sequences and location of human genes throughout chromosomes, ultimately allowing for revolutionary advances in biomedical research and the understanding of human disease (26, 27).

Clinical genetic testing laboratories generally have a robust classification system for variants. Variant interpretation uses evidence such as prior observations of the variant, frequency in the general population, and experimental evidence to determine whether a variant is pathogenic, likely pathogenic, benign, or likely benign (28, 29). When the data are inconclusive, a laboratory will categorize the variant as a "variant of uncertain significance," (VUS). Clinically, pathogenic and likely pathogenic variants are treated in the same way: as positive results. Benign and likely benign variants are not reported due to their clinical irrelevance, and VUS's are reported, with efforts to reclassify and issue reclassification reports as evidence emerges over time.

Positive Results

Generally, a positive result (likely pathogenic or pathogenic (LP/P)) means that the laboratory is confident that the variant in the gene significantly affects the function of that gene's protein product. In the cancer setting, this means that any LP/P variant is one that increases cancer risk. The exact magnitude of that increased risk and for which cancer types varies depending on the gene and sometimes also on the specific variant within the gene.

For many genes, there are evidence-based guidelines, such as those of the National Comprehensive Cancer Network, that outline management of results (4, 5, 9). For some genes, there are no clear guidelines, either because of the rarity of the associated condition or due to limited evidence for the gene's association with increased cancer risk. In these cases, genetic specialists will work with the patient to discuss best management given the available data.

The identification of a pathogenic variant in a family can be lifesaving as demonstrated by the following case example.

Case example

A 42-year-old male, referred to as the consultand, presented to hereditary cancer clinic reporting a recent diagnosis of Lynch syndrome in his maternal half-brother with stage IV colorectal cancer. Lynch syndrome, the most common cause of hereditary colorectal and endometrial cancers, can be due to an inherited pathogenic variant in one of five genes. This particular family had a known pathogenic variant in the *MLH1* gene. Along with colorectal and endometrial cancers, individuals with Lynch syndrome have an increased risk for ovarian, gastric, hepatobiliary tract and urinary tract cancers, amongst others.

As shown in Figure 4.4, the patient's mother died from ovarian cancer and had several siblings with colorectal cancer, with one diagnosed and deceased at age 29. The pattern of Lynch syndrome-associated cancers extended to the patient's maternal grandfather.

Despite the strong family history of cancer, genetic testing was not performed prior to the patient's brother's clinical presentation with stage IV disease. The patient was understandably distressed by his brother's hereditary cancer diagnosis; however, we emphasized the value in having an explanation for the strong family history. Identification of a pathogenic variant had several advantages, including access to targeted therapy for his brother and providing a strategy to quantify cancer risks and initiate appropriate screenings and prophylaxis for our patient and his family members. The stepwise process for family testing, or "cascade testing," is discussed later in "Familial Implications and Cascade Testing."

We initiated genetic testing on our patient, and he was identified to have the familial *MLH1* pathogenic variant. Subsequently, the patient's other siblings underwent testing. His half-sister was identified to have the pathogenic variant and his other half-brother was not. Table 4.4 shows various implications that now apply to the family based on the original identification of Lynch syndrome and follow up testing in family members.

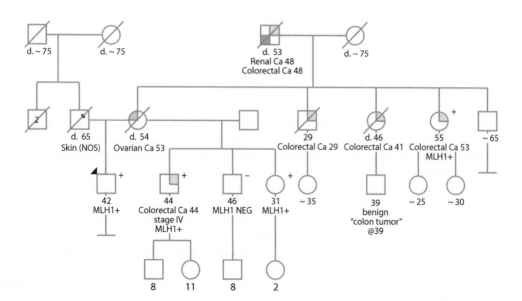

FIGURE 4.4 Example pedigree of a family history with an identified *MLH1* pathogenic variant. *Key:* arrow, consultand; circle, biological female; square, biological male; number within shape = number of individuals; NEG, negative; shading indicates different cancer types; number under shape = current age; d., deceased; slash through symbol = deceased, –/+ represents genetic test results.

TABLE 4.4   Implications of results of original identification of Lynch syndrome and follow up testing in family members

INDIVIDUAL, CANCER DIAGNOSIS, LYNCH SYNDROME STATUS	IMPLICATIONS OF RESULT
Patient, none, positive	• Increased cancer risk • Tailored screening, such as colonoscopy with polypectomy every 1–2 years to significantly reduce colorectal cancer risk
Half-brother, stage IV colorectal, positive	• Explanation for cancer • Targeted therapy such as immune checkpoint inhibitors • Children have a 50% chance to have the pathogenic variant
Half-brother, none, negative	• No increased cancer risk • Testing is not indicated for son
Half-sister, none, positive	• Increased cancer risk • Tailored screening, such as colonoscopy with polypectomy every 1–2 years to significantly reduce colorectal cancer risk • Option for prophylactic hysterectomy and oophorectomy to significantly reduce endometrial and ovarian cancer risk • Daughter has a 50% chance to have the pathogenic variant
Maternal aunt, in survivorship, positive	• Explanation for cancer • Increased risk for additional cancers such as colorectal, ovarian, and endometrial • Colorectal screening may change • Option for prophylactic hysterectomy and oophorectomy to significantly reduce endometrial and ovarian cancer risk • Children have a 50% chance to have the pathogenic variant

The identification of a pathogenic variant can be empowering when there is a strong family history of cancer and there are clinical actions available to prevent and/or significantly reduce cancer risk in surviving family members. Unfortunately, for several of our patient's family members, genetic testing was initiated too late, when the options to prevent cancer no longer existed. Ideally, hereditary cancer syndromes are identified as early as possible so that screening can be initiated and cancer deaths can be prevented.

Negative Results

A negative result requires careful interpretation and highlights the value of involving a genetic counselor in a patient's testing. A negative genetic test result means that no harmful variants were found in the genes analyzed. In some cases, a negative result has a clear meaning and clinical direction. For example, if an individual tests negative for a known familial pathogenic variant, they are most likely at general population risk to develop the cancers associated with that gene. In other cases, a negative result is less informative. There still may be a strong personal and/or family history that suggests an inherited cause to the cancer, despite having no available genetic explanation. For example, the pedigree shown in Figure 4.5 is strongly suggestive of a *BRCA1* or *BRCA2* pathogenic variant, given the pattern of breast (especially early onset), ovarian, pancreatic, and prostate cancer. However, in this case multiple relatives have tested negative on comprehensive cancer panels.

Possible explanations for lack of an identifiable pathogenic variant in families with substantial cancer history may include:

- A pathogenic variant in a gene tested that cannot be detected due to a technical limitation
- A pathogenic variant in a gene not analyzed on the test (either due to incomplete test ordered, or research to date not having identified all genes to test)

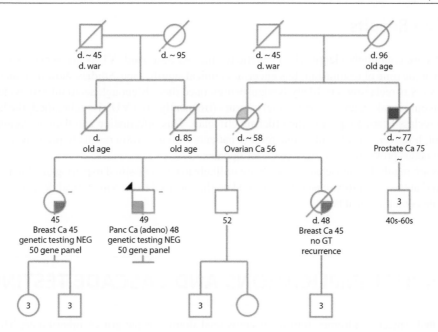

FIGURE 4.5 Example pedigree of a family history that is suggestive of a *BRCA1/2* pathogenic variant but genetic testing is negative. *Key*: arrow, consultand; circle, biological female; square, biological male; number within shape = number of individuals; NEG, negative; GT, genetic testing; shading indicates different cancer types; number under shape = current age; d., deceased; slash through symbol = deceased; –/+ represents genetic test results.

- A complex, multifactorial process whereby several genetic variants in a family, and possibly also environmental factors, increase cancer risk
- Cancers in family members are, coincidentally, sporadic

Generally, a negative result in a strong family history of cancer is more representative of a limitation in current genetic testing capabilities, as opposed to the family not having hereditary contributions to cancer.

In the preceding section, we demonstrated the value of identifying a pathogenic variant for risk stratification of family members, either to return them to general population cancer risks or to identify increased cancer risks and initiate appropriate screening or prophylaxis. Unfortunately, in the case of an uninformative result, we are unable to determine who in the family may have a general population risk for cancer and who may have higher than average risk. Thus, individuals are managed based on personal and family history and recommended to undergo relevant screenings. For example, unaffected females in the family shown here should consider high-risk breast cancer screening incorporating magnetic resonance imaging and the surviving relative with breast cancer may consider a risk-reducing bilateral salpingo-oophorectomy.

Negative results can also have different meanings depending on who in the family was tested. It is always best to test the person in the family who is affected with cancer and thus most likely to have an identifiable pathogenic variant – termed the "informative family member." If an unaffected individual is tested, there are significant limitations. Namely, if they test negative, it is unknown if it was because: (a) there is no identifiable pathogenic variant in the family or (b) there is an identifiable pathogenic variant in the family, but this individual did not inherit it.

Finally, patients sometimes assume that a negative result means that they have no risk of developing cancer in the future. Thus, it is important for clinicians to emphasize that there is still a general baseline population risk for cancer, and that elements such as lifestyle, prior cancer treatments, and family history may increase or decrease that risk.

Uncertain Results

Lastly, VUSs are commonly identified on genetic testing. As described, VUSs are genetic variants with limited data at the time of testing and thus uncertain clinical significance. Studies show that about 90% of the time, a VUS is reclassified to likely benign/benign once there is enough accumulated evidence (30). This can sometimes take a few weeks (rarely) to years (frequently). If a VUS is reclassified, the laboratory will issue a reclassification report to the ordering clinician. This information can then be communicated to the patient; however, it is also advisable for any patients with uncertain results to proactively follow up with their genetics providers every few years for updates.

Patients are regularly counseled that VUS are unlikely to be reclassified to pathogenic but they should be informed that the possibility exists. VUS should neither be used to inform clinical decisions nor to test family members on a clinical basis.

FAMILIAL IMPLICATIONS AND CASCADE TESTING

Most inherited cancer syndromes follow an autosomal dominant pattern of inheritance. This means that cancer genes are not linked to the X or Y chromosomes and thus are equally inherited by men and women. It also means that just one copy of a pair of genes needs to have a pathogenic variant in order to cause the effect (in the case of cancer-associated genes, the effect is increased cancer risk). Because each biological parent passes down one copy of each pair of autosomal (non-sex) genes, when an individual reproduces, they have a 50% chance to pass down the copy of their gene with the pathogenic variant and 50% chance to pass on the copy without the pathogenic variant. Nearly all cancer-associated pathogenic variants are inherited from one parent or the other (rarely *de novo* or brand new in a person). Thus, when a positive result is identified, in most cases patients are counseled that it was inherited, that any full siblings have a 50/50 chance of having it also, and any children or future children also have a 50/50 chance to inherit this same pathogenic variant.

Cascade testing refers to the identification of family members at risk for hereditary conditions after the proband (the person first brought to medical attention for genetic evaluation) is found to have a pathogenic variant on genetic testing (31). There is a logic of testing that will optimally identify at-risk family members and reduce unnecessary genetic testing (Figure 4.6). The ideal cascade testing involves testing a proband's first-degree relatives first. If any one of the first-degree relatives tests positive, then cascade testing involves testing that relative's first degree relatives. If any first-degree relative to the proband tests negative, then testing can stop there for that branch of the family tree.

This is a simplistic view of cascade testing, and several variables exist including relatives who may be deceased, unwilling to test, or do not have access to testing. In these cases, a more distant relative to the proband may be tested, even if a closer relative has not yet been tested.

If one or both of a proband's parents are available, it is advisable that they undergo genetic testing to determine whether the variant was maternally or paternally inherited. The focus of further family member testing can then be narrowed and unnecessary testing avoided.

Genetic counselors assist patients in the process of cascade testing. This includes discussing who should consider genetic testing, ways to communicate to family members, writing family letters, and suggesting ways for family members to access genetic testing. There are many options for genetic counseling and testing, ranging from traditional in-person genetics consults to genetic testing that is ordered online and initiated by the patient. Ideally, family members undergoing genetic testing will have the opportunity to meet with a genetic specialist, such as a genetic counselor. They can find one in their area by using an online service through the National Society of Genetic Counselors in the United States (32). They can also ask their primary care physician or other clinician for a referral or resources.

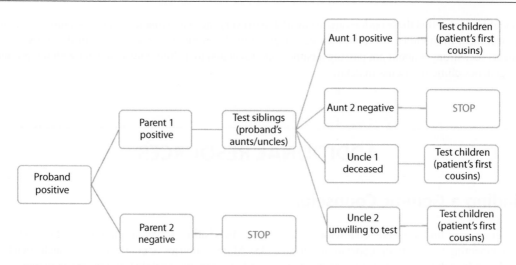

FIGURE 4.6 Example of cascade genetic testing.

Patient-initiated genetic testing is available through some commercial laboratories that will provide tele-health genetic counseling services. Unlike direct to consumer testing, patient-initiated testing is medical grade, requiring involvement of a medical professional. Fortunately, even genetic testing of relatives who live internationally has become much more feasible given the increasing availability of genetics services globally and the ability for laboratories located within the United States to send test kits internationally for family members (15).

In terms of *when* to test relatives, it should be emphasized that genetic testing is rarely ever urgent. For many, but not all hereditary cancer syndromes, there are no risks in childhood and no medical intervention that would be made until adulthood. There are several society statements, such as those of the National Society of Genetic Counselors, that generally recommend against genetic testing for adult-onset conditions in childhood (33, 34). These statements address the lack of medical necessity for testing in childhood, in addition to the ethical principle of autonomy, whereby there is consensus that the individual tested should be of age to consent to testing. A subset of hereditary cancer syndromes does have childhood cancer risks and should be assessed at young ages (for example, Li-Fraumeni syndrome associated with *TP53* pathogenic variants), so it is important to understand the scope of cancer risks for the genetic syndrome identified in the family.

Genetic test results have reproductive implications. As discussed above, with many hereditary cancer syndromes, there is a 50/50 chance for any offspring to inherit the pathogenic variant and associated cancer risks. With certain genes, there is also a risk for a more severe childhood-onset condition if a child inherits one pathogenic variant from each parent (for example, Ataxia Telangiectasia due to biallelic pathogenic variants in the *ATM* gene or Fanconi Anemia due to biallelic pathogenic variants in the *BRCA2* gene). Given these risks, individuals with a pathogenic variant in certain genes will be counseled that their reproductive partner should consider genetic testing for pathogenic variants in the same gene to better define reproductive risks to children.

If a couple wishes to avoid passing certain pathogenic variants to children, the following options exist:

- Use of gamete donor (sperm or egg)
- Preimplantation genetic testing (PGT) – a process requiring in vitro fertilization whereby embryos are created and tested for known pathogenic variant(s); embryos without the pathogenic variant(s) are selected and transferred
- Adoption

It should be noted that these options are not available to everyone due to financial barriers, emotional costs, and technical limitations. There may be significant ethical considerations with some of these options. If patients feel strongly about not passing a pathogenic variant(s) to a child, they can meet with a reproductive genetics clinic to discuss in detail.

ADDITIONAL RESOURCES

Finding a Genetic Counselor

Clinicians may find a genetic counselor in their region by visiting SNPedia: Find a Genetic Counselor and connecting to society or association websites (35). Many countries or continents have such societies, which can be helpful resources to consult when in need of a genetic specialist. Below are examples:

North America

- National Society of Genetic Counselors
- Canadian Association of Genetic Counselors

Europe

- European Society of Human Genetics

Australasia

- Human Genetics Society of Australasia

Asia

- Professional Society of Genetic Counselors in Asia

Africa

- South African Society for Human Genetics

Provider Resources

- American College of Medical Genetics: https://www.acmg.net/
- National Comprehensive Cancer Network: https://www.nccn.org/
- National Society of Genetic Counselors: http://www.nsgc.org

Patient Resources

- Bright Pink – breast and ovarian health organization: http://www.bebrightpink.org/
- Facing Our Risk of Cancer Empowered: https://www.facingourrisk.org/
- Kintalk – hereditary colon cancer: https://kintalk.org/
- National Institutes of Health – Genetics Home Reference: https://medlineplus.gov/genetics/condition/

CONCLUSION

Genetic counseling and testing is an essential aspect of cancer survivorship care. The results of genetic testing can help to explain why a cancer occurred and to stratify a survivor's risk for a future cancer diagnosis. Genetic counseling and testing can inform a personalized cancer risk management plan for survivors and, as importantly, for their cancer-free relatives. Genetic testing is increasingly accessible to cancer survivors due to declining costs and broader insurance coverage. Finally, the survivorship period is an optimal time to incorporate genetically tailored interventions that can reduce subsequent cancer risk.

ACKNOWLEDGMENTS

Miles Picus, M.S. Candidate in Human Genetics & Genetic Counseling, Stanford University School of Medicine.

REFERENCES

1. Schneider K. Collecting and interpreting cancer histories. In: Counseling About Cancer: Strategies for Genetic Counseling. 3rd ed. New York, NY: Wiley-Blackwell; 2012. pp. 221–66.
2. Hampel H, Bennett RL, Buchanan A, Pearlman R, Wiesner GL. A practice guideline from the American College of Medical Genetics and Genomics and the National Society of Genetic Counselors: referral indications for cancer predisposition assessment. Genet Med. 2015;17(1):70–87.
3. PDQ Cancer Genetics Editorial Board. Cancer Genetics Risk Assessment and Counseling (PDQ®): Health Professional Version. In: PDQ Cancer Information Summaries [Internet]. Bethesda (MD): National Cancer Institute (US); 2002 [cited 2020 Sep 30]. Available from: http://www.ncbi.nlm.nih.gov/books/NBK65817/.
4. NCCN Practice Guidelines in Oncology. Genetic/Familial High-Risk Assessment: Breast, Ovarian, and Pancreatic. Version 1.2021; 2020.
5. NCCN Practice Guidelines in Oncology. Genetic/Familial High-Risk Assessment: Colorectal. Version 1.2020; 2020.
6. Blair VR, McLeod M, Carneiro F, Coit DG, D'Addario JL, van Dieren JM, et al. Hereditary diffuse gastric cancer: updated clinical practice guidelines. Lancet Oncol. 2020;21(8):e386–97.
7. Clinical Practice Guidelines for Multiple Endocrine Neoplasia Type 1 (MEN1). The Journal of Clinical Endocrinology & Metabolism | Oxford Academic [Internet]. [cited 2020 Sep 30]. Available from: https://academic-oup-com.laneproxy.stanford.edu/jcem/article/97/9/2990/2536740.
8. Von Hippel-Lindau Disease: Genetics and Role of Genetic Counseling in a Multiple Neoplasia Syndrome | Journal of Clinical Oncology [Internet]. [cited 2020 Sep 30]. Available from: https://ascopubs-org.laneproxy.stanford.edu/doi/full/10.1200/JCO.2015.65.6140.
9. NCCN Practice Guidelines in Oncology Kidney Cancer; Hereditary Renal Cell Carcinomas. Version 1.2021; 2020.
10. Muller M, Guillaud-Bataille M, Salleron J, Genestie C, Deveaux S, Slama A, et al. Pattern multiplicity and fumarate hydratase (FH)/S-(2-succino)-cysteine (2SC) staining but not eosinophilic nucleoli with perinucleolar halos differentiate hereditary leiomyomatosis and renal cell carcinoma-associated renal cell carcinomas from kidney tumors without FH gene alteration. Mod Pathol Off J U S Can Acad Pathol Inc. 2018;31(6):974–83.
11. Knapke S, Nagarajan R, Correll J, Kent D, Burns K. Hereditary cancer risk assessment in a pediatric oncology follow-up clinic. Pediatr Blood Cancer. 2012;58(1):85–9.
12. Singer CF, Balmaña J, Bürki N, Delaloge S, Filieri ME, Gerdes A-M, et al. Genetic counselling and testing of susceptibility genes for therapeutic decision-making in breast cancer – an European consensus statement and expert recommendations. Eur J Cancer Oxf Engl 1990. 2019;106:54–60.
13. Taylor A, Brady AF, Frayling IM, Hanson H, Tischkowitz M, Turnbull C, et al. Consensus for genes to be included on cancer panel tests offered by UK genetics services: guidelines of the UK Cancer Genetics Group. J Med Genet. 2018;55(6):372–7.

14. National Society of Genetic Counselors. Professional Status Survey. 2020;28.
15. Abacan M, Alsubaie L, Barlow-Stewart K, Caanen B, Cordier C, Courtney E, et al. The global state of the genetic counseling profession. Eur J Hum Genet. 2019;27(2):183–97.
16. Bennett RL, French KS, Resta RG, Doyle DL. Standardized human pedigree nomenclature: update and assessment of the recommendations of the National Society of Genetic Counselors. J Genet Couns. 2008;17(5):424–33.
17. Marabelle A, Le DT, Ascierto PA, Di Giacomo AM, De Jesus-Acosta A, Delord J-P, et al. Efficacy of pembrolizumab in patients with noncolorectal high microsatellite instability/mismatch repair-deficient cancer: results from the phase II KEYNOTE-158 study. J Clin Oncol Off J Am Soc Clin Oncol. 2020;38(1):1–10.
18. Tew WP, Lacchetti C, Ellis A, Maxian K, Banerjee S, Bookman M, et al. PARP inhibitors in the management of ovarian cancer: ASCO Guideline. J Clin Oncol Off J Am Soc Clin Oncol. 2020;38(30):3468–93.
19. Schneider K. Genetic testing and counseling. In: Counseling About Cancer: Strategies for Genetic Counseling. 3rd ed. New York, NY: Wiley-Blackwell; 2012. pp. 315–7.
20. Parikh D, Dickerson J, Kurian A. Health disparities in germline genetic testing for cancer susceptibility. Curr Breast Cancer Rep. 2020;12:51–58.
21. Lynce F, Isaacs C. How far do we go with genetic evaluation? Gene, panel, and tumor testing. Am Soc Clin Oncol Educ Book Am Soc Clin Oncol Meet. 2016;35:e72–8.
22. Caswell-Jin JL, Zimmer AD, Stedden W, Kingham KE, Zhou AY, Kurian AW. Cascade genetic testing of relatives for hereditary cancer risk: results of an online initiative. J Natl Cancer Inst. 2019;111(1):95–8.
23. LaDuca H, Polley EC, Yussuf A, Hoang L, Gutierrez S, Hart SN, et al. A clinical guide to hereditary cancer panel testing: evaluation of gene-specific cancer associations and sensitivity of genetic testing criteria in a cohort of 165,000 high-risk patients. Genet Med. 2020;22(2):407–15.
24. Rana HQ, Gelman R, LaDuca H, McFarland R, Dalton E, Thompson J, et al. Differences in TP53 mutation carrier phenotypes emerge from panel-based testing. J Natl Cancer Inst. 2018;110(8):863–70.
25. Lowstuter K, Espenschied CR, Sturgeon D, Ricker C, Karam R, LaDuca H, et al. Unexpected CDH1 mutations identified on multigene panels pose clinical management challenges. JCO Precis Oncol. 2017;(1):1–12.
26. Giani AM, Gallo GR, Gianfranceschi L, Formenti G. Long walk to genomics: History and current approaches to genome sequencing and assembly. Comput Struct Biotechnol J. 2020;18:9–19.
27. Engel LW. The Human Genome Project. History, goals, and progress to date. Arch Pathol Lab Med. 1993;117(5):459–65.
28. Nykamp K, Anderson M, Powers M, Garcia J, Herrera B, Ho Y-Y, et al. Sherloc: a comprehensive refinement of the ACMG–AMP variant classification criteria. Genet Med. 2017;19(10):1105–17.
29. Richards S, Aziz N, Bale S, Bick D, Das S, Gastier-Foster J, et al. Standards and guidelines for the interpretation of sequence variants: a joint consensus recommendation of the American College of Medical Genetics and Genomics and the Association for Molecular Pathology. Genet Med. 2015;17(5):405–23.
30. Mersch J, Brown N, Pirzadeh-Miller S, Mundt E, Cox HC, Brown K, et al. Prevalence of variant reclassification following hereditary cancer genetic testing. JAMA. 2018;320(12):1266–74.
31. Definition of cascade screening – NCI Dictionary of Genetics Terms – National Cancer Institute [Internet]; 2012 [cited 2020 Sep 7]. Available from: https://www.cancer.gov/publications/dictionaries/genetics-dictionary/def/cascade-screening.
32. NSGC Executive Office. Find a Genetic Counselor [Internet]. Available from: https://www.nsgc.org/page/find-a-genetic-counselor.
33. National Society of Genetic Counselors: Blogs: Genetic Testing of Minors for Adult-Onset Conditions [Internet]. [cited 2020 Oct 11]. Available from: https://www.nsgc.org/p/bl/et/blogaid=860.
34. Botkin JR, Belmont JW, Berg JS, Berkman BE, Bombard Y, Holm IA, et al. Points to consider: ethical, legal, and psychosocial implications of genetic testing in children and adolescents. Am J Hum Genet. 2015;97(1):6–21.
35. Find a genetic counselor – SNPedia [Internet]. [cited 2020 Nov 16]. Available from: https://www.snpedia.com/index.php/Find_a_genetic_counselor.

Intimacy and Sexual Health for Cancer Survivors

5

Catherine Benedict, Lauren A. Zimmaro, and Jennifer B. Reese

INTRODUCTION

Between 40% and 100% of cancer survivors experience sexual side effects associated with their treatments.[1] Sexual dysfunction after cancer is associated with significant distress and quality of life deficits.[2,3] Sexual problems are reported by patients of all ages and diagnoses, who are partnered and unpartnered, and irrespective of gender and sexual identity. The effects can be felt in a multitude of ways; survivors feel lost in how to regain their sexual functioning or adapt to changes with respect to body image, sense of self, and sexuality; couples struggle to navigate sexual changes and loss of intimacy in their relationships; survivors who are dating question whether and how to raise the topic with new partners and feel unsure about beginning new sexual relationships. Without intervention, sexual problems often continue well past the completion of cancer treatment and affect long-term survivorship, making it critical that such issues be addressed in patients' care.

Current clinical guidelines from organizations including the National Comprehensive Cancer Network (NCCN) and the American Society for Clinical Oncology (ASCO) state that cancer clinicians should initiate discussions about sexual health with patients, irrespective of age, partnership status, or type of cancer history.[1,4,5] Despite this, most patients are not counseled about risks of treatment-related sexual side effects and report feeling ill-prepared for unexpected challenges when they occur.[6] Patients may wish to talk about sexual problems and treatment options with their healthcare providers but often feel unsure or reluctant to bring it up.

As more patients survive their disease, the screening and management of sexual problems is becoming increasingly relevant to clinicians across disciplines. Primary care physicians, in particular, are likely to encounter long-term survivors whose sexual problems from their cancer treatments never resolved and who could benefit from support.[7] The objective of this chapter is thus to give a brief overview of common sexual problems experienced by cancer survivors and provide guidance to clinicians for addressing these issues with their patients. We first present the common sexual problems experienced by patients based on their cancer treatment history with a review of treatment options. We then review clinical management

DOI: 10.1201/9781003055426-5

strategies including an overview of screening and assessment approaches and tips for effective communication. Discussing sexual health need not be intimidating; even brief, straightforward conversations can go a long way in helping survivors make sense of their sexual side effects and look toward a "new normal." Our hope is that the information in this chapter will prove useful to clinicians who wish to raise the topic of sexual health with the cancer survivors in their practice.

CLINICAL PRACTICE GUIDELINES

- Sexual health and dysfunction resulting from cancer or its treatment should be discussed with all patients, irrespective of age, partnership status, gender/sexual identity, or diagnosis.
- Clinicians should initiate these conversations.
- Discussions should occur early and often throughout cancer care to monitor evolving sexual health concerns.
- Education, interventions, and referrals for specialty care should be provided during the course of treatment and survivorship phase as standard of care.

Source: Based on the American Society of Clinical Oncology (ASCO) clinical guidelines.[1]

Biopsychosocial Framework

According to the biopsychosocial framework (see Figure 5.1), sexual health is a multifaceted construct encompassing physical, emotional, interpersonal, and sociocultural components.[3,8] This framework has several implications for clinical care. First, it suggests that with all the various influences on individuals' sexuality, there is likely to be considerable variability across individual patients' experiences of sexual challenges. Second, the framework underscores the importance of considering the unique factors potentially contributing to patients' symptoms when assessing or managing sexual concerns. Third,

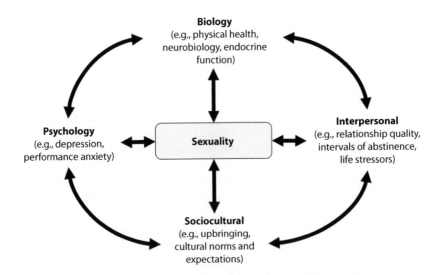

FIGURE 5.1 Biopsychosocial model of sexual function. (Adapted from Rosen RC, Barsky JL. Normal sexual response in women. *Obstet Gynecol Clin North Am.* 2006;33(4):515–526. doi:10.1016/j.ogc.2006.09.005. and Althof SE, Leiblum SR, Chevret-Measson M, et al. Psychological and interpersonal dimensions of sexual function and dysfunction. *J Sex Med.* 2005;2(6):793–800. doi:10.1111/j.1743-6109.2005.00145.x.)

it implies a level of complexity that may feel overwhelming to clinicians, who often lack training in assessment and management of sexual health complaints. It is important that clinicians are aware of the various aspects within the biopsychosocial framework that could be precipitating or maintaining sexual problems for individuals, even if it is out of the clinician's scope of practice to comprehensively manage all of them.

Because the biopsychosocial framework takes into account sociocultural and religious factors, it can be used to address sexual problems from cancer treatments for individuals from different backgrounds. Cultural and religious norms can play a role in patients' experience of sexual changes, personal and inter-personal expectations, willingness to seek help, and the kinds of treatments and management strategies that are acceptable. In many cultures, sexual topics are considered taboo and cause embarrassment or shame, which may prevent patients from initiating discussions with clinicians and seeking medical care. Cultural stereotypes about masculinity and femininity can exacerbate difficulties if identity is strongly routed in ideas of womanhood or manhood that encapsulate sexuality, and cancer treatments interfere with enacting those identities (e.g., loss of breasts after mastectomy; erectile dysfunction due to pelvic radiation/surgery). Language barriers and limited financial resources also affect access to care as well as patients' ability to express their concerns and comfort level communicating about sexual problems. Adjusting language and utilization of certified interpreters may be warranted; although, discussing sensitive topics like sexual function through an interpreter may have implications in itself.

Sexual health is also important to address for individuals from gender and sexual minority groups, who report sexual health needs after cancer but may differ in their experiences and preferences for support. Unfortunately, individuals who identify as lesbian, gay, bisexual, transgender, or queer/questioning (LGBTQ) report higher rates of feeling misunderstood and less satisfied with care across healthcare settings including oncology, compared to those who identify as heterosexual. At the same time, some evidence suggests gay, bisexual, and men who have sex with men are more likely to seek information and support for sexual problems and report greater use of assistive aids for sexual rehabilitation than heterosexual men, including use of medication, penile injection, penile implant, vacuum pump, and nonmedical sexual aids.[9] Clinicians should be prepared to discuss sexual health topics with patients who identify as gender nonconforming or as gender/sexual minorities including LGBTQ. Makadon et al. (2015) provide helpful guidelines for how to ask sexual health history questions during clinical encounters and "dos and don'ts" in taking a sexual history aligned with providing an inclusive and affirmative healthcare environment for LGBTQ patients.[10,11]

COMMON PRESENTING PROBLEMS AND SOLUTIONS

For both men and women, cancer-related sexual dysfunction can present in a number of ways that are often dependent on the treatments patients have received (Table 5.1). First, problems within sexual response are common, including lack of desire, arousal problems, orgasm problems, and pain during sex, leading to reduced sexual satisfaction.[13,14] Second, general side effects of cancer treatments like chemotherapy, such as fatigue, nausea, and general pain, can exacerbate sexual problems like loss of interest in sex. Third, psychosocial factors including underlying depression, anxiety, and body image concerns often contribute to sexual problems or create challenges for treatment. Fourth, with regard to relationships, difficulties in communication between partners and relationship functioning can manifest in the context of sexual problems, and these difficulties can compromise couples' ability to adjust to changes. Patients' partners also may have sexual difficulties either prior to the diagnosis or in relation to the patients' issues, which can further complicate the situation.

Risk factors for sexual problems are listed in Table 5.2. These include physical/health-related and psychosocial factors that directly or indirectly affect sexual function. One risk factor worth considering in detail is advanced stage disease. It is often assumed that patients with advanced stage disease

TABLE 5.1   Sexual problems associated with cancer treatments

TREATMENT	SEXUAL PROBLEMS IN MEN AND WOMEN[a]
Chemotherapy	Side effects include vaginal and rectal mucosal toxicity, gastrointestinal issues, mouth sores, fatigue, nausea and vomiting, weight changes, alopecia and hair loss, among others, all of which can indirectly affect sexual functioning through lowered desire, arousal, and body image problems Gonadotoxic chemotherapies may lead to reproductive problems and indirectly affect sexual health (e.g., through body image problems) • Women may experience premature ovarian failure and menopause symptoms • Men may experience reduced or cessation of spermatogenesis
Endocrine (hormonal) therapy	For women: • Estrogen deprivation (ovarian suppression) is associated with vulvovaginal health changes (dryness, irritation, soreness), vaginal atrophy, and dyspareunia • Increases risk of Genitourinary Syndrome of Menopause (GSM) • *Breast cancer:* Tamoxifen and Aromatase Inhibitors (AIs) associated with menopausal symptoms; AIs lead to more severe symptoms For men: • Hormone treatments can damage the nerves and blood supply and lead to erectile dysfunction • *Prostate Cancer:* androgen deprivation therapy lowers testosterone and often causes erectile dysfunction
Hematopoietic stem cell transplant	Sexual problems may stem from conditioning regimens, graft-versus-host disease (GVHD)–generalized or genital, medications, and cardiovascular complications, combined with psychosocial stressors of disease and treatment For women, lubrication and desire problems are most common For men, erectile dysfunction is most common GVHD after allogenic bone marrow transplant can have systemic and local effects affecting genital and mucous membranes • Vulva and vulvovaginal dryness, itching, scarring, and vaginal stenosis, penile dryness • Structural changes can lead to secondary sexual problems (low libido, dyspareunia, abnormal ejaculation) • Inflammation, rash, and sensitivity in the skin, which may include skin of the vagina and penis
Radiotherapy and brachytherapy	General effects include fatigue and body image concerns *Total body irradiation* can lead to genital tissue sensitivity, vulvovaginal dryness, penile dryness, vaginal atrophy and scarring, as well as gonadal failure and infertility
Radiation to the pelvic area	Vaginal stenosis and shortening, incontinence, vasoconstriction, lymphedema, and loss of genital sensation; infertility risks that can affect sexual health
Radiation to the anal area	Urgency and incontinence that affect comfort level being intimate and sexual self-confidence
Radiation to the breast area	Scarring, burns, lymphedema, and skin thickening
Surgery	Effects of surgery depend on the part of the body affected
Pelvic surgery	Causes structural alterations, nerve damage, and changes in vascularization that may impact sexual response For men, may cause erectile dysfunction
Radical prostatectomy	Erectile dysfunction immediately following surgery with recovery requiring 18 to 24 months Many men will never regain pretreatment levels of erectile function Other problems include ejaculatory dysfunction, orgasmic dysfunction, and loss of penile length

TABLE 5.1 (*Continued*)   Sexual problems associated with cancer treatments

TREATMENT	SEXUAL PROBLEMS IN MEN AND WOMEN[a]
Mastectomy and reconstructive surgery	Feelings of disfigurement, grief surrounding lost breasts, loss of sensation, and dissatisfaction with the appearance and feel of implants or mastectomy scars Body image problems and distress surrounding conceptions of womanhood and femininity May develop post mastectomy reconstruction syndrome characterized by weakness, tightness, or pain in the chest or shoulders ('iron bra' sensation), may continue long after surgery
Colorectal surgeries	Urinary or bowel incontinence and pain that can impact sexual functioning For women, *bladder surgery* can result in nerve damage that leads to problems with lubrication and sexual response
Brain surgery	Range of sexual problems depending on the location and areas affected including loss of libido or sex drive, and arousal and orgasm problems
Head and neck surgery	Physical changes or disfigurement that affects sexual interactions with a partner including kissing and oral sex Body image problems are particularly common

[a] All physical changes may be associated with body image problems, loss of manhood/womanhood, and psychosocial distress.

Source: Peate & Juraskova.[15]

may be unconcerned about sexual function, in light of their morbidity and mortality concerns. Yet many patients nevertheless value intimacy in their relationships and are interested in help for sexual problems and ways to maintain intimacy. For couples, maintaining a sexual relationship and intimacy may be important aspects of keeping a sense of normalcy and closeness in the face of fears about death and dying. Conversations about sexual function should occur with patients with advanced disease or at the end of life just as for patients diagnosed with early stage disease. By contrast, certain factors may buffer against sexual problems including positive prior sexual experiences (e.g., healthy sexual identity), adaptive beliefs and attitudes (e.g., flexible beliefs surrounding sex and sexuality), and aspects of health (e.g., better psychological well-being) and their relationships (e.g., better relationship quality and communication, openness to new ways of achieving intimacy).

Next, we describe common complaints reported by women and men after cancer treatment with an overview of treatment approaches specific to those problems.[7,16] A stepped management approach is recommended for the treatment of sexual dysfunction starting with communication and education and progressing as needed to drug therapy, mildly invasive management, mechanical options, and surgical

TABLE 5.2   Risk factors for sexual problems and distress

- Younger age
- Pre-cancer sexual problems or sexual dissatisfaction
- Body image problems (functioning, appearance)
- Altered femininity/masculinity or threatened sense of womanhood/manhood
- Anxiety, depression, low self-esteem
- Infertility concerns
- Sleep disturbances
- Urinary or bowel incontinence
- Interpersonal issues (e.g., relationship dissatisfaction, partner sexual problems)
- Treatment-induced vasomotor symptoms, changes in genitalia, nerve/vascular damage
- Comorbid medical conditions (e.g., cardiovascular disease, diabetes, arthritis, thyroid problems, inflammatory/irritable bowel disease)
- Medications that may impact hormones and sexual response (antidepressants, oral contraceptives)
- Other general health risk factors (e.g., smoking and obesity)

interventions. Based on the biopsychosocial model of sexuality, treatments may be combined such that biomedical intervention along with psychoeducation and counseling is often optimal. In fact, it is recommended that psychosocial counseling be offered as frontline treatment for all problems with sexual response including desire, arousal, and orgasm.[16] In following sections, attention is given to screening and general clinical management of sexual problems.

Low sexual desire (libido) is an extremely common complaint among women and men affected by cancer. Problems with desire may result from hormonal therapies and be exacerbated by poor body image, altered femininity/masculinity, psychosocial distress, depression, fatigue, and other treatment side effects (e.g., urinary incontinence, nausea, diarrhea, mucositis). Low desire may also be the result of other co-occurring sexual problems and related distress. For instance, if women are experiencing vaginal dryness and discomfort during sexual activity (described further below), their desire for such activity will likely be lessened. Problems with desire are most commonly treated with some form of psychoeducation and counseling to normalize the experience. Mindfulness-based interventions targeting low sexual desire have shown promising results in breast cancer survivors.[17] Two medications have been FDA-approved for treating low sexual desire for premenopausal women. Addyi (flibanserin) is a pill taken once a day that targets serotonin and dopamine receptors.[18,19] Vyleesi (bremelanotide) is an injection self-administered prior to anticipated sexual activity, which targets melanocortin receptors.[20] For postmenopausal women, testosterone therapy is commonly used off-label to improve libido.[21] However, testosterone therapy among breast cancer patients is highly controversial, particularly with hormone-dependent cancer. Testosterone replacement therapy is also recommended for men as treatment for low desire but again, caution should be taken with hormone-dependent cancers such as for men with advanced prostate cancer on androgen deprivation therapy.[22] Hypogonadal men may have more trouble with desire, getting aroused and achieving erections than men with normal hormone levels without sexual stimuli, but may overcome this with the use of additional stimuli such as viewing erotic films and added foreplay.[23] Men should be counseled about the need for extra physical caressing and mental sexual stimulation rather than relying on spontaneous desire. When prescribing medications for low desire, clinicians should consult treating oncologists, discuss potential risks with their patients, and be prudent in recommendations for select patient populations (e.g., breast cancer survivors, those with hormone-dependent cancers).

Vulvovaginal dryness affecting women is defined as a lack of moisture and irritation of the vulva and vagina, occurring both during sexual activity and outside of sexual activity. At its most severe, the vaginal tissue becomes thin and damaged, causing vaginal stenosis. This can cause significant pain and discomfort for women with penetrative intercourse and can also cause irritation and chafing during normal activity. Unresolved vulvovaginal dryness or pain can also interfere with pelvic exams, pelvic floor physical therapy, or dilator therapy. Vaginal moisturizers and lubricants are safe, accessible, and easily administered treatments for vaginal dryness, irritation, and soreness. Counseling about the optimal use of moisturizers and lubricants should be a first step in management, and for some women, to do that may be sufficient to resolve the problem for many women. Low-dose vaginal estrogen therapy to treat urogenital symptoms and vulvovaginal atrophy is highly effective if nonhormonal remedies are inadequate and may be administered as a vaginal ring or tablet by prescription, with the tablets or ring being generally more efficacious compared to topical creams. Caution should be taken when treating women with hormone-dependent breast cancer; guidelines for pharmacologic treatment of women with or at high risk of breast cancer can be found elsewhere.[24] Ospemiphene is a non-estrogen agonist/antagonist that has been shown to increase vaginal lubrication and improve sexual function,[25] though there is limited evidence for safety in cancer survivors.

Painful intercourse (dyspareunia) for women commonly occurs due to changes in vulvovaginal health, such as dryness, described above, or vaginal atrophy related to pelvic radiation or surgery. A pelvic examination is an important part of the clinical assessment of sexual pain.[26] Women tend to naturally tighten vaginal muscles with pain, which can worsen the sensation and can lead to pelvic floor dysfunction, often experienced as anticipatory tightening with sexual activity. Over time, this tightening can develop into secondary vaginismus that makes penetrative sex extremely difficult or impossible. Pelvic floor dysfunction such as this may result from radiation or surgery affecting the pelvic area for gynecologic, colorectal, and anal cancers. Treatments should address vulvovaginal health and aim to improve vaginal tissue quality. Kegel exercises, vaginal dilators (used with a lubricant), and pelvic floor physical therapy are effective treatment approaches. Intravaginal dehydroepiandrosterone (DHEA) ovules are FDA-approved for postmenopausal women with moderate to severe dyspareunia caused by vaginal atrophy, though warnings exist for breast cancer survivors. Other pharmacologic treatments include ospemifene, a systemically administered selective estrogen-receptor modulator (SERM), and topical lidocaine, reviewed elsewhere.[24] There is some evidence that vaginal laser therapy may be effective in the short term for treating dyspareunia and vaginal dryness in cancer survivors with positive effects on overall sexual function and satisfaction, including for women with a history of breast cancer for whom vaginal estrogen may be contraindicated.[27] However, because long-term data on safety and efficacy are lacking, caution is advised when referring women with a cancer history to vaginal laser therapy.[28] Anesthetic gels or lidocaine may also be used to reduce vulvovaginal pain or discomfort during sexual activity. Another management option is the Come Close Ring or the OhNut Protector Ring, which are cushioned rings placed at the base of the penis that serves as a spacer and prevents deep thrusting and penetration. This will not resolve the problem but can help women engage in comfortable sex with a partner. Positions that allow them to have control over the depth and speed of penetration may be most comfortable.

Erectile dysfunction is the most well-studied sexual function complaint for men with cancer and is associated with significant distress including a perceived loss of manhood and anticipatory anxiety leading up to sexual encounters for many men. First-line treatment is typically pharmacologic, followed by mechanical or surgical intervention if needed. Of note, most couples stop using biomedical rehabilitation aids within the first two years,[29] suggesting there are barriers to continued use, and highlighting the importance of promoting sexual activity and intimacy independent of erections. Counseling alongside biomedical intervention may help to improve uptake and adherence, while addressing other underlying sources of distress that may be impacting sexual self-confidence and satisfaction. Erectile dysfunction is most commonly treated with phosphodiesterase type 5 (PDE5) inhibitors (e.g., sildenafil, tadalafil, and vardenafil). The effect of PDE5 inhibitors is an amplification of the normal erectile physiology and depends on intact libido, sexual stimulation, sensory pathways, and other factors that are required for erectile function. Low-dose PDE5 inhibitors, although not successful in producing an erection, help in the healing of the cavernous nerves.[30] Following radical prostatectomy for the treatment of prostate cancer, immediate initiation of erectile dysfunction treatment is critical for successful maintenance of healthy penile tissue.[31] PDE5 inhibitors are not effective for all patients and efficacy is further reduced by poor adherence to intake instructions (i.e., on an empty stomach, two hours before sexual intercourse). "Penile rehabilitation programs" instruct men to achieve medication-assisted erections two to three times per week following radical prostatectomy in the 18- to 24-month recovery period, whether or not the patient intends to have penetrative sex. For men with low testosterone, use of PDE5 inhibitors combined with testosterone therapy leads to greater improvements in erectile function, compared to monotherapy only, particularly for men with more severe hypogonadism.[22,32] Testosterone therapy used alone produces modest improvement in erectile function, up until a threshold of "normal" testosterone level is achieved.

Penile injections have also become a cornerstone of rehabilitation programs, given their increased efficacy relative to oral medications such as PDE5 inhibitors. These injections deliver intracavernosal vasodilators (prostaglandin, phentolamine, and papaverine) at the base of the penis. Since the medication works locally, those men who do not respond to a PDE5 inhibitor have a good chance to responding to penile injections. Pain with administration is minimal.[33] Nevertheless, despite its effectiveness, because many men do not like the idea of doing injections, discontinuation rates are high. For men who prefer to avoid injections, intraurethral suppositories, which contain prostaglandin, and pull blood into the penis to create an erection, may be used, although these tend to be less effective than the injections.

Vacuum devices are another effective option for managing erectile dysfunction. These cylindrical devices are placed over a man's penis and create a vacuum inside that pulls blood into the penis to create an erection. A final option for men with intractable erectile dysfunction is surgery to install an inflatable penile prosthesis. Satisfaction with penile implant surgery tends to be very high, with more than 85% of men reporting satisfaction with the result.[34] Primary care physicians or oncologists may want to refer to a urologist or urology center to manage these treatments.

Orgasm problems (anorgasmia or altered sensation in orgasm) may be experienced by both women and men and is often related to the experience of other co-occurring sexual problems and/or may be a result of hormone imbalances, depression or anxiety, side effects of drugs, or due to nerve damage. Low desire or decreased genital sensation may result in inadequate levels of arousal to achieve orgasm, or orgasms may be experienced as less intense or less enjoyable. For women, addressing any symptoms of vulvovaginal health problems and reducing pain should be treated first and may help resolve orgasm problems. To increase genital stimulation and sensation, sexual aids such as a vibrator can be useful in supporting oxygenated genital blood flow and enhancing genital stimulation. A relatively new treatment for orgasm problems in women is an FDA-approved, non-pharmaceutical clitoral therapy device (EROS Therapy, Urometrics, St. Paul, MN), which is placed over the clitoris and creates a gentle suction, thereby increasing blood flow, vaginal lubrication and stimulation of sensory nerve endings, and greater likelihood of orgasm.[35] For men, problems with orgasms may be a failure to ejaculate or retrograde ejaculation or climacturia (orgasm-associated urinary incontinence). There is limited research to inform the treatment for impaired or absent orgasmic sensation or painful orgasms for men, and treatment is largely based on addressing possible causative factors and the use of psychotherapy.[36] As when treating women, a focused medical history can identify potential etiologies such as medications, penile sensation loss, endocrinopathies, penile hyperstimulation, and psychological etiologies.[37] Treatment for climacturia includes the use of condoms during intercourse, pelvic floor rehabilitation, and behavioral management (e.g., bladder emptying and avoidance of fluid intake before sexual activity).

SCREENING AND ASSESSMENT

Ideally, based on the biopsychosocial framework, assessment should include relevant identifying emotional, relational, and cultural factors influencing cancer-related sexual problems as well as identification of comorbid sexual status. Understanding the timeframe of the development of sexual problems is important, particularly within the context of cancer treatments. It is important to clarify with the patient whether or not they are interested in resuming sexual activity (if stopped) and identify patient driven goals for recovery during the assessment process.

BASIC ASSESSMENT OF SEXUAL CONCERNS

- Current sexual function for each sexual domain (desire, arousal, orgasm, satisfaction)
- Presence of sexual pain
- Sexual and romantic relationships (if applicable)
- Distress about and impact of sexual problem
- Patient expectations and goals for recovery
- Predisposing, precipitating, maintaining, and contextual factors

Source: Adapted from Parish et al.[38]

Scripts for clinicians have been published to guide sexual health discussions.[25,39] Clinicians may start their assessment of sexual health by normalizing the sexual problem and then inquiring about it in a neutral way, such as:

Many [men/women] with cancer experience changes in sexual functioning. Do you have any concerns about your sexual functioning that you would like to discuss or consider treatments for?

As the patient discusses their problems and concerns, empathic listening and open-ended invitations for further disclosure may help the patient feel more comfortable, such as, "Tell me more about... Tell me about a typical sexual experience..." Validated, single-item written screeners have been developed for

TABLE 5.3 Self-reported sexual problems screener

Single-item Screener for Sexual Problems
In the past 12 months, has there ever been a period of 3 months or more than you had any of the following problems or concerns? Check all that apply.

- You wanted to feel more interest in sexual activity
- MEN ONLY: You had difficulty with erections (penis getting hard or staying hard)
- WOMEN ONLY: Your vagina felt too dry, irritated, or sore
- You had pain during or after sexual activity
- You felt anxious about sexual activity
- You did not enjoy sexual activity
- Some other sexual problem or concern
- No sexual problems or concerns

Sexual Symptom Checklist for Women
Please answer the following questions about your overall sexual function:

1. Are you satisfied with your sexual function? Yes/No
2. Do you have any concerns about vaginal health? Yes/No

If not satisfied with sexual function AND/OR concerns about vaginal health, please continue.

3. Do you experience any of the following sexual problems or concerns?
    - Little or no interest in sex
    - Decreased sensation (or loss of sensation)
    - Decreased vaginal lubrication (dryness)
    - Difficult reaching orgasm
    - Pain during sex
    - Vaginal or vulvar pain or discomfort (not during sex)
    - Anxiety about having sex
    - Other problem or concern: _____

4. Would you like more information, resources, and/or would you like to speak with someone about these issues? Yes/No

Source: Flynn et al.[41] and Bober et al.[25]

self-reporting sexual problems (Table 5.3). There are also validated instruments to more formally measure sexual health outcomes.[40]

CLINICAL MANAGEMENT

Although sexual health should ideally be raised early when working with patients diagnosed with cancer, it is never too late to start the discussion. Raising the topic with the patient at any point sends the message that sexual health is an important aspect of care and opens the door for future conversations. Including partners in these discussions can help normalize the issue and convey the importance of addressing the issue jointly. Prior to cancer treatment, anticipatory management to prepare patients for sexual side effects is important to help set expectations and let patients know that treatment options are available if difficulties arise. "Prehabilitation" strategies may be initiated to prevent the occurrence or worsening of sexual problems. As an example, women may be encouraged to start vaginal moisturizers if treatments will involve hormonal changes to prevent or lessen vulvovaginal dryness and irritation. Partners may be included in these conversations, if the patient agrees, to encourage their involvement in a dyadic treatment approach.

TABLE 5.4   Five A's framework

1. Ask	• Ask open-ended, non-judgmental questions about sexual concerns
	• Example:
	"It is common for people to experience changes in their sexual functioning after the treatments you received (such as lower desire or libido, vaginal dryness, or erectile dysfunction). What sorts of changes have you noticed? How have you felt about it?"
2. Advise	• Express to the patient that you are there to help and advise
3. Assess	• Assess sexual health problems efficiently but thoroughly to identity next steps for intervention
4. Assist	• Provide counseling and treatments options, as appropriate
	• Provide information sheets and educational books or websites that are relevant to the presenting problem and needs of the patient
	• Referrals for counseling, pelvic floor physical therapy, urogynecologic care, etc., as appropriate
	• Some patients may be unsure of their readiness to address sexual concerns and may need time to consider their options; plan for follow-up discussions
5. Arrange	• Arrange follow-up and check-in with patients at subsequent visits to assess progress and identify need for more intensive interventions

Source: Adapted from Zhoue et al.[7] and Bober et al.[25]

Frameworks to Guide Communication

Clinicians can draw guidance from the **Five A's Framework** to have these discussions with their patients.[25] The framework is based on five basic components (*ask, advise, assess, assist,* and *arrange*) that can be used to structure conversations to be efficient and flexible in addressing sexual health concerns with patients (Table 5.4). This framework extends the well-known PLISSIT (Permission, Limited information, Specific Suggestions, Intensive Therapy) model. Both the Five A's Framework and the PLISSIT model guide the delivery of information and treatment in a stepped care fashion with increasing intensity.

Educational and Psychosocial Interventions

Although the strategies previously described are often effective in targeting physical manifestations of sexual problems, educational and psychotherapeutic treatments play a central role in addressing the complex nature of sexual functioning for individuals and couples (Table 5.5). Treatment may be enhanced by a combination of pharmacologic treatment, mechanical solutions, physical therapy,

TABLE 5.5   Common targets of psychotherapy for sexual problems

- Educate and increase awareness of sexual response, maladaptive cognitions, patterns of behavior, and sources of sexual difficulties
- Redefine "normal" sexual activity, alter sexual behaviors that are no longer possible or satisfying, and expand sexual behavior repertoire
- Modify negative beliefs about sex or sexual performance to more adaptive beliefs
- Redirect focus from performance to pleasure and sensuality
- Address body image problems and support survivors in reconnecting to their body post cancer treatments and physical changes
- Reduce performance anxiety
- Address barriers to intimacy, while encouraging new definitions of sex and intimacy for couples and an openness to try new sexual activities or positions
- Resolve interpersonal issues that cause or maintain sexual problems such as improving communication skills

and counseling or psychotherapy.[16] Reviews of sexual interventions for cancer patients exist for both women[42–44] and men.[45,46] Caring for patients with sexual problems entails normalizing sexual symptoms and emphasizing their treatability, while validating their emotional and interpersonal experiences. Many patients may never return to baseline levels of sexual functioning, and counseling may be needed to help patients adjust and to support their coping efforts. By the same token, many sexual problems may be improved with simple adjustments (e.g., use of vaginal moisturizer and lubricant, emptying a colostomy bag prior to sex).[47]

As a first step, clinicians may want to provide information about the sexual response cycle and anatomy, effects of cancer treatment on sexual function, and availability of treatment options. Education is a necessary part of treatment to ensure patients understand the full range of potential factors that may be causing, maintaining, or exacerbating sexual problems, not limited to cancer treatment effects.

Psychotherapy in its various forms is a useful treatment for distressing sexual problems for individuals and couples. Cognitive behavioral therapy and mindfulness based cognitive therapy have the most empirical data.[17,48,49] Sex therapy is usually relatively brief (5–20 session) and solution focused, with the goal to increase awareness of difficulties and alter cognitions, emotions, and behaviors in relation to sexual problems. Including the romantic or sexual partner, if desired by the patient, can be helpful to obtain insight about the partner's experiences and needs and to alleviate the burden on patients to relay instructions given in therapy.[50–53] Communication skills training may help patients navigate discussions with their partners, particularly if sexual topics are viewed as embarrassing or shameful.[54] Sensate-focus exercises, which center around non-demand sensual touching, are often used to help couples decrease anxiety and avoidance of sexual interactions, increase personal and interpersonal awareness of one's own and partner's sensations and needs, and improve sexual functioning.[55] There is also strong evidence that couples' therapy can help improve communication, sexual functioning, and intimacy. Patients who are not partnered may want to discuss their concerns about dating and starting new sexual relationships.

Tips for Effective Communication

When embarking on the task of discussing sexual health with patients, it may be helpful to keep the following tips in mind:

- Keep an open, nonjudgmental, and collaborative tone.
- Gain knowledge of the most common problems of patients in your practice and prevailing strategies.
- Identify and maintain a list of referring providers (e.g., mental health professionals, sex therapists/counselors, endocrinologists, pelvic floor or other rehabilitation providers, and gynecologists or urologists).
- Provide patients information about an expected timeline of recovery of sexual function, if known.
- Give patients (and partners, if applicable) clear information on whether and how sexual activity can be engaged in safely during and after treatment.
- Employ ongoing "check in" discussions to provide patients the opportunity to ask questions and receive help when needed.
- Normalize setbacks in sexual recovery and help problem-solve with patients to find new strategies.
- Help patients understand when a return to pre-cancer (baseline) levels of sexual functioning is not possible, and support patients in coping with this loss.
- Include partners in initial discussions of potential sexual side effects as this information can convey to the partner that effects are often physical in nature, rather than a change in desire for the healthy partner.

- Encourage goals that are broader-minded rather than performance-oriented (e.g., achieving intimacy with a partner over having regular orgasms).
- Try sending the message that sex and sexual intimacy encompass more than penetrative intercourse.
- Encourage planning sex for when patients are less fatigued or scheduling it around their treatments.

MULTIDISCIPLINARY CARE

Clinicians should be familiar with local professionals that are able to take referrals for patients in need of specialized treatment of sexual health issues. Having a list of hospital- or community-based practitioners is key to be able to match patients with practitioners that meet their needs. The following disciplines are relevant to the treatment of sexual problems:

- Sexual medicine specialist/therapist
- Urologist, urogynecologist
- Gynecologist, menopause specialist
- Endocrinologist
- Clinical psychologist, couples therapist
- Sexual health counselor, sex therapist

Many of the professional organizations listed have resources for patients, as well as referral directories to find local providers.

PROFESSIONAL ORGANIZATIONS

American Association of Sex Educators Counselors and Therapists (AASECT)
    http://www.aasect.org
American Sexual Health Association (ASHA)
    http://www.ashastd.org
International Society for Sexual Medicine
    http://www.issm.info
International Society for the Study of Women's Sexual Health
    http://www.isswsh.org
North American Menopause Society
    http://www.menopause.org
American College of Obstetricians and Gynecologists
    http://www.acog.org
American Urological Association
    http://auanett.org
American Cancer Society
    http://www.cancer.org
American Society of Clinical Oncology
    http://www.cancer.Net
International Psycho-Oncology Society
    http://www.ipos-society.org

CONCLUSION

Despite the potential complexity of sexual problems experienced by individuals who have been treated for cancer, there is much that can be done to address these issues with patients, leaving good reason to convey a message of hope and optimism. By simply raising the topic of sexual health as a routine practice, clinicians can validate patients' experiences, normalize the occurrence of sexual problems, and set the stage for further evaluation and treatment based on patients' wishes. Along with providing appropriate referrals, offering patients information and access to frontline treatments may engender a greater sense of confidence that they are able to manage their difficulties and participate in their recovery, ultimately achieving a better outcome. We hope that this chapter provides a helpful starting point for clinicians hoping to better understand sexual health after cancer and approach this issue with their patients.

REFERENCES

1. Carter J, Lacchetti C, Andersen BL, et al. Interventions to address sexual problems in people with cancer: American Society of Clinical Oncology Clinical Practice Guideline Adaptation of Cancer Care Ontario Guideline. *J Clin Oncol.* Published online December 11, 2017. doi:10.1200/JCO.2017.75.8995.
2. Schover LR, van der Kaaij M, van Dorst E, Creutzberg C, Huyghe E, Kiserud CE. Sexual dysfunction and infertility as late effects of cancer treatment. *EJC Suppl.* 2014;12(1):41–53. doi:10.1016/j.ejcsup.2014.03.004.
3. Ussher JM, Perz J, Gilbert E, The Australian Cancer and Sexuality Study Team. Perceived causes and consequences of sexual changes after cancer for women and men: a mixed method study. *BMC Cancer.* 2015;15(1):268. doi:10.1186/s12885-015-1243-8.
4. Denlinger CS, Sanft T, Baker KS, et al. Survivorship, Version 2.2018, NCCN Clinical Practice Guidelines in Oncology. *J Natl Compr Canc Netw.* 2018;16(10):1216–1247. doi:10.6004/jnccn.2018.0078.
5. Patient and Survivor Care. ASCO. Accessed December 17, 2020. https://www.asco.org/research-guidelines/quality-guidelines/guidelines/patient-and-survivor-care.
6. Reese JB, Sorice K, Beach MC, et al. Patient-provider communication about sexual concerns in cancer: a systematic review. *J Cancer Surviv.* 2017;11(2):175–188. doi:10.1007/s11764-016-0577-9.
7. Zhou ES, Nekhlyudov L, Bober SL. The primary health care physician and the cancer patient: tips and strategies for managing sexual health. *Transl Androl Urol.* 2015;4(2):218–231. doi:10.3978/j.issn.2223-4683.2014.11.07.
8. Althof SE, Leiblum SR, Chevret-Measson M, et al. Psychological and interpersonal dimensions of sexual function and dysfunction. *J Sex Med.* 2005;2(6):793–800. doi:10.1111/j.1743-6109.2005.00145.x.
9. Ussher JM, Perz J, Rose D, Kellett A, Dowsett G. Sexual rehabilitation after prostate cancer through assistive aids: a comparison of gay/bisexual and heterosexual men. *J Sex Res.* 2019;56(7):854–869. doi:10.1080/00224499.2018.1476444.
10. Makadon HJ, Goldhammer H. Taking a sexual history and creating affirming environments for lesbian, gay, bisexual, and transgender people. *J Miss State Med Assoc.* 2015;56(12):358–362.
11. Hadland SE, Yehia BR, Makadon HJ. Caring for lesbian, gay, bisexual, transgender, and questioning youth in inclusive and affirmative environments. *Pediatr Clin North Am.* 2016;63(6):955–969. doi:10.1016/j.pcl.2016.07.001.
12. Rosen RC, Barsky JL. Normal sexual response in women. *Obstet Gynecol Clin North Am.* 2006;33(4):515–526. doi:10.1016/j.ogc.2006.09.005.
13. Brotto L, Atallah S, Johnson-Agbakwu C, et al. Psychological and interpersonal dimensions of sexual function and dysfunction. *J Sex Med.* 2016;13(4):538–571. doi:10.1016/j.jsxm.2016.01.019.
14. Bober SL, Kingsberg SA, Faubion SS. Sexual function after cancer: paying the price of survivorship. *Climacteric.* Published online May 15, 2019:1–7. doi:10.1080/13697137.2019.1606796.
15. Peate M, Juraskova I. *Principles of Treatment of Sexual Dysfunction.* Oxford: Oxford University Press Accessed October 31, 2020. https://oxfordmedicine.com/view/10.1093/med/9780190934033.001.0001/med-9780190934033-chapter-5.
16. Barbera L, Zwaal C, Elterman D, et al. Interventions to address sexual problems in people with cancer. *Curr Oncol.* 2017;24(3):192–200. doi:10.3747/co.24.3583.
17. Brotto LA, Heiman JR. Mindfulness in sex therapy: applications for women with sexual difficulties following gynecologic cancer. *Sex Relatsh Ther.* 2007;22(1):3–11. doi:10.1080/14681990601153298.

18. U.S. Food & Drug Administration. FDA approves new treatment for hypoactive sexual desire disorder in premenopausal women. *FDA.* Published March 24, 2020. Accessed November 18, 2020. https://www.fda.gov/news-events/press-announcements/fda-approves-new-treatment-hypoactive-sexual-desire-disorder-premenopausal-women.

19. Jaspers L, Feys F, Bramer WM, Franco OH, Leusink P, Laan ETM. Efficacy and safety of flibanserin for the treatment of hypoactive sexual desire disorder in women: a systematic review and meta-analysis. *JAMA Intern Med.* 2016;176(4):453–462. doi:10.1001/jamainternmed.2015.8565.

20. Dhillon S, Keam SJ. Bremelanotide: first approval. *Drugs.* 2019;79(14):1599–1606. doi:10.1007/s40265-019-01187-w.

21. Somboonporn W, Davis S, Seif MW, Bell R. Testosterone for peri- and postmenopausal women. *Cochrane Database Syst Rev.* 2005;(4):CD004509. doi:10.1002/14651858.CD004509.pub2.

22. Corona G, Rastrelli G, Morgentaler A, Sforza A, Mannucci E, Maggi M. Meta-analysis of results of testosterone therapy on sexual function based on international index of erectile function scores. *Eur Urol.* 2017;72(6):1000–1011. doi:10.1016/j.eururo.2017.03.032.

23. Carani C, Bancroft J, Granata A, Del Rio G, Marrama P. Testosterone and erectile function, nocturnal penile tumescence and rigidity, and erectile response to visual erotic stimuli in hypogonadal and eugonadal men. *Psychoneuroendocrinology.* 1992;17(6):647–654. doi:10.1016/0306-4530(92)90023-Z.

24. Faubion SS, Larkin LC, Stuenkel CA, et al. Management of genitourinary syndrome of menopause in women with or at high risk for breast cancer: consensus recommendations from The North American Menopause Society and The International Society for the Study of Women's Sexual Health. *Menopause.* 2018;25(6):596–608. doi:10.1097/GME.0000000000001121.

25. Bober SL, Reese JB, Barbera L, et al. How to ask and what to do: a guide for clinical inquiry and intervention regarding female sexual health after cancer. *Curr Opin Support Palliat Care.* 2016;10(1):44–54. doi:10.1097/SPC.0000000000000186.

26. Coady D, Kennedy V. Sexual health in women affected by cancer: focus on sexual pain. *Obstet Gynecol.* 2016;128(4):775–791. doi:10.1097/AOG.0000000000001621.

27. Jha S, Wyld L, Krishnaswamy PH. The impact of vaginal laser treatment for genitourinary syndrome of menopause in breast cancer survivors: a systematic review and meta-analysis. *Clin Breast Cancer.* 2019;19(4):e556–e562. doi:10.1016/j.clbc.2019.04.007.

28. U.S. Food and Drug Administration. FDA Warns Against Use of Energy-Based Devices to Perform Vaginal "Rejuvenation" or Vaginal Cosmetic Procedures: FDA Safety Communication. *FDA.* Published online November 19, 2018. Accessed January 20, 2021. https://www.fda.gov/medical-devices/safety-communications/fda-warns-against-use-energy-based-devices-perform-vaginal-rejuvenation-or-vaginal-cosmetic.

29. Walker LM, Wassersug RJ, Robinson JW. Psychosocial perspectives on sexual recovery after prostate cancer treatment. *Nat Rev Urol.* 2015;12(3):167–176. doi:10.1038/nrurol.2015.29.

30. McCullough AR, Levine LA, Padma-Nathan H. Return of nocturnal erections and erectile function after bilateral nerve-sparing radical prostatectomy in men treated nightly with sildenafil citrate: subanalysis of a longitudinal randomized double-blind placebo-controlled trial. *J Sex Med.* 2008;5(2):476–484. doi:10.1111/j.1743-6109.2007.00700.x.

31. Fraiman MC, Lepor H, McCullough AR. Changes in penile morphometrics in men with erectile dysfunction after nerve-sparing radical retropubic prostatectomy. *Mol Urol.* 1999;3(2):109–115.

32. Rizk PJ, Kohn TP, Pastuszak AW, Khera M. Testosterone therapy improves erectile function and libido in hypogonadal men. *Curr Opin Urol.* 2017;27(6):511–515. doi:10.1097/MOU.0000000000000442.

33. Nelson CJ, Hsiao W, Balk E, et al. Injection anxiety and pain in men using intracavernosal injection therapy after radical pelvic surgery. *J Sex Med.* 2013;10(10):2559–2565. doi:10.1111/jsm.12271.

34. Falcone M, Rolle L, Ceruti C, et al. Prospective analysis of the surgical outcomes and patients' satisfaction rate after the AMS Spectra penile prosthesis implantation. *Urology.* 2013;82(2):373–376. doi:10.1016/j.urology.2013.04.027.

35. Billups KL, Berman L, Berman J, Metz ME, Glennon ME, Goldstein I. A new non-pharmacological vacuum therapy for female sexual dysfunction. *J Sex Marital Ther.* 2001;27(5):435–441. doi:10.1080/713846826.

36. Clavell-Hernández J, Martin C, Wang R. Orgasmic dysfunction following radical prostatectomy: review of current literature. *Sex Med Rev.* 2018;6(1):124–134. doi:10.1016/j.sxmr.2017.09.003.

37. Jenkins LC, Mulhall JP. Delayed orgasm and anorgasmia. *Fertil Steril.* 2015;104(5):1082–1088. doi:10.1016/j.fertnstert.2015.09.029.

38. Parish SJ, Hahn SR, Goldstein SW, et al. The International Society for the Study of Women's Sexual Health Process of Care for the Identification of Sexual Concerns and Problems in Women. *Mayo Clin Proc.* 2019;94(5):842–856. doi:10.1016/j.mayocp.2019.01.009.

39. Kemertzis M, Ranjithakumaran H, Hand M, et al. Fertility preservation toolkit: a clinician resource to assist clinical discussion and decision making in pediatric and adolescent oncology. *J Pediatr Hematol/Oncol.* 2018;40(3). doi:10.1097/MPH.0000000000001103.

40. Althof SE, Parish SJ. Clinical interviewing techniques and sexuality questionnaires for male and female cancer patients. *J Sex Med.* 2013;10:35–42. doi:10.1111/jsm.12035.

41. Flynn KE, Lindau ST, Lin L, et al. Development and validation of a single-item screener for self-reporting sexual problems in U.S. adults. *J Gen Intern Med.* 2015;30(10):1468–1475. doi:10.1007/s11606-015-3333-3.

42. Candy B, Jones L, Vickerstaff V, Tookman A, King M. Interventions for sexual dysfunction following treatments for cancer in women. *Cochrane Database Syst Rev.* 2016;(2). doi:10.1002/14651858.CD005540.pub3.

43. Kingsberg SA, Althof S, Simon JA, et al. Female sexual dysfunction-medical and psychological treatments, committee 14. *J Sex Med.* 2017;14(12):1463–1491. doi:10.1016/j.jsxm.2017.05.018.

44. Weinberger JM, Houman J, Caron AT, Anger J. Female sexual dysfunction: a systematic review of outcomes across various treatment modalities. *Sex Med Rev.* 2019;7(2):223–250. doi:10.1016/j.sxmr.2017.12.004.

45. Kim P, Clavijo RI. Management of male sexual dysfunction after cancer treatment. *Urol Oncol.* Published online August 26, 2020. doi:10.1016/j.urolonc.2020.08.006.

46. Chung E, Brock G. Sexual rehabilitation and cancer survivorship: a state of art review of current literature and management strategies in male sexual dysfunction among prostate cancer survivors. *J Sex Med.* 2013;10(S1):102–111. doi:10.1111/j.1743-6109.2012.03005.x.

47. Albaugh JA, Tenfelde S, Hayden DM. Sexual dysfunction and intimacy for ostomates. *Clin Colon Rectal Surg.* 2017;30(3):201–206. doi:10.1055/s-0037-1598161.

48. Brotto LA. Mindful sex. *Can J Hum Sex.* 2013;22(2):63–68. doi:10.3138/cjhs.2013.2132.

49. Berner M, Günzler C. Efficacy of psychosocial interventions in men and women with sexual dysfunctions—a systematic review of controlled clinical trials. *J Sex Med.* 2012;9(12):3089-3107. doi:10.1111/j.1743-6109.2012.02970.x.

50. Nelson CJ, Kenowitz J. Communication and intimacy-enhancing interventions for men diagnosed with prostate cancer and their partners. *J Sex Med.* 2013;10 Suppl 1:127–132. doi:10.1111/jsm.12049.

51. Walker LM, King N, Kwasny Z, Robinson JW. Intimacy after prostate cancer: a brief couples' workshop is associated with improvements in relationship satisfaction. *Psycho-Oncology.* 2017;26(9):1336-1346. doi:10.1002/pon.4147.

52. Reese JB, Smith KC, Handorf E, et al. A randomized pilot trial of a couple-based intervention addressing sexual concerns for breast cancer survivors. *J Psychosoc Oncol.* 2019;37(2):242–263. doi:10.1080/07347332.2018.1510869.

53. Reese JB, Zimmaro LA, Lepore SJ, et al. Evaluating a couple-based intervention addressing sexual concerns for breast cancer survivors: study protocol for a randomized controlled trial. *Trials.* 2020;21(1):173. doi:10.1186/s13063-019-3975-2.

54. Badr H. New frontiers in couple-based interventions in cancer care: refining the prescription for spousal communication. *Acta Oncol.* 2017;56(2):139–145. doi:10.1080/0284186X.2016.1266079.

55. Avery-Clark C, Weiner L. Sensate focus in sex therapy and sexual health: the art and science of mindful touch. *J Sex Med.* 2017;14(5):e254–e255. doi:10.1016/j.jsxm.2017.04.256.

Fear of Cancer Recurrence

6

Phyllis Butow and Louise Sharpe

While earlier detection and improved treatments have increased the number of people surviving cancer, those survivors live with a number of physical and psychological sequelae, including fear of cancer recurrence (FCR). Cancer is still seen as an insidious disease, stealthy, hidden, and hard to detect until the damage is done.[1] The propensity of cancer to spread to other parts of the body is associated with fear and dread, eliciting images of tentacles and silent spread.[1] Cancer treatments (particularly chemotherapy) are perceived as toxic and challenging, and are a source of fear in themselves.[2] In a qualitative study of FCR after breast cancer, one woman said: "Chemotherapy was worse than cancer itself. I remember thinking at the end of the treatment if it ever came back I'd just take a tablet and go to heaven. I wouldn't do the chemo again, I wouldn't do it again."[2] Ultimately, cancer is an existential threat, provoking fear of suffering, being a burden on the family, missing key events such as grandchildren growing to adulthood and ceasing to exist.[2]

Such images and fears are hard to overcome, even in the context of ever-improving prognoses and longer survivorship. For people who have already been diagnosed, particularly with a rare or poor prognosis cancer, statistics are not always comforting. Even if their prognosis is good, since their body has already betrayed them once, why would it not do so again? Even if only five in a hundred people have a recurrence, why would they not be amongst the five unlucky ones?[3] While emerging therapies such as immunotherapies are providing hope to those with advanced disease, as yet their long-term outcomes are unknown, and therefore doctors cannot give clear indications of long-term prognosis. For these reasons, all cancer patients and survivors live with uncertainty.

Thus, it is unsurprising that FCR is one of the most significant concerns for people after a cancer diagnosis, and a common reason why survivors seek psychological help or support.[4] FCR has recently been defined by an international expert consensus group as "fear, worry or concern relating to the possibility that cancer will come back or progress."[5] This definition recognizes that FCR can affect all patients who have been diagnosed with cancer, regardless of their prognosis. FCR may impact patients with curable disease who fear recurrence, those with chronic disease who fear relapse, and those with advanced disease who fear further progression.

HOW DOES FCR MANIFEST?

FCR is a normal and understandable response to the uncertainty and existential threat engendered by a cancer diagnosis. Indeed, at low levels, FCR is likely beneficial, motivating adherence to follow-up schedules and a healthy lifestyle. At this mild end of the FCR spectrum, people may experience

DOI: 10.1201/9781003055426-6

occasional thoughts about cancer recurring, with peaks of anxiety at follow-up tests and consultations, or when they experience symptoms, which persist for a few days and then resolve. Mild FCR usually improves over time, as the experience of cancer and its treatment fades and the feared outcome does not occur.

At moderate to severe levels, people experience more frequent thoughts and images about cancer recurrence (perhaps more than once a week, and in the absence of triggers). Commonly they feel unable to control these thoughts, and experience significant anxiety and distress associated with these thoughts. At this level, FCR is no longer beneficial, and is associated with a range of negative psychological impacts (e.g., anxiety, depression, and poor quality of life), such that survivors often seek help to better manage their FCR.

People with severe FCR (regarded as being clinically significant) report constant and intrusive thoughts about cancer and a conviction that cancer will return regardless of actual prognosis. Depending on their coping strategy, they may over-monitor for signs of cancer activity and overuse health services in search of reassurance, or alternatively fearfully avoid screening and follow-up.[5,6] While there has been some disagreement about whether FCR should be regarded as a clinical diagnosis (distinct from other psychological disorders such as anxiety), a recent Delphi study involving international experts in FCR identified the following characteristics of clinically significant FCR: a preoccupation with the cancer returning or progressing, unhelpful coping behaviors; impairment in daily function; clinically significant distress; and an inability to make future plans in case cancer intervenes and disrupts plans.[5] Severe FCR is very disruptive of quality of life, and unlikely to remit without clinical intervention. Patients report a high need for help with FCR, which appears to be currently unmet in routine care.[7,8]

Of note, people with existing psychological diagnoses, such as generalized anxiety disorder or health anxiety appear to be at higher risk of severe FCR.[9,10] Thus, it could be suggested that FCR is simply a sign of anxiety, and does not need to be considered or treated separately. However, the majority of patients with severe FCR do not meet criteria for other psychological disorders, suggesting FCR is a unique and significant mental health issue in its own right.[9] One longitudinal study reported that anxiety was unrelated to FCR when optimism was included in the multivariate model, suggesting a more specific psychological mechanism than in generalized anxiety.[11]

OUTCOMES OF FCR

The high prevalence and severity of FCR is concerning not only because of the distress it causes survivors and its impact on their quality of life,[12] but because it can reduce adherence to follow-up recommendations and increase health service usage and costs.[13–15] For example, in 2,337 American survivors of 10 cancer types who completed a survey at 3 time points (on average 1.3, 2.2, and 8.8 years postdiagnosis), those with high FCR reported lower adherence to physical activity and fruit and vegetable intake recommendations, although the association was weak.[16] Another study found that survivors with high FCR either skipped follow-up and screening (to avoid peaks in FCR) or constantly requested tests and appointments with health professionals (to gain reassurance, albeit short-lived, that their cancer had not returned).[13] The former approach may risk late diagnosis of recurrence (and, as a result, compromise survival), while the latter can burden the health system, and actually contribute to maintaining FCR in the longer term. One study found that those survivors who are highly fearful of recurrence have more visits to the emergency department, and more outpatient vists,[15] supporting findings from other disease settings that fear of disease recurrence increases health costs.[17] Thus, there are reasons at the patient, hospital and health service level for identifying and addressing FCR.

PREVALENCE AND PERSISTENCE OF FCR

Most cancer survivors experience at least mild FCR for a period of time after diagnosis, particularly at the end of treatment. Establishing the prevalence of higher levels of FCR has been complicated by uncertainty regarding cut-offs to distinguish different levels of FCR. The most common measure used to assess FCR is the Fear of Cancer Recurrence Inventory (FCRI) which has a 9-item short-form (FCRI-SF)[18] that can determine severity. Its authors reported that a cut-off of ≥13 on the FCRI-SF provided optimal sensitivity (88%) and specificity (75%) in determining clinical FCR against a clinical interview in a French Canadian cancer sample. However, later studies questioned the utility of this cut-off. Fardell et al.[19] reported on two studies in Australian and Canadian English-speaking samples, both of which identified a cut-off of ≥22 as providing optimal sensitivity and sensitivity. Controversy regarding the optimal cut-off remains, and this probably explains the wide variation in prevalence rates reported across studies.

Across earlier studies investigating FCR prevalence, summarized in a systematic review,[12] 22% to 87% (on average 49%) of cancer survivors reported moderate to high levels of FCR, with more vulnerable groups, such as young women with breast cancer, more likely to report FCR at this level of severity.[13] About 0–15% (on average 7%) of patients reported severe and highly disabling FCR.[12] More recently, greater variability in prevalence has been reported, perhaps reflecting cultural or local issues. For example, Mahendran et al.[20] reported that in a Singapore cancer survivor population, 32% reported severe or pathological FCR, significantly more than earlier reported in Simard et al.'s systematic review.[12]

Longitudinal studies of cancer survivors show that FCR can be long-lasting, and without intervention does not necessarily resolve over time, even when objective risk of recurrence is low.[12] For example, in men on average 11 years post testicular cancer diagnosis (with an excellent prognosis), 24% reported that FCR bothered them quite a bit, and 7% that it bothered them a lot.[21] More recent studies[22–25] have shown FCR declining over time. For example, in the longitudinal American study quoted above,[16] FCR severity decreased over the 8 years of follow-up. However, in those who started with severe FCR, FCR remained higher than in those who started with medium or low FCR, suggesting that this cohort may need help to bring their FCR levels down to more manageable levels.

WHAT FACTORS INCREASE RISK OF FCR?

Diagnosis

FCR has been documented in cancer survivors with varied diagnoses, including breast, colorectal, nasopharynx, head and neck, endometrial and thyroid cancer, melanoma, and Hodgkin's and non-Hodgkin's Lymphoma,[10,12] and in old and young,[26] and is likely a concern for all cancer patients.

Demographic Characteristics and Past Experiences

A systematic review of FCR studies concluded that those who are younger, with higher subjective risk perception, more severe side-effects, and/or other anxiety conditions, are more vulnerable to FCR.[8] Younger patients do not expect a cancer diagnosis, have many life responsibilities, and having lost their sense of invulnerability, may interpret even low risks of recurrence as high and frightening. Those with past experiences which have made them feel unlucky (such as trauma, or a family history of cancer), and those with general anxiety disorder, may have a higher subjective perception of risk and thus be more vulnerable to FCR. Side-effects and symptoms can be a constant reminder of cancer, and a source of worry that they are signs of cancer returning.

Objective Prognosis and Treatment

Interestingly, objective prognostic indicators or markers, such as stage and size of disease, have inconsistently been found to be associated with FCR,[12] perhaps because the amount and detail of prognostic information conveyed to patients varies across health practitioners and settings. A recent paper[27] highlighted that after genomic testing, cancer survivors may be presented with a high and more specific risk of recurrence, or be given the option to omit treatment on the basis of a low risk. Both outcomes could potentially increase FCR, the first because of increased subjective risk and the latter because the safety net of treatment has been taken away. Another longitudinal study of 1,281 German cancer patients (77.5% participation rate) recruited on average 11 months post-diagnosis found that palliative treatment intention, pain and a higher number of physical symptoms, predicted higher FCR, leading the authors to conclude that to some extent, FCR is a realistic response to poorer prognosis and physical decline.[24]

Two recent studies[28,29] found that having adjuvant therapy in addition to surgery increased risk of FCR, perhaps because this made the treatment phase more prolonged and traumatic, and because patients interpret longer, more complex treatment as signifying serious disease while they may struggle to interpret tumor markers. More recently, it has been noted that patients having novel, tailored cancer treatments over long periods may experience higher FCR.[27] For example, targeted tyrosine kinase inhibitors (TKIs) for patients with advanced gastro-intestinal stromal tumors (GIST) or chronic myelogenous leukemia (CML) are given indefinitely, or until treatment intolerance or progression occurs, and for 36 months in those with localized GIST. Further, tests for recurrence or progression are frequent (quarterly) for these therapies, thus triggering peaks of anxiety while awaiting results.

Psychosocial Factors

Conversely, a recent study of FCR in adolescents and young adults found that neither demographic nor medical variables were associated with FCR; rather socio-emotional wellbeing and quality of life predicted FCR.[30] Similar results emerged from the longitudinal German study discussed above.[24] The authors reported that among other variables, lower social support and adverse social interactions predicted higher FCR 1 year after rehabilitation. Perhaps a lack of support leaves survivors more vulnerable to anxiety and worry. Alternatively, survivors and their families may be locked in an unhelpful cycle of negativity, increasing FCR. Cancer caregivers and close members of the survivors' family are just as likely, if not more likely, as the survivor to experience FCR, and the two are intertwined in that high FCR in the caregiver is associated with high FCR in the patient (and vice versa).[31] This suggests that involving caregivers in interventions for FCR may be helpful.

Health Service and Communication Factors

A few studies have shown that satisfaction with health care in survivorship[32,33] and doctor-patient communication influences FCR. Liu and colleagues conducted a systematic review of studies that addressed the relationship between the clinical encounter and FCR.[34] Three studies examined associations between doctor communication coded from audiotaped consultations, and patient-reported FCR.[35–37] These studies found that giving time, space for patients to express emotions and providing information can decrease FCR. Gros and colleagues[36] reported that colorectal cancer patients unsatisfied with information provided during the consultation, and who experienced more interruptions during the consultation, had significantly less decline in FCR from before to after the consultation. Unexpectedly, greater patient perceived empathy conveyed by the doctor to the patient was also associated with less FCR reduction. Liu et al. suggest that this may be because patients with high FCR triggered greater empathy in the clinician, but were also harder to shift in terms of FCR.[34] While Gros and colleagues found no effect of consultation length on FCR levels, Barracliffe and colleagues[35] found that longer consultations and more patient expressions of emotion during consultations with their radiotherapist were associated with greater decline in FCR in breast cancer patients during the course of their adjuvant radiotherapy. Reassuringly, across the studies, open discussion of FCR by health professionals did not trigger increased FCR in patients.

Liu et al. identified five patient surveys exploring factors perceived to increase FCR. In four of the five studies, a common theme identified was that patients desire detailed prognostic information and find that helpful to address FCR. Moreover, those with the highest FCR wanted the most prognostic information. If patients recalled such a discussion about prognosis, they were less likely to over- or under-estimate their recurrence risk, reducing one of the risk factors for FCR (high subjective risk). Those surveyed also indicated a desire for more information about the symptoms of cancer recurrence, so that they could distinguish more effectively between what to worry about, and what to ignore. Only 21% of colorectal cancer patients could name symptoms associated with cancer reappearing while 64% would like to learn more about what these symptoms are.[38]

One study[37] identified revealed that some patients felt uncomfortable raising FCR with their physician, due to fear of appearing ungrateful or damaging the patient-physician relationship by suggesting that their treatment may not have been fully successful. These findings suggest that oncologists can play an important role in preventing and reducing FCR through encouraging open expression of fears and worries, normalizing FCR and providing information that can help patients to maintain realistic risk perceptions and reduce reactivity to unrelated symptoms.

THEORIES OF FCR

If we are to intervene effectively to help survivors better manage their FCR, we need to understand how FCR develops, and the factors maintaining it. This is best done within a theoretical framework which can be tested and refined over time. Three recent systematic reviews by Fardell et al.,[39] Simonelli et al.,[40] and Curran et al.[41] identified theoretical models and frameworks applied to FCR. These included the self-regulation of illness or common sense model,[42] the self-regulatory executive function (S-REF) model,[43] the extended parallel process model (EPPM),[44] the uncertainty theory,[45] a theory of cognitive adaptation,[46] the meaning making model,[47] a social-cognitive processing model,[48] and the threat interpretation model.[49] Maheu et al.[50] note that there is no consensus on the optimal theoretical model of FCR. However, Simonelli et al.,[40] emphasize that what is clear, is that a cancer-specific model (versus general anxiety models) is required to guide interventions, due to the unique aspects of FCR.

The models most commonly applied to FCR are the Commonsense model,[42] uncertainty theory,[45] and metacognitive models (including the S-REF model).[43] Curran et al.,[51] have advocated for the addition of death anxiety to these models, particularly for patients with advanced disease, to account for the central existential fear that dominates FCR. These models will now be discussed in greater detail.

The Commonsense model, developed by Leventhal et al.,[42] posited that those who have past experiences of cancer leading them to believe that cancer is severe, long lasting and out of their control, and who have a poor or inaccurate knowledge base of cure and survival rates, develop a higher risk perception. This, combined with a high emotional response to cancer (including anxiety and remorse over not pursuing more aggressive treatment options), leads to higher FCR.[52] Further, internal cues (such as symptoms) and external cues (such as seeing a health professional, exposure to cancer in the media, and

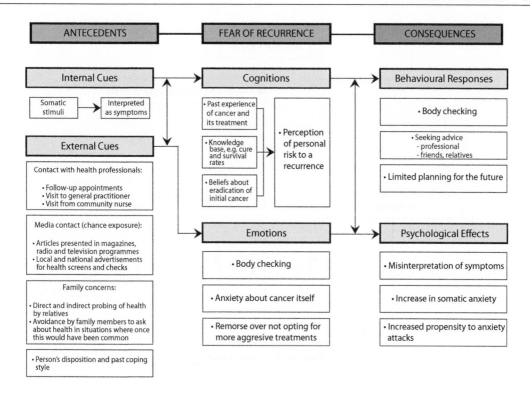

FIGURE 6.1   Summary of initial fear of recurrence formulation.

family raising or avoiding cancer) can increase FCR. FCR then leads to behavioral changes (such as over-checking and seeking reassurance from health professionals) and psychological impacts (such as anxiety and panic attacks). The model was summarized by Lee-Jones & Humphris[52] as shown in Figure 6.1.

While much of this model makes intuitive sense, many of the proposed processes were not well articulated, and the empirical data supporting the model is limited. Furthermore, this primarily cognitive model suggests that FCR develops when the perception of threat is out of proportion to the objective risk. Yet, in the cancer context, the possibility of recurrence is real and enduring, worry about the future is understandable and triggers for worry such as ongoing treatment with hormone or immunotherapy, scans and side-effects are frequent. Moreover, some degree of FCR is likely adaptive as it encourages adherence to follow-up recommendations. Thus, directly challenging the content of people's thoughts about recurrence risk is likely to be suboptimal.

Uncertainty theory[45] notes that uncertainty is inherent to most illnesses, in which processes or outcomes are inconsistent, random, complex and unpredictable, and where tailored information is unavailable. Such uncertainty leaves much room for negative interpretation of risk. Lebel and colleagues[53] further suggest when uncertainty is high, benign physical symptoms are more likely to be interpreted as signs of recurrence, increasing FCR. Furthermore, individuals are known to vary in their tolerance of and attitudes towards uncertainty. Those who view uncertainty as a danger are more likely to see the glass as half empty, increasing subjective risk perception, and are more likely to use negative coping strategies such as reassurance seeking and body checking which tend to maintain FCR. Lebel and colleagues have produced a blended model of FCR, combining elements of the commonsense model and uncertainty theory, shown in Figure 6.2. These authors tested their model in 106 women with breast or gynecological cancer, demonstrating good fit for most of the posited associations.[53]

More recent metacognitive models have built upon these previous conceptualizations and share many commonalities. Metacognitions are thoughts or beliefs about thoughts, such as beliefs about worry. Metacognitive models focus on these underlying beliefs rather than the specific content of the worry.

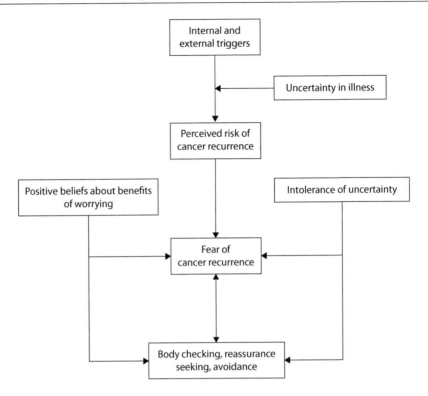

FIGURE 6.2   Blended model of FCR.

For example, Fardell et al.'s.[39] model proposes that for some people, normal worry about recurrence activates an unhelpful style of cognitive processing which increases FCR. These authors propose that people who believe that worry will protect them (e.g., by helping them to identify cancer recurrence early), might cause them harm (e.g., through stress compromising their immune system) or that the worry is uncontrollable, tend to ruminate about their cancer risk, focus their attention on themselves and their symptoms, become very vigilant to threat and try to suppress the worrying thoughts. These concerns are compounded in people who have vulnerability factors (such as prior losses including those related to cancer, or mental health problems). Further, when people have received insufficient or inaccurate information about the risk of recurrence, this also gives rise to the interpretation of higher perceived risk (see Figure 6.3).[39]

Simonelli et al.[40] similarly propose that some people interpret cancer as an ongoing threat (as opposed to others who find meaning or benefit in the experience), leading to rumination, vigilance to signals of threat, and suppression or avoidance of thoughts, exacerbated by contextual and social factors (including the information communicated to them about recurrence). Simonelli's model emphasizes the role of terror management theory and fear of death as a fundamental component of FCR. Heathcote and Ecclestone[49] also suggest that people with ongoing symptoms and side-effects from cancer treatment, such as fatigue or lymphedema, who interpret these as harmful, ruminate about the symptoms and remain vigilant for ongoing signs and symptoms of their cancer returning.

Finally, Curran et al.[51] build on Simonelli's proposition that death anxiety is an essential concept to consider in understanding FCR, commonly absent from other models. Available evidence suggests that death anxiety is common across cancer stages.[54,55] Yalom, who conducted foundational work on death anxiety, views death as a primordial existential concern, along with isolation, meaninglessness and freedom.[56] He proposed that being confronted with the possibility of death brings into focus the ultimate aloneness of facing death, the possible meaninglessness of one's life and the ultimate responsibility one holds for life choices. Yalom suggests that for most people, death anxiety elicits defense mechanisms to reduce anxiety, including avoidance, however these are only partially and temporarily effective. Only

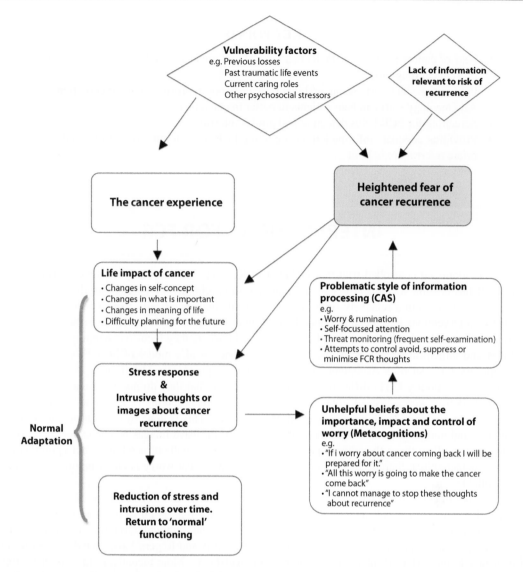

FIGURE 6.3 Cognitive processing model of fear of cancer recurrence. (From Fardell JE, Thewes B, Turner J, et al. Fear of cancer recurrence: a theoretical review and novel cognitive processing formulation. *J Cancer Surviv.* 2016;10(4):663–73.)

when the person is able to transform their fear of death into an opportunity to embrace a more authentic way of living, can anxiety be resolved. Sharpe et al.[57] note that several qualitative studies have confirmed that the core content of FCR often concern fears about death, the process of dying, or the impact on family members should the person die.[58,59] In one study,[60] a patient is quoted as saying:

> I don't want to die now. I think, I feel, there's so much left to do. I want to go on living and I want to watch my little grandchild grow up. I want to live with my family and my husband and my children. It's terrible when you get all full of anxiety about how things are going to be.

Sharpe et al. propose a number of reasons why death anxiety has been omitted from earlier models, including death anxiety in researchers and clinicians themselves, who are not immune to this immutable part of the human condition. However, if patients are to be assisted with FCR, it is important that clinicians and interventions do not model avoidance of such a core issue, themselves.

KEY POINTS

- Fear of cancer recurrence (FCR) is a normal and understandable response to the threat of a cancer diagnosis
- FCR is prevalent, distressing, and if severe, does not improve without intervention
- All Oncology staff can help patients to better manage FCR
- Screening for FCR helps detection and guides referral
- Providing adequate information, normalizing FCR, encouraging disclosure, and appropriate referral are helpful

INTERVENTIONS FOR FCR

The first randomized controlled trial that included FCR as an outcome was published in 2007.[61] Since then, FCR has become a frequently assessed outcome in psychotherapy outcome trials for cancer survivors, but there remain a relatively small number of trials that specifically focus on FCR. However, a number of interventions have been developed based upon the theoretical models described above. Most treatments have either been (a) cognitive behavioral (CBT), where they focus on changing illness-related attitudes and unhelpful behaviors on the basis of Lee-Jones et al.'s model of FCR,[52] or (b) a form of contemporary CBT such as Acceptance Commitment Therapy (ACT), Mindfulness or Metacognitive Therapy. Contemporary CBTs differ from traditional CBT in that they do not challenge the content of unhelpful beliefs or worry. Instead, contemporary CBTs focus on accepting FCR as a normal experience, and try to help people to learn not to engage in their worries. This is done by cultivating an attitude of acceptance and non-judgment towards the fears, worries or intrusive images people experience, so that people learn to allow those thoughts to pass through their mind without needing to act upon them. In addition, metacognitive therapy focuses on dispelling the myth that worry is either helpful, harmful or uncontrollable.

A number of cognitive-behavioral treatments have been shown to be effective in reducing FCR. For example, Herschbach and colleagues[62] found a group-based CBT program to be more effective than a non-randomized control group who did not receive the treatment, although CBT was no more effective in that study than a supportive psychotherapy group. Humphris and Rogers[63] also found a small benefit of their face to face AFTER intervention, compared to usual care. More recently, in the SWORD study, van de Wal and colleagues used a blended CBT approach with five face-to-face sessions and three brief e-consultations and demonstrated that the intervention resulted in moderate to large changes in FCR that were both statistically and clinically significant.[64] However, these studies all used wait-list or usual care comparison groups, and in the only trials with an active control group (supportive psychotherapy in Herschbach's study), CBT fared no better than supportive psychotherapy.

Few of the contemporary CBT approaches that have been developed were specifically developed for the management of FCR. One exception is the ConquerFear program, developed by Butow et al.[65] from the cognitive processing model proposed by Fardell and colleagues.[39] Butow et al.[65] combined components from meta-cognitive therapy (challenging the value placed on, or avoidance of, worry about recurrence) and acceptance commitment therapy. They compared the five session face-to-face ConquerFear intervention with relaxation therapy that was roughly matched for therapist time and attention. Compared to relaxation treatment, ConquerFear produced changes in FCR that were both statistically and clinically significant after treatment and 6 months later. The difference between ConquerFear and relaxation revealed a moderate effect size. Further, analyses confirmed that it was reduction in metacognitions and intrusive thoughts that mediated the relative efficacy of ConquerFear versus relaxation training, confirming the proposed treatment mechanisms.

A 2019 meta-analysis synthesizing the results of the literature to date by Tauber and colleagues[66] identified 23 trials of psychological therapies for FCR. They found moderate evidence to support the use of psychological treatments, with a small overall effect (Hedge's $g = 0.33$). This effect was maintained at follow-up, although the effect size was slightly smaller, and was greater for those with shorter follow-up periods (Hedge's $g = 0.28$). Of the 23 trials included in that meta-analysis, only 8 were of interventions specifically developed for the treatment of FCR, although the difference between FCR-specific interventions (Hedge's $g = 0.44$) and generic interventions (Hedge's $g = 0.26$) was not significantly different. The meta-analysis showed that contemporary CBT (Hedge's $g = 0.42$) was superior to traditional CBT (Hedge's $g = 0.24$).

The results of this meta-analysis confirm that there are at least two efficacious treatment approaches (CBT and contemporary CBT), which have a therapeutic effect on FCR. Available economic analyses suggest that both CBT[67] and contemporary CBT (ConquerFear)[68] are cost-effective options in the management of FCR. The data support that contemporary CBTs are more efficacious and therefore should be the first line of treatment. However, it is important to note that there are gaps in the literature that were identified. Firstly, the majority of studies were with early stage cancer patients (often breast cancer); patients with advanced or recurred disease have largely been omitted from trials, despite the fact that their levels of FCR are at least as high as that of patients with early stage disease, and they have an unmet need for help with FCR. Secondly, with the large numbers of survivors and relatively small psycho-oncology workforce, it is difficult to envisage that all survivors with clinically significant FCR could access treatment face-to-face with a psycho-oncology professional. Thus online options may be needed. While there was good evidence for the efficacy of a blended care approach (van de Wal),[64] this still involved five face-to-face sessions. Unfortunately, a recent large trial of online CBT (the CAREST trial)[69] failed to find any benefit of CBT compared to the wait-list on FCR. However, as yet, contemporary CBTs have not been trialed as online versions, although development and preliminary testing has commenced.[70]

Liu et al.[34] conducted a systematic review of intervention studies conducted by medical or nursing professionals, finding five studies.[63,71–74] Four of these were nurse-led; one coached patients to discuss FCR with their specialist, and three delivered supportive counseling and/or taught strategies to manage FCR. The final intervention trained mixed health professionals to manage FCR through normalization, education and lifestyle strategies. Of the three studies which measured FCR objectively, two demonstrated a significant reduction in FCR in the short term.

Liu et al. went on to develop an 8-minute, oncologist-delivered intervention (CIFeR), comprising normalization of FCR; provision of concrete prognostic information tailored to patient preferences; a take-home education sheet describing red-flag recurrence symptoms, simple strategies to manage worry and links to additional online resources to manage FCR; and psychological referral (if appropriate). A pilot study[75] in which 5 oncologists delivered CIFeR to 62 women with breast cancer found high acceptability, feasibility and potential efficacy. FCR severity and the proportion of women with clinically significant FCR decreased significantly over time. Such approaches are worthy of continued investigation.

IMPLICATIONS FOR ONCOLOGY STAFF

FCR is a critical target for optimal survivorship care. Awareness of FCR can help clinicians to better support their patients, and to identify patients who may benefit from more intensive psychological treatments for high FCR. We recommend screening for FCR, particularly at the end of treatment and during follow-up. There are a number of short, reliable measures now available, such as the 9-item Fear of Cancer Recurrence Inventory (FCRI) severity subscale.[18] Scores ≥22 on this measure suggest a need for specialist psychological input.[19]

It is also useful to directly ask patients if FCR is troubling them. Butow et al.[76] suggest a useful way of encouraging discussion of FCR as follows:

Many people I see worry a lot about their cancer coming back. That's normal and expected after a cancer diagnosis. But if the worry is distressing you, or is starting to stop you getting on with your life, we should do something about it. There are things we can suggest to help you manage these worries. So, has this been a problem for you?

Oncologists can also help by effectively communicating prognosis, the most likely signs and symptoms of a recurrence (as well as those *not* likely to be related to cancer), recommended behaviors to reduce risk (such as exercise and stopping smoking), and standard follow-up schedules and their rationale. Patients and family members can be encouraged to reject pressure to "be positive" and "get back to normal," and rather accept that they may be dealing with FCR for some time. For those with high FCR, direction to appropriate resources, such as booklets and online interventions can be helpful. Examples of online resources are: http://www.cancer.net/survivorship/life-after-cancer/coping-with-fear-recurrence (information and podcast); https://www.mskcc.org/blog/six-tips-managing-fear-recurrence; https://cancer.northwestern.edu/cancerconnections/presentations/McGinty_ShoetoDrop_Mar2015.pdf (powerpoint slides with information and coping strategies). Those with very high or prolonged FCR may need referral to a psycho-oncologist for face-to-face care.

IMPLICATIONS FOR NON-ONCOLOGY STAFF

Other health professionals, such as GPs, are also often confronted with patients experiencing high FCR, perhaps expressing concerns about symptoms and/or requesting additional scans to rule out cancer recurrence. It is helpful to resist referring patients for additional screens and tests unless warranted, as this can maintain a cycle of worry, reassurance seeking, immediate relief and then rising anxiety again. Providing guidance on when to worry about symptoms can reduce excessive requests for scans and tests. Patients can be encouraged to ask themselves: "Have I had this symptom before? What was the outcome then? Is there anything that can explain this symptom (such as a recent prolonged gardening session)?" Symptoms that last more than a week and/or are severe or painful, however, should trigger an appointment with a GP or specialist. As noted above, reassuring patients that FCR is a normal and expected response after a cancer diagnosis is appropriate. It may also be worthwhile to ask the patient what their understanding of their risk of recurrence is. If this is vague, or seems too high, encouraging a return visit to their oncologist for more accurate prognostic information may be helpful. Referral to the resources listed above, or if FCR is persistent, to a psychologist, may also be helpful.

REFERENCES

1. Vrinten C, McGregor LM, Heinrich M, et al. What do people fear about cancer? A systematic review and meta-synthesis of cancer fears in the general population. *Psychooncology*. 2017;26(8):1070–9.
2. Thewes B, Lebel S, Seguin Leclair C, et al. A qualitative exploration of fear of cancer recurrence (FCR) amongst Australian and Canadian breast cancer survivors. *Support Care Cancer*. 2016;24:2269–76.
3. Cartwright LA, Dumenci L, Siminoff L, Matsuyama RK. Cancer patients' understanding of prognostic information. *J Cancer Educ*. 2014;29(2):311–7.
4. Armes J, Crowe M, Colbourne L, et al. Patients' supportive care needs beyond the end of cancer treatment: a prospective, longitudinal survey. *J Clin Oncol*. 2009;27:6172–9.
5. Lebel S, Ozakinci G, Humphris G, Mutsaers B, Thewes B, Prins J, et al. From normal response to clinical problem: definition and clinical features of fear of cancer recurrence. *Support Care Cancer*. 2016;24(8):3265–8.
6. Mutsaers B, Jones G, Rutkowski N, et al. When fear of cancer recurrence becomes a clinical issue: a qualitative analysis of features associated with clinical fear of cancer recurrence. *Support Care Cancer*. 2016;24:4207–18.

7. Ellegaard MB, Grau C, Zachariae R, Bonde Jensen A. Fear of cancer recurrence and unmet needs among breast cancer survivors in the first five years: a cross-sectional study. *Acta Oncol.* 2017;56:314–20.
8. Hodgkinson K, Butow P, Hunt GE, et al. The development and evaluation of a measure to assess cancer survivors' unmet supportive care needs: the CaSUN (Cancer Survivors' Unmet Needs measure). *Psychooncology.* 2007;16:796–804.
9. Thewes B, Bell ML, Butow PN, et al. Psychological morbidity and stress but not social factors influence level of fear of cancer recurrence in young women with early breast cancer: results of a cross-sectional study. *Psychooncology.* 2013;22:2797–806.
10. Mirosevic S, Thewes B, can Herpen C, et al. Prevalence and clinical and psychological correlates of high fear of cancer recurrence in patients newly diagnosed with head and neck cancer. *Head Neck.* 2019; 41(9):3187–200.
11. Llewellyn CD, Weinman J, McGurk M, et al. Can we predict which head and neck cancer survivors develop fears of recurrence? *J Psychosom Res.* 2008;65(6):525–32.
12. Simard S, Thewes B, Humphris G, et al. Fear of cancer recurrence in adult cancer survivors: a systematic review of quantitative studies. *J Cancer Surviv.* 2013;7:300–22.
13. Thewes B, Butow P, Bell ML, et al. Fear of cancer recurrence in young women with a history of early-stage breast cancer: a cross-sectional study of prevalence and association with health behaviours. *Support Care Cancer.* 2012;20:2651–9.
14. Fisher A, Beeken RJ, Heinrich M, et al. Health behaviours and fear of cancer recurrence in 10 969 colorectal cancer (CRC) patients. *Psychooncology.* 2016;25:1434–40. http://dx.doi.org/10.1002/pon.4076.
15. Lebel S, Tomei C, Feldstain A, et al. Does fear of cancer recurrence predict cancer survivors' health care use? *Support Care Cancer.* 2013;21(3):901–6.
16. Séguin Leclair C, Lebel S, Westmaas JL. The relationship between fear of cancer recurrence and health behaviors: a nationwide longitudinal study of cancer survivors. *Health Psychol.* 2019;38(7):596–605. doi:10.1037/hea0000754.
17. Brach M, Sabariego C, Herschbach P, et al. Cost-effectiveness of cognitive-behavioral group therapy for dysfunctional fear of progression in chronic arthritis patients. *J Public Health.* 2010;32(4):547–54.
18. Simard S, Savard J. Screening and comorbidity of clinical levels of fear of cancer recurrence. *J Cancer Surviv.* 2015;9(3):481–91.
19. Fardell J, Jones G, Smith A-B, et al. Exploring the screening capacity of the Fear of Cancer Recurrence Inventory-Short Form for clinical levels of fear of cancer recurrence. *Psychooncology.* 2018;27(s):492–9.
20. Mahendran R, Liu J, Kuparasundram S, et al. Fear of cancer recurrence among cancer survivors in Singapore. *Singapore Med J.* 2020. doi:10.11622/smedj.2020007.
21. Skaali T, Fosså SD, Bremnes R, et al. Fear of recurrence in long-term testicular cancer survivors. *Psychooncology.* 2009;18(12):1273–80.
22. Dunn LB, Langford DJ, Paul SM, et al. Trajectories of fear of recurrence in women with breast cancer. *Support Care Cancer.* 2015;23:2033–43.
23. Halbach SM, Enders A, Kowalski C, et al. Health literacy and fear of cancer progression in elderly women newly diagnosed with breast cancer – a longitudinal analysis. *Patient Educ Couns.* 2016;99,855–62.
24. Mehnert A, Koch U, Sundermann C, Dinkel A. Predictors of fear of recurrence in patients one year after cancer rehabilitation: a prospective study. *Acta Oncologica.* 2013;52:1102–9.
25. Sarkar S, Scherwath A, Schirmer L, et al. Fear of recurrence and its impact on quality of life in patients with hematological cancers in the course of allogeneic hematopoietic SCT. *Bone Marrow Transplant.* 2014;49:1217–22.
26. Sun H, Yang Y, Zhang J, et al. Fear of cancer recurrence, anxiety and depressive symptoms in adolescent and young adult cancer patients. *Neuropsychatr Dis Treat.* 2019; 15: 857–65.
27. Thewes B, Husson O, Poort J, et al. Fear of cancer recurrence in an era of personalized medicine. *JCO 2017;* 2017;35(29):3275–8.
28. Ellegaard MB; Grau C; Zachariae R; Bonde Jensen A. Fear of cancer recurrence and unmet needs among breast cancer survivors in the first five years. A cross-sectional study. *Acta Oncologica.* 2017;56(2):314–20.
29. van de Wal M, van Oort I, Schouten J, et al. Fear of cancer recurrence in prostate cancer survivors. *Acta Oncologica.* 2016;55(7):821–7.
30. Thewes B, Kaal SEJ, Custers JAE, et al. Prevalence and correlates of high fear of cancer recurrence in late adolescents and young adults consulting a specialist adolescent and young adult (AYA) cancer service. *Support Care Cancer.* 2018;26:1479–87. https://doi.org/10.1007/s00520-017-3975-2.
31. Hodges LJ, Humphris G. Fear of recurrence and psychological distress in head and neck cancer patients and their carers. *Psychooncology.* 2009;18(8):841–8.
32. Koch-Gallenkamp L, Bertram H, Eberle A, et al. Fear of recurrence in long-term cancer survivors—do cancer type, sex, time since diagnosis, and social support matter? *Health Psychol.* 2016;35(12):1329.
33. van de Wal M, van de Poll-Franse L, Prins J, Gielissen M. Does fear of cancer recurrence differ between cancer types? A study from the population-based PROFILES registry. *Psychooncology.* 2016;25(7):772–8.
34. Liu JJ, Butow P, Beith J. Systematic review of interventions by non-mental health specialists for managing fear of cancer recurrence in adult cancer survivors. *Support Care Cancer.* 2019;27(11):4055–67.
35. Barracliffe L, Yang Y, Cameron J, et al. Does emotional talk vary with fears of cancer recurrence trajectory? A content analysis of interactions between women with breast cancer and their therapeutic radiographers. *J Psychosom Res.* 2018;106:41–8.
36. Gros SE, Nitzsche A, Gloede TD, et al. The initial clinical interview – can it reduce cancer patients' fear? *Support Care Cancer.* 2015;23(4):977–84.

37. Ozakinci G, Swash B, Humphris G, et al. Fear of cancer recurrence in oral and oropharyngeal cancer patients: an investigation of the clinical encounter. *Eur J Cancer Care.* 2018;27(1). https://doi.org/10.1111/ecc.12785.

38. Papagrigoriadis S, Heyman B. Patients' views on follow up of colorectal cancer: implications for risk communication and decision making. *Postgrad Med J.* 2003;79:403–7.

39. Fardell JE, Thewes B, Turner J, et al. Fear of cancer recurrence: a theoretical review and novel cognitive processing formulation. *J Cancer Surviv.* 2016;10(4):663–73.

40. Simonelli LE, Siegel SD, Duffy NM. Fear of cancer recurrence: a theoretical review and its relevance for clinical presentation and management. *Psychooncology.* 2017;26(10):1444–54.

41. Curran L, Sharpe L, Butow P. Anxiety in the context of cancer: a systematic review and development of an integrated model. *Clin Psychol Rev.* 2017;56:40–54.

42. Leventhal H, Diefenbach M, Leventhal EA. Illness cognition: using common sense to understand treatment adherence and affect cognition interactions. *Cognit Ther Res* 1992;16:143–63.

43. Wells A, Matthews G: Modelling cognition in emotional disorder: the S-REF model. *Behav Res Ther.* 1996;34:881–8.

44. Witte K. Fear control and danger control: a test of the extended parallel process model (EPPM). *Commun Monogr.* 1994;61(2):113–34.

45. Mishel MH. Uncertainty in illness. *J Nurs Scholarsh.* 1988;20(4):225–31.

46. Taylor SE. Adjustment to threatening events: a theory of cognitive adaptation. *Am Psychol.* 1983;38:1161–73.

47. Neimayer RA. *Meaning reconstruction and the experience of loss.* Washington, DC: American Psychological Association; 2001.

48. Lepore SJ. A social-cognitive processing model of emotional adjustment to cancer. In Baum A, Andersen BL (Eds). *Psychological interventions for cancer.* Washington, DC: American Psychological Association; 2001. pp. 91–116.

49. Heathcote LC, Eccleston C. Pain and cancer survival: a cognitive-affective model of symptom appraisal and the uncertain threat of disease recurrence. *Pain.* 2017;158(7):1187–91.

50. Maheu C, Hébert M, Louli J, et al. Revision of the fear of cancer recurrence cognitive and emotional model by Lee-Jones et al. with women with breast cancer. *Cancer Rep.* 2019;2(4):e1172. https://doi.org/10.1002/cnr2.1172.

51. Curran L, Sharpe L, MacCann C, et al. Testing a model of fear of cancer recurrence or progression: the central role of intrusions, death anxiety and threat appraisal. *J Behav Med.* 2020;43:225–36. https://doi.org/10.1007/s10865-019-00129-x.

52. Lee-Jones C, Humphris G, Dixon R, Hatcher MB. Fear of cancer recurrence—a literature review and proposed cognitive formulation to explain exacerbation of recurrence fears. *Psychooncology*;1997:6:95–105.

53. Lebel S, Mahey C, Tomei C et al. Towards the validation of a new, blended theoretical model of fear of cancer recurrence. *Psychooncology.* 2018;27(11):2594–601.

54. Cella DF, Tross, S. Death anxiety in cancer survival: a preliminary cross-validation study. *J Pers Assess.* 1987;51(3):451–61. http://dx.doi.org/10.1207/s15327752jpa5103_12.

55. Sigal JJ, Ouimet MC, Margolese R, et al. How patients with less-advanced and more-advanced cancer deal with three death-related fears: an exploratory study. *J Psychosoc Oncol.* 2007;26(1):53–68. http://dx.doi.org/10.1300/J077v26n01_04.

56. Yalom ID. *Existential psychotherapy.* New York, NY: Basic Books; 1980.

57. Sharpe L, Curran L, Butow P, Thewes B. Fear of cancer recurrence and death anxiety. *Psychooncology.* 2018;27:2559–65.

58. Cesario SK, Nelson LS, Broxson A, Cesario AL. Sword of Damocles cutting through the life stages of women with ovarian cancer. *Oncol Nurs Forum.* 2010;37(5):609–17. https://doi.org/10.1188/10.ONF.609–617.

59. Johnson Vickberg SM. Fears about breast cancer recurrence. *Cancer Pract.* 2001;9(5):237–43.

60. Oxlad M, Wade TD, Hallsworth L, Koczwara B. I'm living with a chronic illness, not… dying with cancer': a qualitative study of Australian women's self-identified concerns and needs following primary treatment for breast cancer. *Eur J Cancer Care.* 2008;17(2):157–66.

61. Cameron LD, Booth RJ, Schlatter M, et al: Changes in emotion regulation and psychological adjustment following use of a group psychosocial support program for women recently diagnosed with breast cancer. *Psychooncology.* 2007;16:171–80.

62. Herschbach P, Book K, Dinkel A, et al. Evaluation of two group therapies to reduce fear of progression in cancer patients. *Support Care Cancer.* 2010;18:471–9.

63. Humphris GM, Rogers SN. AFTER and beyond: cancer recurrence fears and a test of an intervention in oropharyngeal patients. *Soc Sci Dent.* 2012;2:29–38.

64. van de Wal M, Thewes B, Gielissen M, et al. Efficacy of a blended cognitive behaviour therapy for high fear of recurrence in breast, prostate and colorectal cancer survivors: the SWORD study, a randomized controlled trial. *Journal of Clinical Oncology* 2017;35(19): 2173–83.

65. Butow PN, Turner J, Gilchrist J, et al. A randomized controlled trial (RCT) of a psychological intervention (Conquer Fear) to reduce clinical levels of fear of cancer recurrence in breast, colorectal and melanoma cancer survivors. *J Clin Oncol.* 2017;35(36):4066–77.

66. Tauber NM, O'Toole MS, Dinkel A, et al. Effect of psychological intervention on fear of cancer recurrence: a systematic review and meta-analysis. *J Clin Oncol.* 2019;37(31):2899–915.

67. Burm R, Thewes B, Rodwell L, et al. Long-term efficacy and cost-effectiveness of blended cognitive behavior therapy for high fear of recurrence in breast, prostate and colorectal Cancer survivors: follow-up of the SWORD randomized controlled trial. *BMC Cancer.* 2019;19(1):1–13.

68. Shih STF, Butow P, Bowe SJ, et al. Cost-effectiveness of an intervention to reduce fear of cancer recurrence: the ConquerFear randomized controlled trial. *Psychooncology.* 2019;28(5):1071–9.

69. van Helmondt SJ, van der Lee ML, van Woezik RAM, et al. No effect of CBT-based online self-help training to reduce fear of cancer recurrence: first results of the CAREST multicenter randomized controlled trial. *Psychooncology*. 2020;29(1):86–97.
70. Smith AB, Bamgboje-Ayodele A, Butow P, et al. Development and usability evaluation of an online self-management intervention for fear of cancer recurrence (iConquerFear). *Psychooncology*. 2020;29(1): 98–106.
71. Shields CG, Ziner KW, Bourff SA, et al. An intervention to improve communication between breast cancer survivors and their physicians. *J Psychosoc Oncol*. 2010;28(6):610–29.
72. Cox A, Bull E, Cockle-Hearne J, et al. Nurse led telephone follow up in ovarian cancer: a psychosocial perspective. *Eur J Oncol Nurs*. 2008;12(5):412–7.
73. Berrett-Abebe J, Cadet T, Nekhlyudov L, et al. Impact of an interprofessional primary care training on fear of cancer recurrence on clinicians' knowledge, self-efficacy, anticipated practice behaviors, and attitudes toward survivorship care. *J Cancer Educ*. 2018;34:505–11.
74. Davidson J, Malloch M, Humphris G. A single-session intervention (the Mini-AFTERc) for fear of cancer recurrence: a feasibility study. *Psychooncology*. 2018;27(11):2668–70.
75. Liu J, Bui KT, Serafimovska A, et al. CIFeR: a novel clinician-lead Intervention to address Fear of cancer Recurrence (FCR) in breast cancer survivors. *JCP Oncol Pract* 2021:OP2000799. doi:10.1200/OP.20.00799.
76. Butow P, Sharpe L, Thewes B, et al. Fear of cancer recurrence: a practical guide for clinicians. *Oncologist*. 2018; 32(1):32–8.

Personalized Symptom Management for Cancer Survivorship

7

Doris Howell, Martin Chasen, and
Anish Singh Jammu

INTRODUCTION

Worldwide the number of cancer survivors, defined as people with cancer during active treatment (early survivorship) or after treatment (post-treatment survivorship), is growing due to earlier detection, better treatments, and population aging (1). This has led to an unprecedented number of individuals living with the long term and late effects of cancer as a chronic illness (2). In 2018, there were approximately 43.8 million survivors diagnosed within the previous 5 years; and 7.8 million lived with disability (3). While many cancer survivors recover their health within 6–12 months after treatment (4), many continue to experience ongoing medical, mental, and social health challenges and significant symptom burden that disrupts functioning in daily life and negatively impacts on quality of life (QOL) (5). USA population-based data shows adult cancer survivors have poor physical and mental health compared to those without cancer (Figure 7.1) (3) and worse QOL. Worse QOL is directly associated with symptom burden (6). Adult survivors of childhood cancer experience similar long term and late effects, psychological morbidity, and less than optimal QOL (7).

During early survivorship patients experience a range of adverse treatment effects that can persist as long-term symptoms, including bone loss, hearing loss, musculoskeletal issues (myalgias and arthralgias), cognitive impairment, altered bladder, bowel and sexual functioning; and comorbidities arising from late effects (i.e., metabolic syndrome, cardiovascular disease, impaired endocrine, pulmonary and neurological effects, subsequent cancers, etc.) that can be disabling (8). Other issues such as premature menopause and loss of fertility, and body image concerns can add to distress and further restricts the individual's ability to live a normal life. Chronic physical symptoms (lasting 6 months or more) including fatigue, neuropathic pain, and insomnia are common across breast, colorectal, and prostate cancers (9). Many of these symptoms interact as symptom clusters (i.e., fatigue, insomnia, depression) likely due to shared biological mechanisms adding to burden and the complexity of symptom management (10). In addition to

DOI: 10.1201/9781003055426-7

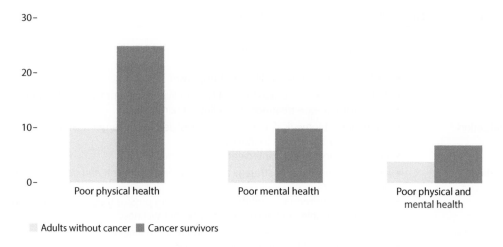

FIGURE 7.1 Health-related quality of life in survivors compared to adults without cancer. (From Lebel S, Ozakinci G, Humphris G, Mutsaers B, Thewes B, Prins J, et al. From normal response to clinical problem: definition and clinical features of fear of cancer recurrence. *Support Care Cancer.* 2016;24:3265–3268.)

physical symptoms, survivors may grapple with psychological problems such as depression, anxiety and post-traumatic stress disorder as a long-term problem (11, 12). Fear of cancer recurrence or progression, a specific type of anxiety, also can occur both before and after treatment (13). Long term physical and emotional symptoms can disrupt functioning in daily life, occupational or career goals (i.e., return to work or work productivity), marital and family relationships, and lead to financial distress (14). Children may also experience emotional and behavioral problems in response to cancer in a parent that can disrupt family functioning (15). Of particular concern, the complexity of cancer and problems such as depression and multimorbidity can impair participation in self-management of symptoms and healthy behaviors, which is associated with worse mortality (16, 17).

Given the wide range of survivorship issues and the inter-individual and personal factors that contribute to variability in illness and symptom burden, a personalized symptom management approach is paramount. Inter-individual variability in type and intensity of symptoms is dependent on complex genomic and bio-behavioral pathways that contribute to symptoms and their persistence, histopathology, pathophysiological pathways, type of cancer (i.e., dysphagia and trismus in head and neck cancer), disease stage, treatment type and modality (systemic chemotherapy, immunotherapy, radiotherapy or combined) and whether treatment is ongoing (hormonal therapy, oral cancer therapies), or a combination of these factors (8, 18, 19). Personal factors also contribute to individual variability in symptom burden including age (younger), sex/gender (female sex), where a person lives (rural or urban), social support (i.e., isolation), and other social determinants of health (i.e., culture/ethnicity/race, marginalization, education, health literacy, economic) (20). Thus, personalized symptom management must consider the "whole" person experience of living with symptoms and cancer as a chronic disease, which is what individuals want and desire when they are ill (21).

In this chapter, we focus on personalized symptom management in cancer survivorship from the lens of personalized cancer medicine known as the 4Ps (predictive, personalized, preventive, and participatory) (22) and now labeled the 5Ps to include the psycho-cognitive aspect of an individual's response to illness (23) (Table 7.1). We emphasize the role of patient-reported outcomes and digital technology for enabling *personalized, predictive, and preventive* symptom care; and the *participatory* component that focuses on survivor activation in self-management of symptoms and health that is critical for mitigating symptom morbidity and optimizing QOL.

TABLE 7.1   Components of P5's personalized cancer medicine

Prediction	• Detect the risk for disease development • Determine disease progression • Recognize prodromal signs • Understand individual likelihood of response
Prevention	• Reduce likelihood of disease/disability by individualizing preventive measures • Move from disease treatment to wellness maintenance
Personalization	• Use genetic, biomedical, environment, lifestyle data to target health care delivery, and treatments to individuals • Tailor each decision and intervention to the individual
Participation	• Involve the individual in strategy aimed to predict, prevent, and personalize the process of care • Increase the individual's confidence to shift from passive receiver of care to an active, responsible, and aware driver of his/her wellness
Psycho-cognitive	• How individuals act to prevent, cope, and react to illness • Decisions about different therapeutic options • How to interact with health care providers and adhere to treatment

PERSONALIZATION OF CARE USING PATIENT REPORTED OUTCOME DATA

Patient-generated health data (PGHD) are health-related data created, recorded, or gathered by or from patients (or family members) to help address a health concern (24). PGHD data is derived from health histories, biometric data (i.e., fit-bit, telehealth monitoring devices), symptoms, lifestyle behaviors (smoking, physical activity, diet, and nutrition), and other data (i.e., environmental and personal). Collection of PGHD has been aided through the rapid evolution of digital health technologies (i.e., web-based platforms, apps or wearable devices, patient portals, mobile health devices (m-Health)) for tailoring supportive care and the patients desire to be engaged in managing their own health (25). PGHD including health monitoring devices and patient reported outcomes (PROs) are shifting care towards personalized symptom management as they enable better prediction and prevention of symptoms and coaching to engage survivors in full monitoring of their health.

Herein, we focus specifically on PROs as providing essential information for enabling personalized symptom management. PROs are defined as those outcomes that "matter" to patients (i.e., QOL) that are distinct, but complementary to disease-focused outcomes such as survival and mortality (26); and are now a performance metric in value-based health care (27). PRO is an umbrella term for "any report that comes directly from the patient about a health condition and its treatment" (28). PRO data may focus on specific aspects of disease or treatment such as symptom experience, physical, psychosocial, or existential distress, mental health disorders, overall functioning and sexual functioning, phases of cancer treatment, cancer type specific or generic, and/or multidimensional health-related quality of life (HRQOL) outcomes. For example, a pan Canadian framework for PRO measurement (PROM), labeled the PROMs-Cancer Core, was identified based on a scoping review of the literature and a Delphi stakeholder consensus with patients, clinicians, and health care administrators. This framework has been used to guide development and standardization of PROs monitored and tracked for use in routine care in Canadian cancer systems (Figure 7.2) (29).

PROs are more reflective of underlying health status than physician reports and facilitate discussion of burdensome symptoms and QOL issues and solidify survivors' participation in shared decision-making and treatment planning when used in clinical care (30). PRO data is also critical for ensuring the "voice" of patients/survivors is represented at all levels of health care decision-making (31). PROs can improve

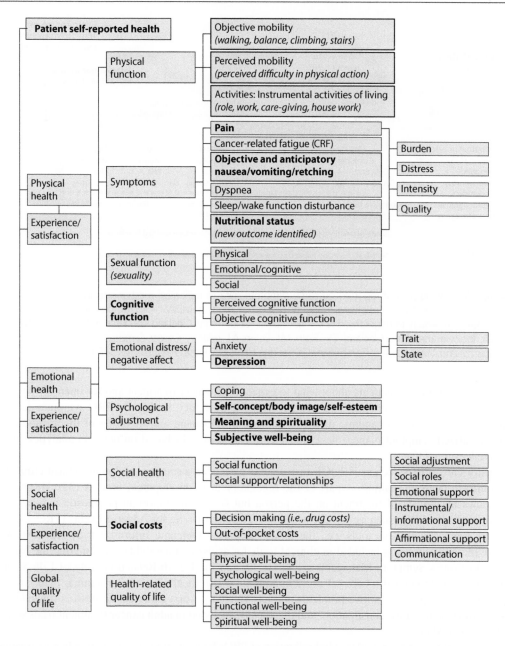

FIGURE 7.2 PROMs cancer core framework. (From Howell D, Fitch M, Bakker D, Green E, Sussman J, Mayo S. et al. Core domains for a person-focused outcome measurement system in cancer (PROMS-Cancer Core) for routine care: a scoping review and Canadian Delphi Consensus. *Value Health.* 2013;16(1):76–87. doi: 10.1016/j. jval.2012.10.017. PMID: 23337218.)

understanding of the "whole" person impact of cancer and treatment for personalizing care, and when used by clinicians can translate into better patient experience and health outcomes (32). Additionally, the integration of "real-time" PRO data with biological and genomic data (Figure 7.3) can improve symptom prediction and knowledge of symptom pathways that can inform testing of therapeutic agents to disrupt these pathways and possibly prevent symptoms (33, 34). Longitudinal symptom tracking of PROs electronically in "real-time" contributes to prediction of the natural evolution of chronicity and related risk factors and the "true" pattern of symptom trajectories between regular clinic visits (35). This data can

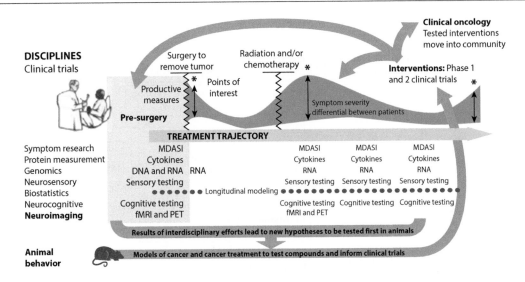

FIGURE 7.3   Linking patient reported outcome symptom data to biological mechanisms in "Real-time." DNA = deoxyribonucleic acid; fMRI = functional magnetic resonance imaging; MDASI = MD Anderson Symptom Inventory; PET = positive emission tomography; RNA = ribonucleic acid. (From Cleeland CS, Fisch MJ, Dunn AJ. Symptom research: looking ahead. In: Cleeland CS, Fisch MJ, Dunn AJ, editors. *Cancer Symptom Science: Measurement, Mechanisms, and Management.* Cambridge: Cambridge University Press; 2011. p. 341–348.)

be used to better inform patients about what to expect with cancer treatment and for intensifying proactive support at critical timepoints along the survivorship trajectory. Linking of PRO symptom data with underlying biological and genomic data can improve development and targeting of therapeutic agents for personalized symptom management; and identification of risks based on big data analytics such as machine learning (36).

Historically, PROs such as HRQOL instruments have been a standard endpoint in most clinical trials to inform decision-making as part of the regulatory drug development process (37). HRQOL not only shows the impact of treatment on the person but is also an important prognostic indicator (38). Symptom specific PROs such as the Chemotherapy Toxicity Criteria for Adverse Events (PRO-CTCAE) (39) and computer adaptive tools, i.e., the Patient Reported Outcome Information System (PROMIS) (40) are increasingly being included in clinical trials for assessing tolerability (41). In 2011, the National Cancer Institute's Symptom Management and Health and the Health-Related Quality of Life Steering Committee, recommended a core set of 12 symptoms – specifically fatigue, insomnia, pain, anorexia (appetite loss), dyspnea, cognitive problems, anxiety (includes worry), nausea, depression (includes sadness), sensory neuropathy, constipation, and diarrhea be included in adult cancer treatment trials where a PRO is measured (42).

Less attention has been paid to standardization of PROs for screening and evaluation in post-treatment cancer survivorship follow-up care or for remote monitoring. However, core symptoms of depression, anxiety, pain, fatigue, cognitive problems, fear of cancer recurrence or progression, physical functioning, financial distress, overall QOL and health status are recommended (43, 44) (Table 7.2). Additionally, core outcome sets have been identified by the International Consortium for Health Outcome Measurement (ICHOM) for breast, lung, prostate, and colorectal cancer for use from diagnosis to treatment completion and long-term survivorship with recommended use of the European Organization for Research and Treatment Consortium-QOL Questionnaire supplemented with cancer or symptom specific modules (connect.ichom.org). An example for breast cancer is shown in Figure 7.4. Other PROs are also important to measure in cancer survivorship include self-efficacy, self-management capacity, empowerment, and adherence to recommended health behaviors, but these are seldom included in PRO information systems for routine monitoring and follow-up. Examples of these measures are shown in Table 7.3.

TABLE 7.2   Recommended core patient reported outcomes for survivorship

EARLY SURVIVORSHIP-DURING ACUTE TREATMENT	POST-TREATMENT AND LONG-TERM SYMPTOMS
Health-related QOL	Health-related QOL
Fatigue	Fatigue
Insomnia	Insomnia
Pain	Pain
Anorexia	Health Behaviors
Nausea	Fear of Recurrence
Depression	Depression
Sensory Neuropathy	Sensory Neuropathy
Constipation	Sexual Function
Diarrhea	Bowel/Bladder Dysfunction
Anxiety	Anxiety
Cognitive Problems	Cognitive Problems
Performance Status	Health Status
	Physical Functioning and Disability
	Financial Distress

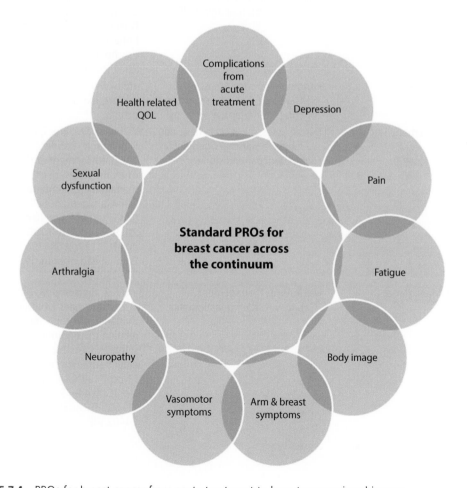

FIGURE 7.4   PROs for breast cancer from acute treatment to long-term survivorship care.

TABLE 7.3   Example of PROs for measuring self-management capacity, self-efficacy, and empowerment

PRO MEASURES	DESCRIPTION	SOURCE
Self-Efficacy for Managing Chronic Disease Scale (6-item scale) (SECDS)	Respondents rate their confidence to perform six self-management behaviors (1 = "not at all confident" to 10 = "totally confident"). A mean score is calculated (range 1 to 10).	Stanford Patient Education Research Center. Self-efficacy for managing chronic disease 6-item scale. 2013. http://www.selfmanagementresource.com/resources/evaluation-tools/english-evaluation-tools
Cancer Survivors Self-Efficacy Scale	Same items as the SECDS; added 5 additional items specific to survivor self-management behaviors.	Foster C, Breckons M, Hankins M, Fenlon D, Cotterell P. Developing a scale to measure self-efficacy to self-manage problems following cancer treatment. sychooncology. 2013;22(S1):16.
Cancer Behavior Inventory-Brief (CBI-B)	14 items measure level of confidence for maintaining independence and positive attitude; participating in medical care; coping and stress management; managing affect.	Heitzmann CA, Merluzzi TV, Jean-Pierre P, Roscoe JA, Kirsh KL, Passik SD. Assessing self-efficacy for coping with cancer: development and psychometric analysis of the brief version of the Cancer behavior inventory (CBI-B). Psychooncology. 2011;20:302–12.
Symptom Management Self-Efficacy	Range of Tools for Measuring Self-Efficacy: PROMIS short forms or computer adaptive versions	https://www.healthmeasures.net/explore-measurement-systems/promis
The Self-Management Self-Test (SMST).	5-item assessment scale designed to measure self-management competence in individuals	Wehmeier PM, Fox T, Doerr JM, Schnierer N, Bender M, Nater UM. Development and validation of a brief measure of self-management competence: The Self-Management Self-Test (SMST). Ther Innov Regul Sci. 2019 Jul 14:2168479019849879. doi: 10.1177/2168479019849879. Epub ahead of print. PMID: 31303020.
Medication Management Capacity	Medication Management Capacity (MMC) questionnaire	Sino CG, Sietzema M, Egberts TC, Schuurmans MJ. Medication management capacity in relation to cognition and self-management skills in older people on polypharmacy. J Nutr Health Aging. 2014 Jan;18(1):44–49. doi: 10.1007/s12603-013-0359-2. PMID: 24402388.

TABLE 7.3 (*Continued*)   Example of PROs for measuring self-management capacity, self-efficacy, and empowerment

PRO MEASURES	DESCRIPTION	SOURCE
Healthy Lifestyle and Self-Management Behaviors	Self-Management of Chronic Conditions (PRISM-CC), an inventory for assessment of self-management behaviors in chronic diseases. Usually measured based on American Cancer Society Guidelines as an assessment of behaviors.	Packer T, Kephart G, Audulv Å, et al. Protocol for development, calibration and validation of the Patient-Reported Inventory of Self-Management of Chronic Conditions (PRISM-CC). BMJ Open 2020;10:e036776. doi: 10.1136/bmjopen-2020-036776. Example: Physical activity measured using the following variables: (1) the frequency of moderate and vigorous physical activity (per week) and (2) the duration (in minutes) of each physical activity reported. Smoking; self-report of current smoking status (current smoker, former smoker, or lifelong abstainer). Alcohol behavior is self-reported as lifetime abstainer (<12 drinks in lifetime) with identification of number of drinks per week (limit is one/week for females; 2 per week for males)
Cancer Patient Empowerment Questionnaire (CPEQ)	CPEQ is 67 items, measuring 3 dimensions of empowerment: (A1) empowerment outcomes consisting of three components: (A1) the intrapersonal-, (A2) interactional-, and (A3) behavioral component, (B) empowerment facilitators (enablement), and (C) the value of empowerment.	Eskildsen NB, Ross L, Bulsara C. et al. Development and content validation of a questionnaire measuring patient empowerment in cancer follow-up. Qual Life Res 2020;29:2253–2274. https://doi.org/10.1007/s11136-020-02483-9.
Health Education Impact Questionnaire (heiQ)	Measures social integration and support, health service navigation, constructive attitudes and approaches, skill and technique acquisition, and emotional distress.	Maunsell E, Lauzier S, Brunet J, Pelletier S, Osborne R, Campbell H. Health-related empowerment in cancer: validity of scales from the Health Education Impact Questionnaire. Cancer 2014;120.
Patient Activation Measure (PAM)-Brief	13 item measure of knowledge, skills and confidence in managing chronic disease across four levels of activation (low to high).	Hibbard JH, Stockard J, Mahoney ER, Tusler M. Development of the Patient Activation Measure (PAM): conceptualizing and measuring activation in patients and consumers. Health Serv Res. 2004;39(4 Pt 1):1005–1026. doi: 10.1111/j.1475-6773.2004.00269.

IMPLEMENTATION OF PROS CAN LEAD
TO IMPROVED HEALTH OUTCOMES

Systematic reviews and meta-analysis have shown that electronic PRO data collection is acceptable to patients and clinicians, enables early identification of emotional distress and mental health problems, i.e., depression, improves patient and clinician communication about symptoms and QOL, improves clinician prescribing for symptom management, and reduces intensity and interference of symptoms (45–47). PRO data is highly valued by health care providers in clinical practice and for opening a dialogue about QOL issues and for addressing sensitive topics such as sexual functioning in prostate cancer survivors (48). However, implementation of PROs in "real-world" cancer settings has lagged uptake in clinical trials (49). Ontario cancer programs (n = 14) with over a decade of experience in implementing PROs for physical and emotional symptom screening in routine care and as a performance metric (50) have shown positive effects using Ontario population-based data on reducing emergency department visits in early stage breast and mixed cancer populations exposed to PROs (51, 52). Additionally, a survival advantage was shown in advanced cancer populations compared to matched controls using Ontario population-based data (53). Barbera and colleagues (53), observed that the probability of survival within the first year was higher among those exposed to routine screening and longitudinal reporting with the Edmonton Symptom Assessment System (ESAS) compared to those who were not (81.9% vs. 76.4% at 1 year, 68.3% vs. 66.1% at 3 years, 61.9% vs. 61.4% at 5 years, P-value < 0.0001); and was associated with a decreased mortality risk (HR: 0.48, 95% CI: 0.47–0.49).

Measurement of PROs alone will not improve health outcomes unless clinicians act on the data. Evidence-based implementation strategies alongside targeted training of clinicians in how to interpret and use PROs for personalized symptom management, champions to facilitate practice change, leadership support, and performance accountability are essential for uptake of PROs in "everyday" care (54). The use of these implementation strategies in a multi-site quality improvement collaborative that also focused on training clinicians in use of PROs for personalized symptom management in Ontario and Quebec showed "real-world" impact of PROs for reducing health care utilization, emotional distress, and improving levels of patient activation (55, 56). Our person-centered care process for integration of PROs in the clinical encounter that emphasizes tailoring of symptom management to PRO symptom reports; and participatory communication by clinicians to foster engagement of patients in symptom self-management is depicted in Figure 7.5. The term PRO-cision has been coined for an approach that uses PRO data for personalization in routine care with a number of steps identified as key to implementation such as early engagement of clinicians in selecting PROs, targeted training of clinicians, and easily interpretable PRO data displays (57).

In our implementation study testing PRO implementation in "real-world" cancer settings we identified a number of strategies necessary for facilitating PRO implementation (55). Key strategies were recently summarized and endorsed in a pan-Canadian consensus meeting by clinicians, patients/families and other key stakeholders (58). The top five key strategies are summarized in Table 7.4. As noted, clear pathways for personalizing symptom care linking evidence-based recommendations from guidelines to PRO scores is essential for a quality response as depicted in Figure 7.6. Thus, we linked best practice interventions to ESAS symptom cut-off scores of mild (1–3), moderate (4–6), severe (7–10), and care pathways to inform patient management (Figure 7.7a, b) (59). The PRO-based pathways for fatigue, insomnia, and emotional distress (anxiety, depression) management are disseminated by the Canadian Association of Psychosocial Oncology (www.capo.ca), the International Psychosocial Oncology Society (www.ipos.ca) and adapted for use by the American Society of Clinical Oncology (ASCO) (60) and for remote telephone triage protocols for symptoms in Canadian cancer care (61).

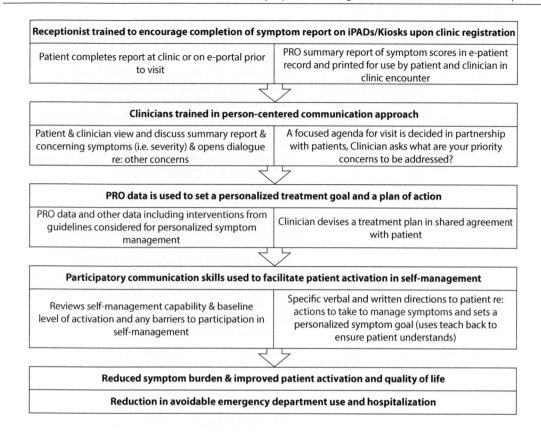

FIGURE 7.5   Care process for a personalized response to PRO data in routine care.

PERSONALIZING SYMPTOM MANAGEMENT IN CANCER SURVIVORSHIP CARE

Given the beneficial effects of PRO data during routine cancer treatment there are important benefits of PROs for identification of problems as part of screening and/or evaluating the effects of clinical interventions (i.e., rehabilitation) on outcomes in cancer survivorship. However, the evidence of benefits is less clear in post-treatment survivor populations and implementation more challenging due to infrequent monitoring and variability in models of survivorship FU care. A scoping review in survivorship care identified only four studies of routine use of PROs in breast cancer survivors for distress screening (62).

A practical example of PROs for personalized symptom management can be observed at the William Osler Health System Cancer Survivorship Clinic (WOHS-CSC) in Ontario led by Dr. Martin Chasen. Unmet needs of cancer survivors increase along the cancer treatment trajectory, thus, best practices in survivorship care requires "effective and timely identification of the needs of cancer survivors, integration of interdisciplinary care planning, coordination with community resources, and more efficient communication between health care providers" (63).

The WOHS-CSC serves a diverse patient population in Brampton, Ontario. Based on 2016 census data from Statistics Canada, 73.3% of the population identify as a member of a visible minority group including, but not limited to, South Asian, Black, Filipino, Latin American, and Chinese (64). The local

TABLE 7.4　Five key strategies for implementation of PRO data for personalization and tailoring of care

Select Relevant PROs	• Engage clinicians/patients/survivors in selecting valid/reliable PROs that are meaningful (generic or condition specific or combination) and considers health literacy and diversity (language, race/ethnicity/culture). • Electronic completion at critical time points across the trajectory and use a display of scores that facilitate interpretation and scores needing attention. • PROs (short) for screening for cases and augment with multidimensional measures for efficiency in assessment and evaluation of treatment impact.
Integrate PROs in clinical work flow	• Ensure completion and integration of PROs in electronic health record and print to ensure use in clinical encounter unless computer access in clinics. • Map clinical care processes and identify who will respond to PRO scores (i.e., nurse counsels on fatigue scores) and automate referral for "red-flags." • Integrate PROs into portals for completion prior to/or between visits-assign who will respond between visits (i.e., telephone triage nurse). • Use effective implementation strategies, i.e., peer champions to foster uptake.
Educational outreach	• Train clinicians in interpretation of PRO scores and use in personalizing care and addressing "what matters most" in goals for visit and care. • Educate patients/survivors in how to interpret PRO scores and their use in symptom monitoring/evaluating the effect of self-management strategies; and how to use in communicating with clinical team and treatment change. • Include education as part of all new staff orientation programs and communicate importance to patients as part of care mandate.
Align PRO scores to care pathways	• Link PRO scores to evidence-based interventions to ensure a quality response. PROs to select goals for symptom management (i.e., reduction that makes a difference in functioning). • Align patient education resources to PROs being monitored and self-management actions to be taken. • Link PRO scores to genomic and biological data to enable future risk prediction in models of survivorship care.
Establish accountability for PROs use	• Set targets for PROs completion as a performance metric for cancer programs. • Use PRO data in audit and feedback and multidisciplinary team rounds. • Establish indicators for PRO performance and include in quality improvement programs. • Administrative leaders and program heads assume governance for the PROs program and integrate within digital strategy.

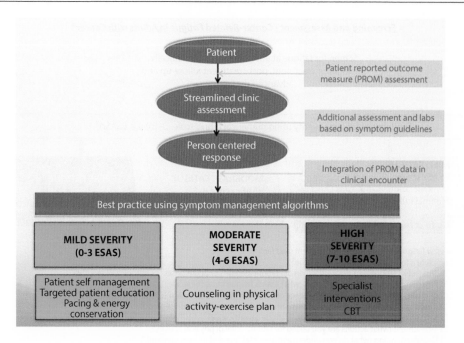

FIGURE 7.6   Framework for a quality clinician response to patient reported outcomes.

community served by WOHS is diverse in terms of languages spoken, religion, and socioeconomic status (65). All patients from the WOHS Oncology Department are eligible to be referred to the Survivorship Clinic by their oncologists.

At the WOHS CSC, survivorship care needs are assessed through PROs at referral. During this initial interview, survivors are introduced to the processes & functions of the clinic and also complete their survivorship care plan details and PROs using ESAS (66), the Distress Thermometer (DT) (67), and the Canadian Problem Checklist (CPC) (68). PRO scores are examined, and areas of concern or improvement are discussed with the multidisciplinary team to personalize and tailor psychological, social, informational, emotional, and/or practical support to the distinct needs of each survivor across socioeconomic strata.

A study of the impact of the WOHS CSC, published in 2019, demonstrates the outcome of PRO utilization for personalized symptom management in a real-world cancer survivorship context (69). Statistical analysis of ESAS and DT scores was conducted to determine effectiveness of the clinic approach on patient-reported symptoms and distress over time. From the baseline to follow-up visit, a statistically significant decline in symptom scores was observed for seven of the 9 ESAS symptoms (pain, tiredness, nausea, depression, anxiety, drowsiness, appetite, well-being, and shortness of breath) (Figure 7.8). In clinical terms, the statistically significant decline for specific symptoms can be attributed to personalized symptom management with tailoring of symptom and supportive care to the individual in routine FU visits based on PRO and other assessment data. The DT provides clinic patients with the opportunity to quantify their distress and highlight causes from the adjoining problem checklist. While a statistically significant decline in distress was observed among the overall study population from the baseline to follow-up visit, an extremely significant decline in distress was noted among high risk patients with a baseline DT $\geq$4 (Figure 7.9). The observed decline in distress may be attributed to the active intervention of the clinic to address the individually identified causes of distress; and was independent of the total number of visits individual patients made to the clinic. Specifically, the greater decline in distress among the high-distress population may be associated with consistent, proactive referral to psychosocial specialists and other resources (i.e., peer support) as part of care tailoring. The

Screening and Assessment - Cancer-Related Fatigue in Adults with Cancer*

Screen for fatigue at entry to system, periodically throughout treatment, post-treatment follow-up and advanced disease[1]

Tiredness of fatigue severity using numerical rating scale (0-10) (i.e. ESASr)[2]

MILD FATIGUE
ESASr score 1-3
Minimal fatigue symptoms
Minimal interference in self care, daily activity, work
Go to care pathway 1

MODERATE FATIGUE
ESASr score 4-6
Go to care pathway 2

SEVERE FATIGUE
ESASr score 7-10
Go to pathway 3

☐ Review fatigue severity scores with patient (and family)
☐ Complete a focused assessment of fatigue
    ☐ O-onset of fatigue and duration (when did fatigue begin) ○ acute onset ○ chronic (>3 months)
    ☐ P-perpetuating or provoking factors (what makes fatigue better or worse?)
    ☐ Q-quality of fatigue (describe experience of fatigue in own words; how distressing is fatigue)
    ☐ R-referral or radiation (other symptoms with fatigue? i.e. sleep, depressed mood)
    ☐ S-severity of fatigue (use of quantitative fatigue severity scale)
    ☐ T-treatment (what actions are you taking for fatigue, level of physical activity?)
    ☐ U-understanding (what do you understand about fatigue and its management?)
    ☐ I-interference (How is fatigue affecting your activities of daily living? [work, social life, concentration, memory, mood, physical activity levels)
    ☐ V-value (what is your goal/expectations for this symptom?)

Complete a comprehensive assessment of fatigue (laboratory tests and physical exam)

    ☐ Treatment complications ○ anemia ○ infection ○ fever
    ☐ Nutritional deficiencies (caloric intake, weight loss/gain)
    ☐ Fluid and electrolyte imbalances [sodium, calcium potassium, magnesium]
    ☐ Medications ○ opioids ○ antihistamines ○ antidepressants ○ alcohol/recreational drug use
    ☐ Comorbid conditions (cardiac, pulmonary, metabolic, endocrine, hepatic or renal insufficiency)
    ☐ Other symptoms/side-effects ○ pain (see ESASr score - ≥ 4 see pain guidelines)
                       ○ depression (see ESASr score - ≥ 4 see depression guidelines)
                       ○ anxiety (see ESASr score - ≥ 4 see anxiety guidelines)
                       ○ sleep disturbances (see ESASr score - ≥ 4 see sleep guidelines)
    ☐ Activity level changes ○ decreased physical activity ○ decreased exercise pattern

Conduct physical exam
    ☐ Gait   ☐ Posture   ☐ Range of motion
    ☐ Eyes (conjunctival pallor if anemic)
    ☐ Oral assessment   ○ cheliosis ○ angular chelitis ○ angular stomatitis
    ☐ Muscle wasting
    ☐ Tachycardia   ☐ Shortness of breath ○ at rest ○ on exertion
    ☐ *****Typical symptoms of fatigue:** tiredness, disproportionate to recent activity; impairment of ADLs/disturbance in quality of life; diminished concentration or attention; significant distress or negative mood to feeling fatigued (e.g., sad, frustrated, irritable); sleep disturbance (insomnia or hypersomnia); sleep perceived as non-restorative; decreased motivation or interest in usual activities.

FIGURE 7.7   (a) Algorithms linking PRO symptom severity scores to clinical assessment. (b) Linking PRO scores to care pathways for evidence-based interventions.

WOHS Cancer Survivorship Clinic demonstrates the "real-world" impact of PRO utilization in personalizing symptom management as part of routine survivorship care.

Survivors receiving care through the WOHS-CSC are transitioned to the care of their family physician when their survivorship care needs are deemed manageable in consultation with the patient and their family. The WOHS-CSC actively coordinates education sessions and provides detailed follow-up schedules for discharged survivors, in order to support family physicians in providing appropriate care. While

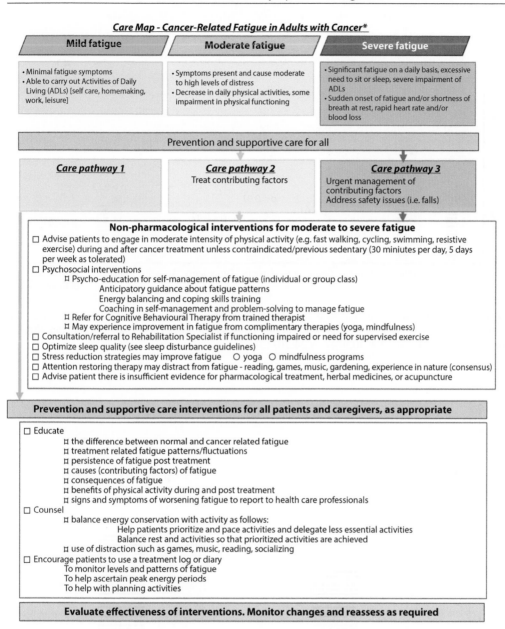

Care Map - Cancer-Related Fatigue in Adults with Cancer*

Mild fatigue	Moderate fatigue	Severe fatigue
• Minimal fatigue symptoms • Able to carry out Activities of Daily Living (ADLs) [self care, homemaking, work, leisure]	• Symptoms present and cause moderate to high levels of distress • Decrease in daily physical activities, some impairment in physical functioning	• Significant fatigue on a daily basis, excessive need to sit or sleep, severe impairment of ADLs • Sudden onset of fatigue and/or shortness of breath at rest, rapid heart rate and/or blood loss

Prevention and supportive care for all

Care pathway 1	*Care pathway 2* Treat contributing factors	*Care pathway 3* Urgent management of contributing factors Address safety issues (i.e. falls)

Non-pharmacological interventions for moderate to severe fatigue

☐ Advise patients to engage in moderate intensity of physical activity (e.g. fast walking, cycling, swimming, resistive exercise) during and after cancer treatment unless contraindicated/previous sedentary (30 miniutes per day, 5 days per week as tolerated)
☐ Psychosocial interventions
　　⊠ Psycho-education for self-management of fatigue (individual or group class)
　　　Anticipatory guidance about fatigue patterns
　　　Energy balancing and coping skills training
　　　Coaching in self-management and problem-solving to manage fatigue
　　⊠ Refer for Cognitive Behavioural Therapy from trained therapist
　　⊠ May experience improvement in fatigue from complimentary therapies (yoga, mindfulness)
☐ Consultation/referral to Rehabilitation Specialist if functioning impaired or need for supervised exercise
☐ Optimize sleep quality (see sleep disturbance guidelines)
☐ Stress reduction strategies may improve fatigue　○ yoga　○ mindfulness programs
☐ Attention restoring therapy may distract from fatigue - reading, games, music, gardening, experience in nature (consensus)
☐ Advise patient there is insufficient evidence for pharmacological treatment, herbal medicines, or acupuncture

Prevention and supportive care interventions for all patients and caregivers, as appropriate

☐ Educate
　　⊠ the difference between normal and cancer related fatigue
　　⊠ treatment related fatigue patterns/fluctuations
　　⊠ persistence of fatigue post treatment
　　⊠ causes (contributing factors) of fatigue
　　⊠ consequences of fatigue
　　⊠ benefits of physical activity during and post treatment
　　⊠ signs and symptoms of worsening fatigue to report to health care professionals
☐ Counsel
　　⊠ balance energy conservation with activity as follows:
　　　　Help patients prioritize and pace activities and delegate less essential activities
　　　　Balance rest and activities so that prioritized activities are achieved
　　⊠ use of distraction such as games, music, reading, socializing
☐ Encourage patients to use a treatment log or diary
　　To monitor levels and patterns of fatigue
　　To help ascertain peak energy periods
　　To help with planning activities

Evaluate effectiveness of interventions. Monitor changes and reassess as required

FIGURE 7.7 *(Continued)*

family physicians are encouraged to request return referrals to the clinic for any immediate concerns, patients and their families are also able to access the clinic directly if any additional support or guidance is required. Building personalized follow-up care pathways that include GPs in survivorship care will be essential to address the needs of a burgeoning survivor population; and PRO data linked to other factors will help to identify risk factors to determine the most appropriate provider (70). Cross-sectional surveys show that general practitioners (GPs) value PROs and use them for shared decision making and to direct patient discussions, which may promote continuity between oncologist and GPs in survivorship care, but integration of electronic records across care sectors is needed (71).

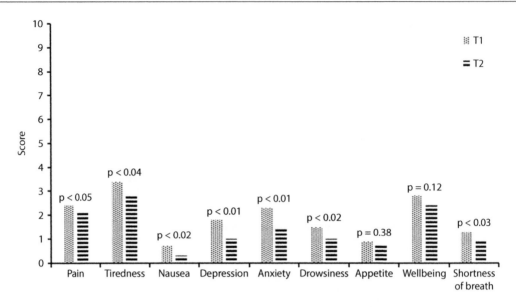

FIGURE 7.8 Mean ESAS scores at baseline (T1) and follow-up visit (T2) (n = 168). (From Chasen M, Hollingshead S, Conter H, Bhargava, R. Quality of life for patients surviving cancer: are we moving ahead?. *Curr Oncol.* 2017;24(3);151–152. doi: 10.3747/co.24.3671.)

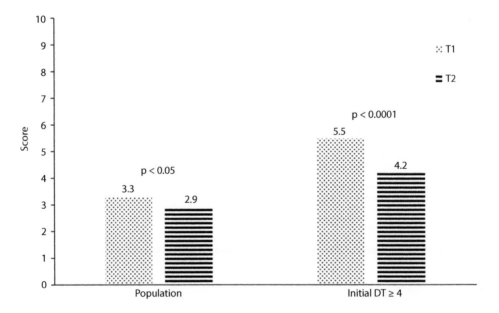

FIGURE 7.9 Mean DT scores for clinic population (n = 176) and those with initial DT ≥ 4 (n = 74): baseline visit (T1) and follow-up visit (T2). (From Jammu A, Chasen M, van Heest R. Hollinshead S, Kaushik D, Gill H, Bhargava R. Effects of a Cancer Survivorship Clinic—preliminary results. *Support Care Cancer.* 2020;28;2381–2388. doi: 10.1007/s00520-019-05067-7.)

Personalized Survivorship Care Plans

Personalizing symptom management in survivorship care can also be facilitated through the use of electronic survivorship care plans (e-SCP). Our team at the Princess Margaret Cancer Centre, Toronto, Canada developed an e-SCP that pulled data from synoptic disease and treatment summaries and other sources in

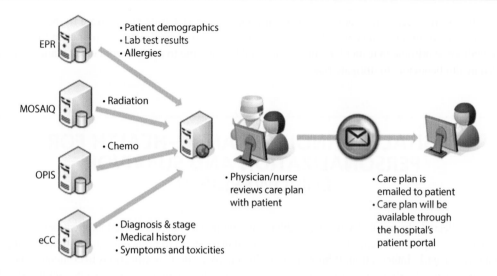

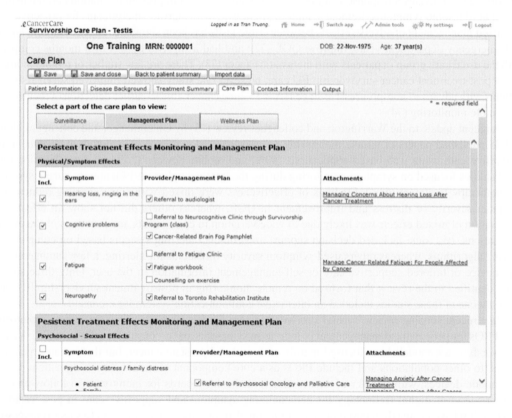

FIGURE 7.10 Electronic survivorship care plan personalized to expected persistent symptoms: (a) algorithm; (b) programmed planning.

the electronic health record to automate population of the e-SCP (Figure 7.10). A personalized symptom report was summarized in the e-SCP based on type of cancer, and treatment received (e.g., ototoxicity with platinum-based regimes). Oncologists checked and signed-off on the pre-populated e-SCP and specifically checked the surveillance regimes to ensure accuracy and personalization to the individual's risks of disease recurrence (i.e., advanced stage testicular cancer). Clinic nurses were trained to provide personalized counseling of survivors for managing persistent post-treatment symptoms and late effects (i.e., metabolic syndrome in testicular cancer) that could occur, and to provide guidance regarding recommended health behaviors to mitigate risks.

DIGITAL TECHNOLOGY AND E-HEALTH FOR PERSONALIZATION AND SURVIVOR EMPOWERMENT

PRO data collected electronically through tablets, mobile phones, or web-based applications for remote monitoring can shift cancer care from reactive (acute management) to proactive care to reduce symptom burden through early intervention. Remote monitoring enables "alert" notifications to clinicians via alerting systems when adverse events or symptoms are clinically significant (i.e., exceed a pre-set threshold of severity). This activates a response from the clinical team designed to prevent escalation and intensification of burdensome symptoms. Remote symptom monitoring with alerting of clinicians for proactive, personalized management of adverse effects between clinic visits has been shown to reduce symptom burden and emergency department visits, improve QOL (72); and had a survival benefit of 5 months compared with the usual care group in patients with metastatic cancer (73). There are few studies of remote monitoring in post-treatment cancer survivorship FU care, however one study showed improved survival among patients with advanced non-progressive stage IIA to IV lung cancer, due to earlier detection of recurrences via remote monitoring (74).

A recent update to the Warrington and colleagues review (75) by Oldenmenger and colleagues identified 35 published papers of remote monitoring for personalization of cancer symptom management and supportive care using web-based applications (40%) and mobile devices (26%) or a combination (76). Most studies focused on symptom monitoring during the treatment phase (91%), mainly during systemic chemotherapy treatment (63%). Findings of effectiveness were mixed with some showing reduction in symptom severity or distress and improvement in QOL, whereas others did not show an effect. The observation of mixed effects was likely due to wide variation in components and functions of the mobile applications, i.e., some included decision support and clinician alerting systems based on complex risk scoring algorithms, whereas others used symptom severity thresholds for alerting, a few automated self-care advice or tailored supportive care or self-management information to the user. Only three studies were identified in the review that focused on remote monitoring in post-treatment survivorship FU care; and only one of these studies included an interactive communication system for e-consult.

In a recent scoping review, virtual survivorship care models were identified for remote monitoring with PROs for personalized management of long-term symptoms and e-consult for follow-up (77). Virtual survivorship care models have focused mainly on breast and prostate cancer, but there is an urgency to expand to other populations and include PROs as a core component of monitoring using patient portals and mobile devices; with transfer of data to electronic health records for monitoring in follow-up care. Other reviews of digital technology for personalizing symptom and supportive care in post-treatment survivorship have primarily focused on dissemination of information and education to support empowerment or engagement of survivors in managing some aspect of long-term symptoms or health (i.e., weight management and/or exercise) (78, 79). Studies for remote monitoring identified by Oldenmenger (76) and in other reviews (77–79) targeting post-treatment cancer survivors are summarized in Table 7.5.

An integrative review of the literature identified the antecedents, attributes and consequences of empowerment that may provide a useful framework for designing future mobile health platforms for cancer survivors (80) (Figure 7.11). Empowerment is an important psychological resource for survivors' effective management of sequelae of cancer and for regaining a sense of control (81).

TABLE 7.5 Digital technology for remote monitoring and virtual follow-up in survivorship

TARGET	FUNCTIONS	PRO	STUDY TYPE/ POPULATION	SIGNIFICANT EFFECTS	REFERENCE
Remote symptom monitoring	Symptom assessment/ education via a web-based platform	Memorial Symptom Assessment Scale (MSAS)	Breast cancer (n = 59). RCT	No effects	Wheelock AE, Bock MA, Martin EL, Hwang J, Ernest ML, Rugo HS, et al. SIS. NET: a randomized controlled trial evaluating a web-based system for symptom management after treatment of breast cancer. Cancer. 2015; 121(6):893–899.
Remote symptom monitoring	Symptom monitoring, education focused on self-management	European Organization for Research and Treatment Consortium (EORTC)	Post-treatment survivors (n = 320) RCT	QOL	Vander Hout A, van Uden-Kraan CF, Holtmaat K, Jansen F, Lissenberg-Witte BI, Nieuwenhuijzen GAP, et al. Role of eHealth application Oncokompas in supporting self-management of symptoms and health-related quality of life in cancer survivors: a randomised, controlled trial. Lancet Oncol. 2020; 21(1):80–94.
Remote pain monitoring	Pain monitoring, education, e-consult and self-management support	Pain Intensity Scale	Country: Netherlands Post-treatment survivors (n = 100) Feasibility, RCT	Symptom reduction	Oldenmenger WH, Baan MAG, Van der Rijt CCD. Feasibility of monitoring patients' cancer-related pain via the internet. 9th Congress of the European Pain Federation EFIC; 2015; Vienna, Austria.
Remote monitoring of symptoms and PSA by clinical nurse specialists	PROMs submitted via a web-platform and prostate specific antigen (PSA)– transferred directly from the lab and monitored by Clinical Nurse Specialists; appointments booked online as needed; alerting of oncologist	Prostate specific measure and PSA	Prostate cancer (n = 627)	Improved survivorship needs, self-management activation, QOL, psychological well-being and satisfaction with care	Frankland, J. et al. Follow-up care after treatment for prostate cancer: evaluation of a supported self-management and remote surveillance programme. BMC Cancer 2019;19;368

(Continued)

TABLE 7.5 (Continued)   Digital technology for remote monitoring and virtual follow-up in survivorship

TARGET	FUNCTIONS	PRO	STUDY TYPE/POPULATION	SIGNIFICANT EFFECTS	REFERENCE
Tele-rehabilitation	Instant messaging and video calls with research staff; 8-week tailored exercise program	Physical activity	Post-treatment breast cancer survivors (n = 81)	Improved global health status, physical and cognitive function, arm symptoms, pain severity/interference	Galiano-Castillo, N. et al. Telehealth system: a randomized controlled trial evaluating the impact of an internet-based exercise intervention on quality of life, pain, muscle strength, and fatigue in breast cancer survivors. Cancer 2016;122:3166-3174
Remote monitoring, self-management education and cognitive behavioral therapy	Web-based system to support self-management and psychological adjustment (cognitive behavioral therapy)	Emotional distress scale online reporting	Breast cancer survivors (n = 150) RCT	Less emotional distress	Berg SW van den, et al. BREATH: web-based self-management for psychological adjustment after primary breast cancer – results of a multicenter randomized controlled trial. JCO 2015; 33(25): 2763-2771.
Remote monitoring and tailored self-management information	Web-based, interactive tailoring of information to needs; online sharing, diaries; e-consult with nurses	Global symptom distress	Leukemia and lymphoma-followed into rehabilitation (n = 145) RCT	Improved symptom distress	Ruland CM, Holte HH, Roislien J, Heaven C, Hamilton GA, Kristiansen J, et al. Effects of a computer-supported interactive tailored patient assessment tool on patient care, symptom distress, and patients' need for symptom management support: a randomized clinical trial. JAMA 2010;17(4):403–410.
Remote monitoring	Mobile phones, Algorithm supporting alerting system; tiered self-management resources	Chemotherapy toxicities	Solid tumor populations (n = 1312) Matched controls	Less urgent care visits	Girgis A, Durcinoska I, Arnold A, Descallar J, Kaadan N, Koh ES, et al. Web-based patient-reported outcome measures for personalized treatment and care (PROMPT-Care): multicenter pragmatic nonrandomized trial. J Med Internet Res. 2020 Oct 29;22(10): e19685. doi: 10.2196/19685. PMID: 33118954; PMCID: PMC7661255.

Virtual follow-up	Video-based medical consultation and with a clinical nurse specialist	Empowerment/ emotional distress scale	Breast cancer (n = 109)	No change in empowerment or distress	Visser A, van Laarhoven HW, Govaert PH, Schlooz MS, Jansen L, van Dalen T, Prins JB. Group medical consultations in the follow-up of breast cancer: a randomized feasibility study. J Cancer Surviv. 2015 Sep;9(3):450–461. doi: 10.1007/s11764-014-0421-z. Epub 2015 Jan 13. PMID: 25579623.
Virtual follow-up	Nurse-led virtual consultation and multidisciplinary team, electronic survivorship care plan	No remote monitoring of symptoms element-measured self-efficacy	Childhood cancer survivors (n = 27) Single arm prospective study	Improved self-efficacy in 6-month follow-up; satisfaction	Signorelli C, Wakefield CE, Johnston KA, Fardell JE, McLoone JK, Brierley ME, et al. Re-Engage: a novel nurse-led program for survivors of childhood cancer who are disengaged from cancer-related care. J Natl Compr Canc Netw. 2020 Aug;18(8):1067–1074. doi: 10.6004/jnccn.2020.7552. PMID: 32755982.

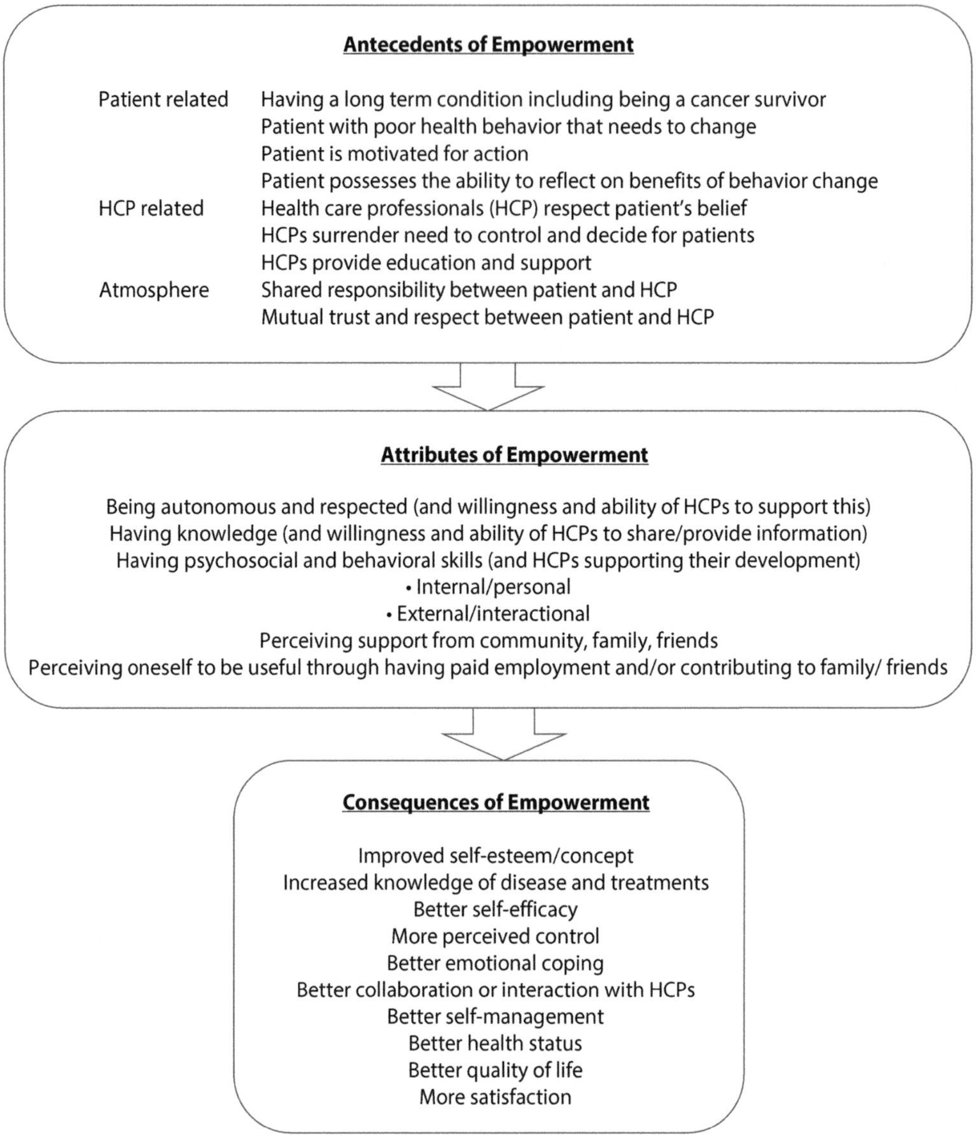

Antecedents of Empowerment

Patient related   Having a long term condition including being a cancer survivor
                    Patient with poor health behavior that needs to change
                    Patient is motivated for action
                    Patient possesses the ability to reflect on benefits of behavior change
HCP related   Health care professionals (HCP) respect patient's belief
                    HCPs surrender need to control and decide for patients
                    HCPs provide education and support
Atmosphere   Shared responsibility between patient and HCP
                    Mutual trust and respect between patient and HCP

Attributes of Empowerment

Being autonomous and respected (and willingness and ability of HCPs to support this)
Having knowledge (and willingness and ability of HCPs to share/provide information)
Having psychosocial and behavioral skills (and HCPs supporting their development)
• Internal/personal
• External/interactional
Perceiving support from community, family, friends
Perceiving oneself to be useful through having paid employment and/or contributing to family/ friends

Consequences of Empowerment

Improved self-esteem/concept
Increased knowledge of disease and treatments
Better self-efficacy
More perceived control
Better emotional coping
Better collaboration or interaction with HCPs
Better self-management
Better health status
Better quality of life
More satisfaction

FIGURE 7.11 Components of cancer survivor empowerment for information technology. (From Groen WG, Kuijpers W, Oldenburg HAS, Wouters MWJM, Aaronson NK, van Harten WH. Empowerment of cancer survivors through information technology: an integrative review. *J Med Internet Res.* 2015;17(11):e270. doi: 10.2196/jmir.4818.)

PERSONALIZATION OF SUPPORT TO ACTIVATE SURVIVORS IN SYMPTOM SELF-MANAGEMENT

The *participation* component of personalized medicine, defined as building the confidence of patients (self-efficacy) and shifting their role from passive recipients of care to active partners, aware and responsible as drivers of optimal health/wellness (23), is essential to personalized symptom management.

Survivors hold responsibility for enacting disease (i.e., adherence to life-long hormonal treatment in breast cancer) and symptom specific self-management (SM) behaviors (i.e., exercise to reduce chronic fatigue) to reduce symptom burden, maintain health, and prevent/mitigate late effect risks (82). Unfortunately, they may experience a long and painful trial-and-error process to identify effective strategies to manage long term symptoms as they seldom receive targeted instruction during or after treatment in SM (83). This can result in poor adherence to health behaviors (84) and makes them potentially vulnerable to worse health and survival.

Defining Self-Management and Self-Management Support

Effective SM is a continuous dynamic process that encompasses the capability to monitor one's condition and to affect the cognitive, behavioral, and emotional responses required to maintain health and a satisfactory QOL (85). This can be challenging given the dynamic nature of cancer and consequently survivors feel vulnerable and may lack confidence (self-efficacy) for initiating the self-management behaviors necessary to recover health after treatment (86). Thus, self-management support (SMS) provided by clinicians is considered essential to enable and empower patients to adjust to living with cancer as a chronic illness. SMS is defined as "the systematic provision of education and supportive interventions by health care staff to increase patients' skills and confidence in managing their health problems, including regular assessment of progress and problems, goal setting, and problem-solving support (87)."

SMS goes beyond typical knowledge-based education to coaching health behavior change and building of the patient's core disease self-management skills and self-efficacy as the key mechanism for promoting effective medical, emotional, and lifestyle management of chronic disease (88) (Figure 7.12). SMS also helps patients in developing, refining, and utilizing core disease management skills (problem-solving, decision-making, utilizing resources, collaborating with health care providers, goal-setting and action planning, and self-tailoring (i.e., adapting SM behaviors to daily life and situational context)) (89).

SMS includes education, involvement of patients in decision-making, coaching adjustment of behaviors and medications in daily life. SMS also facilitates effective application of behaviors to manage symptoms, cope with stress/psychosocial distress (anger, depression, acceptance, anxiety, biographical disruption, fear of recurrence), and lifestyle behaviors (including exercise) to maintain health and mitigate late effect risks (90). A pragmatic behavioral counseling framework for personalizing SMS coaching,

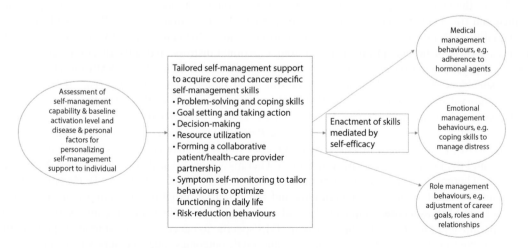

FIGURE 7.12 Process and tasks of self-management mediated by self-efficacy.

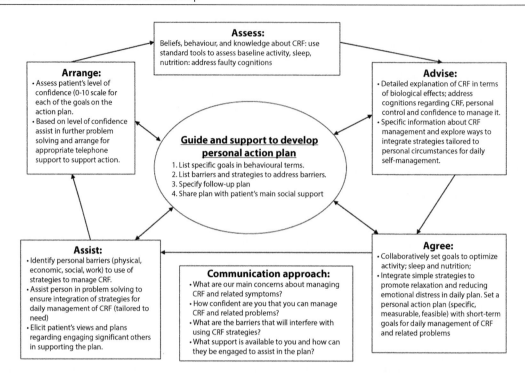

FIGURE 7.13   5As behavior change counseling framework applied to cancer fatigue.

labeled the 5As (assess, advise, agree, assist, and arrange) is recommended (91). An example of the application of this framework for cancer-related fatigue (CRF) is shown in Figure 7.13; and includes assessment of cognitive-perceptions aligned with the psycho-cognitive element of the 5Ps framework since illness and symptom perceptions can influence symptom response and perpetuate persistence of CRF post-treatment (92). The intensity of CRF is essentially reduced by the self-management behaviors that survivors enact, i.e., exercise, energy conservation and pacing, and reframing of cognitions, which are shown to be effective in reducing CRF (93). A 5Ps framework can be integrated within routine clinical practice and helps to systematize the coaching process and can be completed in rapid, episodic ambulatory care visits within about 20–30 minutes.

While the evidence regarding the efficacy of SMS interventions in cancer survivorship is more limited and fragmented in comparison to other chronic diseases, Boland and colleagues identified six high quality SMS intervention studies from an initial yield of 2633 citations with small effect size differences shown for fatigue, physical functioning, emotional distress, and self-efficacy in three studies (exercise, psychosocial interventions) (94). A meta-analysis of Internet-based SMS targeting CRF in cancer survivors also showed reduced fatigue (the Brief Fatigue Index, relative risk$=0.74$, 95% confidence interval (CI; 0.69, 0.79), $P<0.01$; the Cancer Fatigue Scale or the Multidimensional Fatigue Scale, weighted mean difference$=-10.15$, 95% CI (-11.42, -8.89), $P<0.01$; and related symptoms of Anxiety, relative risk$=1.07$, 95% CI (0.55, 2.05), $P<0.01$; Depression scale, relative risk$=0.70$, 95% CI (0.60, 0.81), $P<0.01$; the Pittsburgh Sleep Quality Index, relative risk$=0.46$, 95% CI (0.33, 0.62), $P<0.01$; and the Function Assessment of Cancer Therapy – General scale or the Function Assessment of Cancer Therapy – Breast, weighted mean difference$=13.76$, 95% CI (3.38, 24.14), $P<0.01$.) (95).

Healthy lifestyle behavior interventions and rehabilitation programs targeting cancer survivors that integrate SMS as a core component have also shown positive effects on function, weight loss, and fitness parameters (96, 97). A recent review in SMS specific to cancer survivorship identified 21 studies with mixed-evidence of effect on symptom and QOL outcomes, due to heterogeneity in intervention components (98). Personalizing SMS for effective illness and symptom management requires a comprehensive assessment of the individuals' self-management capability (99). Additionally, tailoring of support is needed to address the multiple factors that can impact on survivors ability to participate in SM (i.e., older or young adults, multi-morbidity, marginalization, other health disparities, sex/gender differences, low health literacy, and cognitive overload and/or impairment, etc.) or just being too ill or overwhelmed (89).

Personalized SMS targeting cancer pain has become a prominent focus for tailoring of information and enablement strategies that support patients in management of pain in daily life (100). This includes motivating patients to take an active role in managing pain, enhancing their self-efficacy to solve problems caused by pain, and incorporating pain-relieving strategies into daily life. Personalized SMS should target the individual's capability (psychological and physical capacity to engage in the activity), motivation (cognitive processes that energize and direct behavior) and opportunity (external factors that make enacting the behavior possible or prompt it) (101). Personalized symptom goals as an outcome of SMS (i.e., goal setting and action planning) may be a relevant target for interventions and evaluating their therapeutic effect as an individualized response criterion (102, 103). For example, patients are asked to describe, on a 0 to 10 scale, the level/intensity of pain that will allow the patient to achieve comfort in physical, functional, and psychosocial domains (103).

Participatory Communication Skills to Promote Survivor Involvement in Care

Participatory and person-centered communication skills are a vital skill for promoting involvement and activation of survivors in self-management of cancer and health. Consequently, both patients/survivors and clinicians require training to achieve documented benefits of improved patient satisfaction, treatment adherence, psychological well-being, provision of information by providers, patient participation in self-management, and clinical outcomes as shown in other chronic diseases (i.e., reduction in hypertension in congestive heart failure and A1C levels in diabetes) (104).

A systematic review of 32 intervention studies focused on training patients in communication skills identified three behavioral categories critical to operationalizing patients' level of engagement or active participation in health care interactions including: (1) information seeking and verifying behaviors (e.g., asking questions), (2) assertive statements (e.g., articulating values, beliefs, treatment preferences), (3) expressing emotions or concerns (105). Although findings of effectiveness were mixed, communication training of patients is a potentially effective tool for promoting patient participation in health care, however, further research is needed to establish effects on health outcomes.

Clinician training in participatory communication skills to promote patient-centered care defined as "respecting and responding to patients' wants, needs and preferences, so that they can make choices in their care that best fit their individual circumstances," was identified as a priority by the National Cancer Institute in 2007 (NCI) (106). The NCI identified six essential functions of person-centered communication including fostering healing relationships, exchange of information, responding to patients' emotions, managing uncertainty, making informed decisions, and enabling patient self-management. A narrative review identified the best practices and skills aligned with the NCI six core functions (107), which was modified based on motivational interviewing communication skills (108) that are also necessary for promoting survivor involvement in self-management and behavior change (Table 7.6).

Patient-centered communication skills are multidimensional and complex and will require use of best practices in promoting clinicians application of these skills in routine care including practice and feedback with standardized patients, videotaping with clinical supervision, and ongoing coaching and mentorship, and infrastructure such as the use of quality indicators for assessment of performance and for quality improvement (e.g., audit and feedback) (104).

Communicating evidence for decision-making is a specific skill and has strong synergies with SMS that are facilitated through a collaborative partnership in which health professionals and survivors work

TABLE 7.6 Person-centered, participatory communication skills for clinicians to promote activation in self-management

FUNCTIONS OF THE MEDICAL INTERVIEW	ROLES AND RESPONSIBILITIES OF THE CLINICIAN	SKILLS
Fostering the relationship	• Establish rapport and connection. • Discuss mutual roles/responsibilities and role of patient as partner. • Express caring and commitment. • Respect patients beliefs and perceptions, privacy and autonomy.	• Engage open communication (e.g., what has this been like for you?). • Use appropriate language. • Use active listening skills (open-ended questions, affirmations, reflections, summarizations) (OARS).
Gathering information	• Assess illness and wellness needs using a holistic, biopsychosocial assessment framework. • Ascertain from the person, needs to be addressed in the clinical visit – prioritize "what matters most." • Identify patients agenda for visit and negotiate areas for patient education.	• Use open-ended questions to explore full effect of illness. • Review PRO data with patient and elicit other concerns and perspective on symptom scores. • Elicit full set of concerns and the patients' perspective of problems and possible solutions (e.g., what do you think can be done?). • Use tools such as Ask-Tell-Ask.
Providing information	• Assess patients informational needs and learning style. • Tailor information to learning style and health literacy, age, cognitive impairment. • Share only necessary information building on current understanding-avoid telling all assumed to "keep patient safe." • Ask permission to share information building on current understanding. • Identify and build on strengths.	• Avoid jargon. • Use simple strategies/tools to ascertain patient learning style. • Provide uncomplicated explanations and instructions. • Encourage questions and check understanding. • Emphasize key messages. • Use strategies such as teach-back (e.g., can you tell me what you understand are the steps you should take to manage _____?
Decision-making	• Prepare person for deliberate involvement in decision-making. • Enable and support patient decision-making that aligns with health values and preferences. • Advise re: specific decision steps for tailoring behaviors based on symptom monitoring (i.e., exercise to avoid exacerbation of severe fatigue).	• Encourage patient participation in decision-making. • Outline choices using lay language. • Explore patient preferences and understanding. • Use evidence-based decision-support tools and resources for support.

TABLE 7.6 (*Continued*)   Person-centered, participatory communication skills for clinicians to promote activation in self-management

FUNCTIONS OF THE MEDICAL INTERVIEW	ROLES AND RESPONSIBILITIES OF THE CLINICIAN	SKILLS
Enabling disease and treatment-related behavior	• Assess patient's capacity for self-management and barriers to active participation in managing health. • Elicit change talk and help patient to focus on priorities for change. • Identify a realistic change goal and actions to take to manage illness. • Arrange for specific support (i.e., exercise or nutrition specialist). • Set a goal/action plan and follow-up.	• Assess patients readiness to change health behaviors-use agenda setting tools to focus. • Recognize change talk and roll with resistance. • Elicit patients goals and realistic actions to manage specific problems or adopt healthy behavior goals. • Brainstorm solutions/ideas for behaviors building on strengths. (i.e., what worked to quit smoking in past).
Responding to emotions	• Facilitate patient expression of emotional consequences of illness (positive emotion-focused coping). • Promote problem-focused coping skills; and strategies to manage uncertainty. • Identify psychological distress and engage specialists to address as necessary.	• Acknowledge (normalize) and explore feelings and concerns. • Express empathy. • Support patients navigation skills to peer and health system support-facilitate connection as needed. • Teach patients problem-solving process.

Source: Modified from Hales King A & Hoppe RB. (Ref. 107); Epstein RM & Street RL. (Ref. 106); Rollnick S, Miller R, Butler CR. (Ref. 108).

together to identify and enact decisions and plans that are jointly agreed on the basis of both medical evidence and what matters most to individuals. Epstein and colleagues proposed a number of additional skills required of clinicians for discussing evidence including: (1) an ability to communicate complex information in simple language and terms, (2) tailoring the amount and pace of information to needs and preferences, using diagrams and other approaches that facilitate comprehension, considering the values of patients while weighing choices, explanation of probability and outcome of each option, evaluation of internet information patients bring with them, fostering an environment conducive to open questioning by patients (i.e., time to question and take in the information), checking patient understanding and negotiation (109). Decision-making specific to self-management also includes preparation and specific instructions to survivors in making daily decisions to adjust and tailor their behaviors based on symptom self-monitoring that can maximize functioning in day-to-day living.

SUMMARY AND FUTURE RESEARCH

Poorly controlled symptoms are a major threat to quality cancer care, avoidable health care utilization, diminished QOL, and survival. Personalized symptom management that addresses elements of precision medicine and the "whole" person impact of cancer and treatment are essential in survivorship care. As noted by Hood, while the starting point for personalized cancer medicine may be genes, individualized health care only becomes possible when clinicians understand and address the "totality" of individuals in the context of the life cycle and the human experience of illness not merely disease (23). PROs use in routine care can enable proactive, preventive, predictive, and personalization of symptom care in cancer survivorship. The participatory component of personalized symptom management requires greater attention since activation of survivors in disease and health management is key to better health outcomes and likely survival. Application of all elements of the precision medicine framework is necessary for personalized symptom management and a more concerted effort is needed to ensure the integration of SMS in routine cancer survivorship care as a core element of precision care.

REFERENCES

1. Miller KD, Nogueira L, Mariotto AB, Rowland JH, Yabroff KR, Alfano CM, Jemal A, Kramer JL, Siegel RL. Cancer treatment and survivorship statistics, 2019. *CA Cancer J Clin.* 2019 Sep;69(5):363–385. doi: 10.3322/caac.21565.
2. Phillips JL, Currow DC. Cancer as a chronic disease. *Collegian.* 2010;17(2):47–50. doi: 10.1016/j.colegn.2010.04.007.
3. Jemal A, Torre L, Soerjomataram I, Bray F, editors. *The Cancer Atlas*, 3rd ed. Atlanta, GA: American Cancer Society, 2019. Available from: http://canceratlas.cancer.org.
4. Bubis LD, Davis L, Mahar A, Barbera L, Li Q, et al. Symptom burden in the first year after cancer diagnosis: an analysis of patient-reported outcomes. *J Clin Oncol.* 2018;36(11):1103–1111. doi: 10.1200/JCO.2017.76.0876.
5. Alfano CM, Rowland JH. Recovery issues in cancer survivorship: a new challenge for supportive care. *Cancer J.* 2006;12:432–443.
6. Huang I-C, Hudson MM, Robison LL, Krull KR. Differential impact of symptom prevalence and chronic conditions on quality of life of cancer survivors and non-cancer individuals: a population study. *Cancer Epidemiol Biomark Prev.* 2017;26(7):1124–1132. doi: 10.1158/1055-9965.
7. Bhakta N, Liu Q, Ness KK, et al. The cumulative burden of surviving childhood cancer: an initial report from the St Jude Lifetime Cohort Study (SJLIFE). *Lancet.* 2017;390:2569–2582.
8. Leach CR, Weaver KE, Aziz NM, Alfano CM, Bellizzi KM, Kent EE, et al. The complex health profile of long-term cancer survivors: prevalence and predictors of comorbid conditions. *J Cancer Surviv.* 2015;9(2):239–251.
9. Gegechkori N, Haines L, Lin JJ. Long term and latent side effects of specific cancer types. *Med Clin North Am.* 2017;101(6):1053–1073.
10. Bjerkeset E, Röhrl K, Schou-Bredal I. Symptom cluster of pain, fatigue, and psychological distress in breast cancer survivors: prevalence and characteristics. *Breast Cancer Res Treat.* 2020;180(1):63–71. doi: 10.1007/s10549-020-05522-8.
11. Niedzwiedz CL, Knifton L, Robb KA, Srinivasa VK, Smith DJ. Depression and anxiety among people living with and beyond cancer: a growing clinical and research priority. *BMC Cancer.* 2019;19:943. doi: 10.1186/s12885-019-6181-4.
12. Götze H, Friedrich M, Taubenheim S. et al. Depression and anxiety in long-term survivors 5 and 10 years after cancer diagnosis. *Support Care Cancer.* 2020;28:211–220. doi: 10.1007/s00520-019-04805-1.
13. Lebel S, Ozakinci G, Humphris G, Mutsaers B, Thewes B, Prins J, et al. From normal response to clinical problem: definition and clinical features of fear of cancer recurrence. *Support Care Cancer.* 2016;24:3265–3268.
14. Carrera PM, Kantarjian HM, Blinder VS. The financial burden and distress of patients with cancer: understanding and stepping-up action on the financial toxicity of cancer treatment. *CA Cancer J Clin.* 2018;68(2):153–165. doi: 10.3322/caac.21443.
15. Thastum M, Watson M, Kienbacher C, et al. Prevalence and predictors of emotional and behavioural functioning of children where a parent has cancer: a multinational study. *Cancer.* 2009;115:4030–4039.
16. Gobeil-Lavoie A, Chouinard M, Danish A, Hudon C. Characteristics of self-management among patients with complex health needs: a thematic analysis review. *BMJ Open.* 2019;9:e028344. doi: 10.1136/bmjopen-2018-028344.
17. Karavasiloglou N, Pestoni G, Wanner M, Faeh D, Rohrmann S. Healthy lifestyle is inversely associated with mortality in cancer survivors: results from the Third National Health and Nutrition Examination Survey (NHANES III). *PLOS ONE.* 2019;14(6):e0218048. doi: 10.1371/journal.pone.0218048.
18. Yeh CT, Wang L-S. Potential pathophysiological mechanism of cancer-related fatigue and current management. *Formos J Surg.* 2014;(47):173–182.
19. Bortolato B, Hyphantis TN, Valpione S, Stubbs B, Pavlidis N, Carvalho AF. Depression in cancer: the many biobehavioural pathways driving tumor progression. *Cancer Treat Rev.* 2016;52:58–70.
20. Alcaraz KI, Wiedt TL, Daniels EC, Yabroff KR, Guerra E, Wender RC. Understanding and addressing social determinants to advance cancer health equity in the United States: a blueprint for practice, research, and policy. *CA Cancer J Clin.* 2020;70:31–46. doi: 10.3322/caac.21586.

21. Cherny NI, de Vries EGE, Emanuel L, Fallowfield L, Francis PA, Gabizon A. Words matter: distinguishing personalized medicine and biologically personalized therapeutics. *JNCI.* 2014;106(12):1–5.

22. Flores M, Glusman G, Brogaard K, Price ND, Hood L. P4 medicine: how systems medicine will transform the healthcare sector and society. *Per Med.* 2013;10(6):565–566. doi: 10.2217/pme.13.57.

23. Gorini A, Pravettoni G. P5 medicine: a plus for a personalized approach to oncology. *Nat Rev Clin Oncol.* 2011; doi: 10.1038/nrclinonc.2010.227.c1.

24. Office of the National Coordinator for Health Information Technology. Consumer eHealth: Patient-Generated Health Data; 2014. http://www.healthit.gov/policy-researchers-implementers/patient-generated-health-data.

25. Nasi G, Cucciniello M, Guerrazzi C. The performance of mHealth in cancer supportive care: a research agenda. *J Med Internet Res.* 2015;17(2):e9. doi: 10.2196/jmir.3764.

26. Squitieri L, Bozic KJ, Pusic AL. The role of patient-reported outcome measures in value-based payment reform. *Value Health.* 2017 Jun;20(6):834–836. doi: 10.1016/j.jval.2017.02.003. Epub 2017 Mar 22. PubMed PMID: 28577702.

27. Lipscomb J, Donaldson MS, Hiatt RA. Cancer outcomes research and the arenas of application. *J Natl Cancer Inst Monogr.* 2004;(33):1–7. doi: 10.1093/jncimonographs/lgh038. PMID: 15504917.

28. FDA. Patient-reported outcome measures: use in medical development to support labeling claims; 2009. www.fda.gov/downloads/Drugs/GuidanceComplianceRegulatoryInformation/Guidances/UCM193282.pdf.

29. Howell D, Fitch M, Bakker D, Green E, Sussman J, Mayo S. et al. Core domains for a person-focused outcome measurement system in cancer (PROMS-Cancer Core) for routine care: a scoping review and Canadian Delphi Consensus. *Value Health.* 2013;16(1):76–87. doi: 10.1016/j.jval.2012.10.017. PMID: 23337218.

30. Xiao C, Polomano R, Bruner DW. Comparison between patient-reported and clinician-observed symptoms in oncology. *Cancer Nurs.* 2013;36:E1.

31. LeBlanc TW, Abernethy AP. Patient-reported outcomes in cancer care-hearing the patient voice at greater volume. *Nat Rev Clin Oncol.* 2017;14(12):763–772.

32. Howell D, Liu G. Can routine collection of patient-reported outcome data actually improve person-centered health? *Healthcare Pap.* 2012;17(4):42–47.

33. Cleeland CS, Fisch MJ, Dunn AJ. Symptom research: looking ahead. In: Cleeland CS, Fisch MJ, Dunn AJ, editors. *Cancer Symptom Science: Measurement, Mechanisms, and Management.* Cambridge: Cambridge University Press; 2011. pp. 341–348.

34. Yeh CT, Wang L-S. Potential pathophysiological mechanisms of cancer-related fatigue and current management. *Formos J Surg.* 2014;(47):173–182.

35. Geisinger JM, Wintner LM, Zabernigg A, Gamper E-M, Oberguggenberger AS, Sztankay MJ, et al. Assessing quality of life on the day of chemotherapy administration underestimates patients' true symptom burden. *BMC Cancer.* 2014;14:758. doi: 10.1186/1471-2407-14-758.

36. Martin LJ, Smith SB, Khoutorsky A, Magnussen CA, Samoshking A, Sorge RE, et al. Epiregulin and EGFR interactions are involved in pain processing. *J Clin Invest.* 2017;127(9):3353–3366. doi: 10.1172/JCI87406.

37. Kyte DG, Draper H, Ives J, Liles C, Gheorghe A, Mercieca-Bebber R, et al. Patient reported outcomes (PROs) in clinical trials: is 'in-trial' guidance lacking? A systematic review. *PLOS ONE* 2013;8(4):e60684. doi: 10.1371/journal.pone.0060684.

38. Gotay CC, Kawamoto CT, Bottomley A. The prognostic significance of patient-reported outcomes in cancer clinical trials. *Artic J Clin Oncol.* 2008;26:1355–1363.

39. Kluetz PG, Chingos DT, Basch EM, Mitchell SA. Patient-reported outcomes in cancer clinical trials: measuring symptomatic adverse events with the National Cancer Institute's patient-reported outcomes version of the common terminology criteria for adverse events (PRO-CTCAE). *Am Soc Clin Oncol Educ Book* 2016;35:67–73.

40. Cella D, Riley W, Stone A, Riley W, Stone A, Rothrock N, et al. The Patient-Reported Outcomes Measurement Information System (PROMIS) developed and tested its first wave of adult self-reported health outcome item banks: 2005–2008. *J Clin Epidemiol.* 2010;63:1179–1194.

41. Kluetz PG, Kanapuru B, Lemery S, Johnson LL, Fiero MH, Arscott K, et al. Informing the tolerability of cancer treatments using patient-reported outcome measures: summary of an FDA and Critical Path Institute Workshop. *Value Health.* 2018 Jun;21(6):742–747. doi: 10.1016/j.jval.2017.09.009. Epub 2017 Nov 7. PMID: 29909880.

42. Reeve BB, Mitchell SA, Dueck AC, Basch E, Cella D, Reilly CM, et al. Recommended patient-reported core set of symptoms to measure in adult cancer treatment trials. *J Natl Cancer Inst.* 2014;106(7):129. doi: 10.1093/jnci/dju129.

43. Brittaney-Belle E, Chen G, Chen RC. Patient-reported outcomes in cancer survivorship, *Acta Oncologica.* 2017;56(2):1 66–173. doi: 10.1080/0284186X.2016.1268265.

44. Ramsey I, Corsini N, Hutchinson AD, Marker J, Eckert M. A core set of patient-reported outcomes for population-based cancer survivorship research: a consensus study. *J Cancer Surv.* 2020. doi: 10.1007/Cas11764-020-00924-5.

45. Kotronoulas G, Kearney N, Maguire R, Harrow A, Di Domenico D, Croy S, MacGillivray S. What is the value of the routine use of patient-reported outcome measures toward improvement of patient outcomes, processes of care, and health service outcomes in cancer care? A systematic review of controlled trials. *J Clin Oncol.* 2014 May 10;32(14):1480–1501. doi: 10.1200/JCO.2013.53.5948.

46. Bottomley A, Reijneveld JC, Koller M, Flechtner H, Tomaszewski KA, Greimel A. Current state of quality of life and patient-reported outcomes research. *Eur J of Cancer.* 2019;121:55–63. doi: 10.1016/j.ejca.2019.08.016.

47. Damman OC, Jani A, de Jong BA, Becker A, Metz MJ, de Bruijne MC, et al. The use of PROMs and shared decision-making in medical encounters with patients: an opportunity to deliver value-based health care to patients. *J Eval Clin Pract.* 2020;26(2):524–540. doi: 10.1111/jep.13321.

48. Brundage MD, Barbera L, McCallum F, Howell D. A pilot evaluation of the expanded prostate cancer index composite for clinical practice (EPIC-CP) tool in Ontario. *Qual Life Res.* 2018;28(3):771–782. doi: 10.1007/s11136-018-2034-x.

49. Anachkova M, Donelson S, Ska Licks AM, et al. Exploring the implementation of patient-reported outcome measures in cancer care: need for more 'real-world' evidence results in the peer reviewed literature. *J Patient-Reported Outcomes.* 2018;2(64):1–21.

50. Barbara L, Moody L. A decade in review: Cancer Care Ontario's approach to symptom assessment and management. *Med Care.* 2019;57:S80–S84.

51. Barbera L, Sutradhar R, Howell D. Sussman J, Seow H, Dudgeon D, et al. Does routine symptom screening with ESAS decrease ED visits in breast cancer patients undergoing adjuvant chemotherapy?. *Support Care Cancer* 2015;23:3025–3032. doi: 10.1007/s00520-015-2671-3.

52. Barbera L, Atzema C, Sutradhar R, Seow H, Howell D, Husain A, Sussman J, Earle C, Liu Y, Dudgeon D. Do patient-reported symptoms predict emergency department visits in cancer patients? A population-based analysis. *Ann Emerg Med.* 2013 Apr;61(4):427–437.e5. doi: 10.1016/j.annemergmed.2012.10.010.

53. Barbera L, Sutradhar R, Seow H, Earle CC, Howell D, Mittmann N, Thiruchelvan O. Impact of standardized Edmonton Symptom Assessment System use on emergency department visits and hospitalization: results of a population-based retrospective matched cohort analysis [published online ahead of print, 2020 May 28]. *J Clin Oncol Pract.* 2020:JOP1900660. doi: 10.1200/JOP.19.00660.

54. Mooney K, Berry DL, Whisenant M, Sjooberg D. Improving cancer care through patient experience: how to use patient-reported outcomes in practice. *Am Soc Clin Oncol Educ Book.* 2017;37:695–704.

55. Howell D, Rosberger Z, Mayer C, Faria R, Hamel M, Snider A. et al. Personalized symptom management: a quality improvement collaborative for implementation of patient reported outcomes (PROs) in 'real-world' oncology multisite practices. *J Patient Rep Outcomes.* 2020;4(1):47. Published 2020 Jun 17. doi: 10.1186/s41687-020-00212-x.

56. Howell D, Li M, Sudrahar R, Gu S, Iqbal J, O'Brien M, et al. Integration of patient reported outcomes (PROs) for personalized symptom management in 'real-world' oncology practices: a population-based cohort comparison study of impact on health care utilization. *Support Care Cancer.* 2020 Oct;28(10):4933–4942. doi: 10.1007/s00520-020-05313-3. Epub 2020 Feb 4. PMID: 32020357.

57. Brundage MD, Wu AW, Rivera YM, Snyder C. Promoting effective use of patient-reported outcomes in clinical practice: themes from a "Methods Tool kit" paper series. *J Clin Epidemiol.* 2020 Jun;122:153–159. doi: 10.1016/j.jclinepi.2020.01.022.

58. Ahmed S, Barbera L, Bartlett SJ, Bebb DG, Brundage M, Bryan S, et al. A catalyst for transforming health systems and person-centred care: Canadian national position statement on patient-reported outcomes. *Curr Oncol.* 2020 Apr;27(2):90–99. doi: 10.3747/co.27.6399.

59. Howell D, Keshevarz H, Broadfield L, Hack T, Hamel M, et al. A pan Canadian practice guideline for screening, assessment, and management of cancer-related fatigue in adults. Version 2, 2015. Toronto: Canadian Partnership Against Cancer and the Canadian Association of Psychosocial Oncology. Available at: https://capo.ca/resources/Documents/Guidelines/3APAN-~1. PDF. Accessed Sept 15, 2020.

60. Bower JE, Bak K, Berger A, Breitbart W, Escalante CP, Ganz PA, et al. Screening, assessment, and management of fatigue in adult survivors of cancer: an American Society of Clinical Oncology clinical practice guideline adaptation. *J Clin Oncol.* 2014 Jun 10;32(17):1840–1850. doi: 10.1200/JCO.2013.53.4495.

61. Stacey D, Carley M. The pan-Canadian Oncology Symptom Triage and Remote Support (COSTaRS)-Practice guides for symptom management in adults with cancer. *Can Oncol Nurs J.* 2017;27(1):92–98.

62. Riis CL, Bechmann T, Jensen PT, Coulter A, Steffensen KD. Are patient-reported outcomes useful in post-treatment follow-up care for women with early breast cancer? A scoping review. *Patient Relat Outcome Meas.* 2019;10:117–127. doi: 10.2147/PROM.S195296.

63. Chasen M, Hollingshead S, Conter H, Bhargava, R. Quality of life for patients surviving cancer: are we moving ahead?. *Curr Oncol.* 2017;24(3);151–152. doi: 10.3747/co.24.3671.

64. Statistics Canada. *Census Profile, 2016 Census [Brampton] [Internet].* Ottawa: Statistics Canada; 2016 [cited 2020 Nov 07]. Available from: https://www12.statcan.gc.ca/census-recensement/2016/dp-pd/index-eng.cfm.

65. Statistics Canada. *Census Profile, 2016 Census [Brampton] [Internet].* Ottawa: Statistics Canada; 2016 [cited 2020 Nov 07]. Available from: https://www12.statcan.gc.ca/census-recensement/2016/dp-pd/index-eng.cfm.

66. Bruera E, Kuehn N, Miller MJ, Selmser P, Macmillan K. The Edmonton Symptom Assessment System (ESAS): a simple method for the assessment of palliative care patients. *J Palliative Care.* 1991;7(2):6–9.

67. Hegel MT, Collins ED, Kearing S, Gillock KL, Moore CP, Ahles TA. Sensitivity and specificity of the Distress Thermometer for depression in newly diagnosed breast cancer patients. *Psychooncology.* 2008;17(6):556–560.

68. Bultz BD, Groff SL, Fitch M, Blais MC, Howes J, Levy K, Mayer C. Implementing screening for distress, the 6th vital sign: a Canadian strategy for changing practice. *Psychooncology.* 2011;20:463–469.

69. Jammu A, Chasen M, van Heest R. Hollinshead S, Kaushik D, Gill H, Bhargava R. Effects of a Cancer Survivorship Clinic—preliminary results. *Support Care Cancer.* 2020;28;2381–2388. doi: 10.1007/s00520-019-05067-7.

70. Alfano CM, Jefford M, Maher J, Birken SA, Mayer DK. Building personalized cancer follow-up care pathways in the United States: lessons learned from implementation in England, Northern Ireland, and Australia. *Am Soc Clin Oncol Educ Book*. 2019 Jan;39:625–639. doi: 10.1200/EDBK_238267.

71. Turner GM, Litchfield I, Finnikin S. et al. General practitioners' views on use of patient reported outcome measures in primary care: a cross-sectional survey and qualitative study. *BMC Fam Pract*. 2020;21:14. doi: 10.1186/s12875-019-1077-6.

72. Basch E, Deal AM, Dueck AC, et al. Overall survival results of a trial assessing patient-reported outcomes for symptom monitoring during routine cancer treatment. *JAMA*. 2017;318(2):197–198. doi: 10.1001/jama.2017.7156.

73. Denis F, Basch E, Septans AL, Bennouna J, Urban T, Dueck AC, Letellier C. Two-year survival comparing web-based symptom monitoring vs routine surveillance following treatment for lung cancer. *JAMA*. 2019 Jan 22;321(3):306–307. doi: 10.1001/jama.2018.18085.

74. Denis F, Viger L, Charron A, Voog E, Dupuis O, Pointreau Y, Letellier C. Detection of lung cancer relapse using self-reported symptoms transmitted via an internet web-application: pilot study of the sentinel follow-up. *Support Care Cancer*. 2014;22(6):1467–1473.

75. Warrington L, Absolom K, Conner M, Kellar I, Clayton B, Ayres M, Velikova G. Electronic systems for patients to report and manage side effects of cancer treatment: systematic review. *J Med Internet Res*. 2019 Jan 24;21(1):e10875. doi: 10.2196/10875.

76. Oldenmenger WH, van den Hurk CJG, Howell D. Utilizing technology to managing symptoms. In: Charalambous A, editor. *Developing and Utilizing Digital Technology in Healthcare for Assessment and Monitoring*. New York, NY: Springer Publishing; 2020.

77. Pham Q, Hearn J, Gao B, Brown I, Hamilton RI, Berlin A, Caffazo AJ, Fiefer A. Virtual care models for cancer survivorship. *npj Digit Med*. 2020;3:113. doi: 10.1038/s41746-020-00321-3.

78. Aapro M, Bossi P, Dasari A, Fallowfield L, Gascón P, Geller M, Jordan K, Kim J, Martin K, Porzig S. Digital health for optimal supportive care in oncology: benefits, limits, and future perspectives. *Support Care Cancer*. 2020 Oct; 28(10):4589–4612. doi: 10.1007/s00520-020-05539-1. Epub 2020 Jun 12. PMID: 32533435; PMCID: PMC7447627.

79. Roberts AL, Fisher A, Smith L, Heinrich M, Potts HWW. Digital health behaviour change interventions targeting physical activity and diet in cancer survivors: a systematic review and meta-analysis. *J Cancer Surviv*. 2017 Dec;11(6):704–719. doi: 10.1007/s11764-017-0632-1. Epub 2017 Aug 4. PMID: 28779220; PMCID: PMC5671545.

80. Groen WG, Kuijpers W, Oldenburg HAS, Wouters MWJM, Aaronson NK, van Harten WH. Empowerment of cancer survivors through information technology: an integrative review. *J Med Internet Res*. 2015;17(11):e270. doi: 10.2196/jmir.4818.

81. McCorkle R, Ercolano E, Lazenby M, Schulman-Green D, Schilling LS, Lorig K, Wagner EH. Self-management: enabling and empowering patients living with cancer as a chronic illness. *CA Cancer J Clin*. 2011 Jan–Feb;61(1):50–62. doi: 10.3322/caac.20093.

82. Girgis A. The role of self-management in cancer survivorship care. *Lancet Oncol*. 2020 Jan;21(1):8–9. doi: 10.1016/S1470-2045(19)30715-6.

83. Rutherford C, Müller F, Faiz N. King M, White K. Patient-reported outcomes and experiences from the perspective of colorectal cancer survivors: meta-synthesis of qualitative studies. *J Patient Rep Outcomes*. 2020;4:27. doi: 10.1186/s41687-020-00195-9.

84. Tollosa DN, Tavener M, Hure A, James EL. Adherence to multiple health behaviours in cancer survivors: a systematic review and meta-analysis. *J Cancer Surviv*. 2019 Jun;13(3):327–343. doi: 10.1007/s11764-019-00754-0.

85. Creer TL, Holroyd KA. Self-management of chronic conditions. In Baum A, Newman S, Weinman J, West R, McManus C, editors. *Cambridge Handbook of Psychology, Health and Medicine*. UK: Cambridge University Press, 2006.

86. Foster C, Fenlon D. Recovery and self-management support following primary cancer treatment. *Brit J Cancer*. 2011;105:S21–S28.

87. Adams K, Greiner AC, Corrigan JM, editors. Report of a summit. In *The First Annual Crossing the Quality Chasm Summit: A Focus on Communities*. Washington, DC: National Academies Press, 2004.

88. Howell D, Harth T, Brown J, Bennett C, Boyko S. Self-management education interventions for patients with cancer: a systematic review. *Support Care Cancer*. 2017 April;25(4):1323–1355. doi: 10.1007/s00520-016-3500-z.

89. Howell D, Mayer DK, Fielding R, Eicher M, Verdonck-de Leeuw IM, Johansen C, et al. Management of cancer and health after the clinic visit: a call to action for self-management in cancer care. *J Natl Cancer Inst*. 2020 Jun 11 [Online ahead of print] djaa083. doi: 10.1093/jnci/djaa083.

90. Howell DD. Supported self-management for cancer survivors to address long-term biopsychosocial consequences of cancer and treatment to optimize living well. *Curr Opin Support Palliat Care*. 2018 Mar;12(1):92–99. doi: 10.1097/spc.0000000000000329.

91. Glasgow RE, Davis CL, Funnell MM, Beck A. Implementing practical interventions to support chronic illness self-management. *Jt Comm J Qual Saf*. 2003 Nov;29(11):563–574. doi: 10.1016/s1549-3741(03)29067-5.

92. Teel CS, Meek P, McNamara AM, Watson L. Perspectives unifying symptom interpretation. *Image J Nurs Sch*. 1997;29(2):175–181. doi: 10.1111/j.1547-5069.1997.tb01553.x.

93. Mustian KM, Alfano CM, Heckler C, Kleckner AS, Kleckner IR, Leach CR, Mohr D, Palesh OG, Peppone LJ, Piper BF, Scarpato J, Smith T, Sprod LK, Miller SM. Comparison of pharmaceutical, psychological, and exercise treatments for cancer-related fatigue: a meta-analysis. *JAMA Oncol*. 2017 Jul 1;3(7):961–968. doi: 10.1001/jamaoncol.2016.6914.

94. Boland L, Bennett K, Connolly D. Self-management interventions for cancer survivors: a systematic review. *Support Care Cancer*. 2018 May;26(5):1585–1595. doi: 10.1007/s00520-017-3999-7.

95. Kim SH, Kim K, Mayer DK. Self-management intervention for adult cancer survivors after treatment: a systematic review and meta-analysis. *Oncol Nurs Forum*. 2017 Nov 1;44(6):719–728. doi: 10.1188/17.ONF.719-728.

96. Demark-Wahnefried W, Rogers LQ, Alfano CM, Thomson CA, Courneya KS, Meyerhardt JA, et al. Practical clinical interventions for diet, physical activity, and weight control in cancer survivors. *CA Cancer J Clin*. 2015 May–Jun;65(3):167–189. doi: 10.3322/caac.21265.

97. Lawn S, Zrim S, Leggett S, Miller M, Woodman R, Jones L, Kichenadasse G, Sukumaran S, Karapetis C, Koczwara B. Is self-management feasible and acceptable for addressing nutrition and physical activity needs of cancer survivors? *Health Expect*. 2015 Dec;18(6):3358–3373. doi: 10.1111/hex.12327.

98. Cuthbert CA, Farragher JF, Hemmelgarn BR, Ding Q, McKinnon GP, Cheung WY. Self-management interventions for cancer survivors: a systematic review and evaluation of intervention content and theories. *Psychooncology*. 2019 Nov;28(11):2119–2140. doi: 10.1002/pon.5215.

99. Hibbard JH, Greene J, Sacks R, Overton V, Parrotta CD. Adding a measure of patient self-management capability to risk assessment can improve prediction of high costs. *Health Aff (Millwood)*. 2016 Mar;35(3):489–494. doi: 10.1377/hlthaff.2015.1031.

100. Mokhallalati Y, Mulvey MR, Bennett MI. Interventions to support self-management in cancer pain. *Pain: Clin Updates*. 2018:3:e690. doi: 10.1097/PR9.0000000000000690.

101. Michie S, van Stralen MM, West R. The behaviour change wheel: a new method for characterizing and designing behaviour change interventions. *Implement Sci*. 2011;6;42. https://doi.org/10.1186/1748-5908-6-42.

102. Hui D, Bruera E. A personalized approach to assessing and managing pain in patients with cancer. *J Clin Oncol*. 2014 Jun 1;32(16):1640–1646. doi: 10.1200/JCO.2013.52.2508.

103. Watanabe YS, Miura T, Okizaki A, Tagami K, Matsumoto Y, Fujimori M, Morita T, Kinoshita H. Comparison of indicators for achievement of pain control with a personalized pain goal in a comprehensive cancer center. *J Pain Symptom Manage*. 2018 Apr;55(4):1159–1164. doi: 10.1016/j.jpainsymman.2017.12.476.

104. Levinson W, Lesser CS, Epstein RM. Developing physician communication skills for patient-centered care. *Health Aff (Millwood)*. 2010 Jul;29(7):1310–1318. doi: 10.1377/hlthaff.2009.0450.

105. D'Agostino TA, Atkinson TM, Latella LE, Rogers M, Morrissey D, DeRosa AP, Parker PA. Promoting patient participation in healthcare interactions through communication skills training: a systematic review. *Patient Educ Couns*. 2017 Jul;100(7):1247–1257. doi: 10.1016/j.pec.2017.02.016. Epub 2017 Feb 16. PMID: 28238421; PMCID: PMC5466484.

106. Epstein RM, Street RL. *Patient Centered Communication in Cancer Care: Promoting Health and Reducing Suffering*. Bethesda, MD: National Cancer Institute/National Institute of Health Publication; 2007. Publication 07-6225. Available online: https://healthcaredelivery.cancer.gov/pcc/monograph.html.

107. King A, Hoppe RB. "Best practice" for patient-centered communication: a narrative review. *J Grad Med Educ*. 2013;5(3):385–393. doi: 10.4300/JGME-D-13-00072.1.

108. Rollnick S, Miller R, Butler CR. *Motivational Interviewing in Health Care: Helping Patients Change Behavior*. New York, NY: Guilford Press; 2008.

109. Epstein RM, Alper BS, Quill TE. Communicating evidence for participatory decision making. *JAMA*. 2004;291(19):2359–2366. doi: 10.1001/jama.291.19.2359.

Psychosocial and Behavioral Interventions for Symptom Management in Cancer Survivors

8

Roberto M. Benzo, Blanca Noriega Esquivels, and Frank J. Penedo

INTRODUCTION

In this chapter, we provide a review of various psychosocial and behavioral interventions for symptom management in cancer survivors. We also describe common symptoms experienced by cancer patients, theoretical models used to guide the interventions, and different interventions based on either the unit of care, (e.g., individual, dyadic, group, etc.), delivery mode (e.g., in-person, self-administered, group-based, technology-based, etc.), specific cancer types (solid tumor vs. hematologic), and populations (older adults, racial/ethnic minorities, rural communities).

The Lasting Effect of Cancer Treatment

The National Cancer Institute (NCI) and other organizations define an individual as a "cancer survivor" from the time of diagnosis through the remainder of their life [1]. Cancer survivorship care involves attention to a person's health and well-being, and addressing the physical, mental, emotional, social, and financial needs of survivors following primary treatment [1]. These organizations also include family members, caregivers, friends and the community as part of the survivorship experience. During this experience, patients may undergo curative or long-term maintenance therapies, may develop recurrences or secondary cancers, or enter remission, all of which have an impact on physical, psychosocial, and financial well-being and health-related quality of life (HRQoL) – a multidimensional construct that taps into several areas of function (Figure 8.1) [2]. The survival benefits associated with early

DOI: 10.1201/9781003055426-8

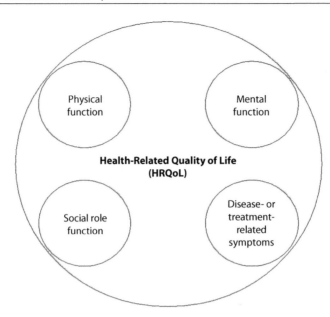

FIGURE 8.1 Health-related quality of life is made up of four dimensions: physical, mental, social, and disease-/treatment-related symptoms.

detection and treatment efficacy which account for a growing number of cancer survivors, can be offset by commonly experienced chronic and debilitating symptoms that compromise HRQoL [2]. Fatigue, pain, and sleep disturbance are common, further compromise HRQoL and can negatively impact health behaviors.

Symptom Burden and Health Related Quality of Life

Symptom burden can be measured using various patient-reported outcomes (PROs) measures that tap into specific indicators such as fatigue, pain, depression and anxiety, or more comprehensive and multi-dimensional measures of PROs such as HRQoL [3]. In addition to the presence or absence of the symptom, survivors are asked to report various dimensions such as: intensity, distress, prevalence, frequency, consequences, and quality [4]. Fatigue, pain, sleep disruptions, and emotional distress (e.g., anxiety and depression) are commonly experienced symptoms. More than 40% of cancer survivors experience simultaneously occurring symptoms (symptom cluster) of pain, fatigue, and sleep disturbances [2]. A review published by Wu and Harden (2015) reported that fatigue is the most frequently reported symptom among cancer survivors, with a prevalence ranging from 9% to 100% [5]. Concurrent with fatigue, survivors report disrupted sleep patterns as one of the top five concerns across various cancers [6]. Even after treatment, disrupted sleep is often the most severe symptom experienced during extended and long-term survivorship [5]. In contrast, there are less data available on depression/mood disturbance and pain, and even less on cognitive limitation during extended and long-term survivorship [5]. Nonetheless, estimates are that about one third of cancer patients, at some point during the cancer continuum report clinically elevated levels of depression, anxiety or an adjustment disorder. When physical and emotional symptoms are unattended they can impact multiple aspects of HRQoL, leading to poorer treatment adherence and satisfaction, increased use of the healthcare system and other resources [2, 7]. On the other hand, adequate symptom management is associated with better HRQoL among survivors and caregivers, greater treatment compliance and potentially better clinical outcomes such as survival [8].

The Challenges of Symptom Management

Symptom management interventions have been developed to prevent and/or manage symptoms. Some of this work has focused on gaining an understanding of the physiology and psychological mechanisms that may drive symptoms. For example, Guimond et al. found that maladaptive emotional regulation (suppression and avoidance of emotions) was a possible psychological mechanism underlying psychological symptoms in breast cancer patients [9]. Some have mapped the underlying biological pathways through which poor emotional regulation can impact physical symptoms. For example, elevated inflammatory biomarkers (e.g., interleukin-6 and TNF-α) have been linked to depression on the one hand, and persistent fatigue among breast cancer survivors on the other [10] – a phenomenon known as "sickness behavior." Thus, advancing our understanding of these mechanisms is vital as they could serve as intervention targets and/or biomarkers that drive symptom response in symptom management programs. Some approaches to manage symptoms have involved pharmacologic treatments such as analgesics, sedatives, and psychostimulants. However, these approaches have had limited success and pharmacotherapy can lead to further exacerbation of other symptoms or produce new ones (e.g., the use of opioids to control pain may also cause fatigue) [11]. Notably, non-pharmacologic interventions, such as exercise, mindfulness-based stress reduction programs and cognitive-behavioral therapy, can have a positive impact on a person's social support, self-esteem, emotional distress, physical function, and overall HRQoL [2, 12].

THEORETICAL MODELS INFORM SYMPTOM MANAGEMENT INTERVENTIONS

Conceptual and theoretical frameworks in cancer survivorship have informed our understanding of how sociodemographic, cultural, clinical, stress, psychosocial, lifestyle, and biological factors may uniquely or interactively impact key outcomes such as symptom burden (e.g., pain, fatigue, depression, sleep, cognition), HRQoL and disease activity (e.g., progression, recurrence, secondary cancers and cancer, and all-cause mortality). Multiple behavior change theories have been used to guide symptom management interventions including, but not limited to: Stress and Coping Theory [13], Self-efficacy Theory [14], Chronic Care Model [15], Social Cognitive Theory [16], Problem Solving Theory [17], Self-regulatory Theory [18], Motivational Interviewing [19], and Uncertainty in illness [20]. For example, social cognitive theory constructs have been used to guide the promotion of exercise, which has been shown to reduce fatigue and improve HRQoL. Parelkar et al. used the transactional model of stress and coping to examine the relationship between self-reported efforts to manage stress and the uptake of health behaviors across several lifestyle behavior domains [21]. Data from a national, population-based, cross-sectional survey of 2,888 survivors found that participants who took a more active approach in controlling their stress were more likely to make changes in the physical, psychosocial, and preventative health behaviors, compared to those who used more passive stress-coping approaches. The Chronic Care Self-Management Model targets creating a partnership between clinicians and survivors, to empower them to assume a more active role in managing their symptoms and achieving their goals in survivorship care [15]. The aim of self-management is to empower survivors to report and manage late and long-term effects of treatment, seek support when needed, and engage in lifestyle changes that promote healthy living. This model acknowledges survivors' goals and preferences and fosters their confidence in their ability to perform care activities by using effective self-management strategies such as problem-solving, decision-making, goal setting, enhancing communication, monitoring progress, and resource utilization. Biobehavioral models address behavioral, psychosocial, and biological mechanisms that may impact symptom burden, and techniques to modify such mechanisms. For example, cognitive-behavioral stress management interventions combined cognitive behavioral therapy (CBT) techniques with relaxation training to achieve increased stress awareness (e.g., how stress impacts emotions and physical symptoms), and each anxiety reduction, coping, social support and communication skills to improve both physiological (e.g., reduced inflammation) and psychosocial (e.g., improved mood) adaptation, on the one hand, and better HRQoL and lower symptom burden, on the other [22].

Types of Psychosocial Interventions

In the following sections we describe various types of psychological and behavioral symptom management interventions available to cancer care and primary care clinicians. These interventions can be sorted by the mode of delivery, types of cancer, cancer stage, and target population. These interventions typically aim to minimize the negative impacts of the disease and promote positive adjustment, and can do so by focusing on:

- Guiding treatment decisions and preparation
- Teaching adaptive coping skills such as planning and problem solving
- Improving social support seeking behaviors and reducing social isolation
- Modifying maladaptive cognitions and negative health behaviors
- Improving communication with clinicians, family members, and caregivers
- Promoting adherence to recommendations and healthy lifestyle behaviors

INTERVENTION FORMATS

Individual Support and Self-Management Interventions

Individual support interventions are delivered on a one-on-one basis. These interventions can be delivered in-person, by telephone, video conference, or via an eHealth or mHealth application. These programs typically include evidence-based therapy. This approach allows the patient to receive individualized attention and support, resulting in a more tailored intervention relative to a group therapy approach. A limitation of this approach is that it is resource intensive (e.g., time, money), thus limiting its reach in helping cancer survivors. Self-management interventions provide the necessary skills to assist survivors adopt health behaviors to promote healthier lifestyles. Self-management interventions typically aim to increase the patient's knowledge of the disease, improve their understanding of the health care system and resources available to them, and teach them problem-solving and decision-making skills. PROs (e.g., symptoms, HRQoL) are the most common type of outcomes in self-management interventions; however, other studies have included outcomes such as number of health care visits [23], physical fitness [24, 25], biological outcomes (e.g., IL-6, C reactive protein, TNF receptor type II) [24], disease progression, and overall survival [26, 27]. Self-management interventions can range anywhere from a single session to 12-months in length, and can be delivered across different modes (e.g., print, web-based, in-person, group-based).

Group Interventions

Group-based interventions offer various advantages over individual-level interventions. From a feasibility perspective, group formats allow for efficient delivery of evidence-based programs that maximize reach and are not resource intensive (e.g., one group leader can deliver a program to 8–10 participants at a time). A group-based approach can also provide therapeutic benefits to patients. Groups provide supportive and nurturing therapeutic settings where survivors can express their feelings to others who share similar experiences, learn from others and gain a sense of "community" and "universality" specific to their cancer experience with subsequent reductions in psychological distress [28]. During group sessions cancer survivors can speak with others who share similar experiences in regard to treatment, side-effects, symptoms, and feelings of uncertainty. Involvement in group interventions may also reduce social isolation and loneliness which is common after cancer treatment.

Many mindfulness-based and other stress reduction interventions have used a group-based approach, and have been linked to reductions in stress, anxiety, depression, fatigue and, improvements in HRQoL, including post-traumatic growth among cancer survivors [29]. Bower et al examined the effect of a mindfulness-based intervention for younger breast cancer survivors compared to a wait list control group in a randomized controlled clinical trial [24]. The mindfulness-based intervention was designed to reduce stress, depression, and inflammation. The interventions consisted of six weekly two-hour group sessions with content focused on mindfulness, relaxation, mind body connection, and guided practices of meditation and gentle movement exercises (e.g., mindful walking). The intervention also included a psychoeducational component for cancer survivors [24]. Participation in the mindfulness-based intervention led to significant reductions in perceived stress, pro-inflammatory gene expression, inflammatory signaling, and marginal reductions in depressive symptoms. Participants in the intervention group also reported reductions in fatigue, sleep disturbance, and increased feelings of peace and meaning and positive affect post intervention [24].

Patient-Caregiver Dyadic Interventions

Family members often serve as caregivers and play an important role in supporting cancer patients [30]. Research has shown that in addition to cancer survivors, family caregivers also experience physical and psychological symptoms, and face both social and spiritual concerns due to caregiving stress [31]. Moreover, caregiving stress has been linked to high levels of psychological distress (i.e., anxiety, depression) fatigue, sleep impairments, compromised immune function, poor health-related behaviors, and greater morbidity [32–35]. Given these unfavorable outcomes, researchers have begun to develop symptom management interventions that target both patients and caregivers.

A recent meta-analysis, including 23 RCTs and 2317 patient-caregiver dyads, found that interventions for caregiver-patient dyads were associated with improvements in various psycho-social dimensions of patient HRQoL, relatedness, marital functioning, depression, and anxiety in caregivers [30]. Psychoeducational-based interventions are the most common types of patient-caregiver dyad interventions and have been linked to improvements in individual psychological well-being and relationship functioning [30].

MODES OF DELIVERY

One important consideration in the development and implementation of symptom management interventions is the mode of delivery (in-person, self-administered, technology-based). Many of these interventions address physical (e.g., pain, nausea, sexual health issue, constipation, etc.) or psychological

CALL-OUT BOX: CARING FOR THE INFORMAL CAREGIVER

Informal caregivers are typically individuals who share a strong personal connection to the person with cancer, such as a spouse/partner, close relative, or friend. Caregivers may provide assistance with most aspects of everyday life. Common tasks that informal caregivers perform in addition to their existing responsibilities (e.g., finances, housekeeping, etc.) include administration of medications, management of symptoms, monitoring for disease- and treatment-related side effects, wound care (e.g., post-surgical care), and catheter or line care (e.g., PICC, nephrostomy, gastrotomy) [34].

Informal caregivers encounter their own stresses and psychological burden associated with the physical and emotional toll that come with providing care to a cancer patient. Informal caregivers receive little preparation, training, or support to learn and perform their caregiving role, which can further exacerbate cancer-related distress and lead to negative outcomes (e.g., sleep disruption, depression, financial difficulties) [34]. Strategies for preparing the cancer caregiver include caregiver education, improving communication between patient/caregiver and the medical team, empowering the caregiver to deliver holistic care, and supporting caregiver self-care. Pasacreta et al. found that a 6-hour caregiver education program led by nurses and social workers improved caregivers knowledge and confidence about caregiving [36].

symptoms (e.g., anxiety, depression, etc.), or both. In the following sections we provide a brief description of the various delivery approaches.

In-Person

The most traditional and common mode of delivering an intervention is in-person. An in-person approach requires participants to have access to reliable transportation, sufficient time (e.g., scheduling, transport, wait times associated with a clinical visit), and a healthcare system with the necessary specialists. Symptom management interventions delivered to cancer survivors using an in-person approach generally focus on improving outcomes such as QOL, pain, sleep, and relationship functioning.

There is a growing evidence base that supports using psychological and behavioral interventions to reduce or mitigate the symptom burden of cancer survivors. Dalton and colleagues developed a tailored CBT program and evaluated if it was more effective than either standard CBT or usual care in patients with cancer-related pain [37]. Those undergoing CBT were required to attend five 50-minute in-person treatment sessions. Compared to the standard CBT condition, participants in the tailored CBT condition experienced significant improvement from pre- to post-intervention in worst pain, least pain, less interference of pain with sleep, less confusion, less pain with activities, walking, relationships, and sleep.

Other types of interventions that have shown efficacy in reducing pain contain structured exercise programs. Jarden et al. developed an intervention for patients undergoing hematopoietic stem cell transplantation, which consisted of a supervised four- to six-week structured exercise program, progressive muscle relaxation, and psychoeducation, in addition to standard treatment and care [38]. Results showed that participants assigned to the intervention experienced a significant reduction in mucositis, cognitive, gastrointestinal, and functional symptom clusters.

Self-Administered

Self-administered interventions are those where the patient is responsible for going through the materials in their own time (self-directed), mostly in a structured manner, and may include educational components, behavior change techniques (e.g., promotion of physical activity, dietary quality, etc.), and

IMPLICATION FOR PRACTICE: MANAGING CANCER-RELATED SYMPTOMS

Patients with cancer typically experience multiple symptoms although current practice guidelines address single symptoms. Treatment recommendations are made without consideration of how strategies for mitigating individual symptoms may influence others, or how these treatments interact with one another. In a recent review intended for a nursing audience, Kwekkeboom et al. reviewed symptom management strategies and identified a substantial number with potential benefit across multiple symptoms, including pharmacological and non-pharmacological approaches [39]. The authors propose that shifting the practice paradigm from single to multi-symptom assessment and management begins with nursing evaluations. Four key messages from their review include the following:

- Multi-symptom assessment scales can serve to identify co-occurring symptoms.
- Integration of multi-symptom PRO assessments may be completed prior to clinical appointments.
- Clinicians can select recommended symptom management strategies that are effective for several symptoms.
- Clinicians can triage patients to either psychosocial, behavioral, and/or pharmacologic interventions based on PRO's and in-depth assessments.

stress-management skills. Approximately 17–75% of cancer survivors experience cancer-related cognitive impairments. In a pilot study, a self-administered home-based computerized (mHealth) cognitive training program was compared to usual care among men ($n = 60$) with advanced prostate cancer on androgen deprivation therapy [40]. All participants were screened for at least mild cognitive impairment. Participants in the intervention group were instructed to use BrainHQ (www.brainhq.com), which is an online platform with various visual attention and information processing exercises, for one-hour/day, five-days/week for a total of 8-weeks. Although the intervention was deemed feasible and acceptable, the findings were mixed. Participants reported significant improvements in reaction times but not memory [40].

Technology Based (e.g., eHealth, mHealth, Telehealth)

Over the past few decades, there has been an increased use of technology in symptom management interventions. Health information technologies are those that support the collection, aggregation, and management of health information [41]. The term eHealth (i.e., electronic health) is an umbrella term that refers to the use of information and communication technologies in health-related services and processes [42]. eHealth covers a wide variety of applications such as electronic health records, electronic medication overview, and telemedicine-related services. Often, the terms telemedicine, telehealth, and tele-oncology are used interchangeably with eHealth. While telemedicine is embedded within eHealth, it refers specifically to information and communication technologies that support the delivery of health services to patients from a different physical location [42]. Within eHealth, mHealth is the use of mobile and wireless devices (e.g., computers, tablets, and smartphones) that support patient care, education, and research.

The role of eHealth in cancer survivorship

The increasing use of eHealth has transformed patient-centered cancer care through the expansion of assessments and interventions that are increasingly more dynamic, ecologically valid, and assisted by technology. eHealth can be used to improve patient-provider communication, enhance symptom and toxicity assessment and management, and increase patient engagement across the care continuum [43]. In addition, eHealth may help us overcome barriers such as facilitating cancer care access for underserved groups (e.g., minorities, low income, etc.) or rural communities that lack access to cancer survivorship care. Ultimately, the use of these technologies may allow us to improve our ability to collect PROs and implement system-level changes (e.g., reduce visits to emergency departments, hospital readmissions, and improve satisfaction with treatment).

Perhaps one of the most important uses of eHealth is to collect PROs, which are defined as "any report of the status of a patient's health that comes directly from the patient" [1], and are absent of any interpretation by a clinician or anyone else. PROs include descriptions of a patient's symptoms, satisfaction with care, physical and mental function, adherence to prescribed medication or therapy, perceived value of treatment, HRQoL, and measures of emotional, spiritual, and social well-being. Facilitating the collection of PROs using eHealth technologies, may assist health-care providers and patients to better understand their survivorship experience and help guide them in the development of an effective and customized cancer survivorship care plan.

Integration of PROs with health information technologies can provide benefits for cancer patients, healthcare providers, and healthcare systems [43]. One example of a PRO is the Patient Reported Outcomes Measurement Information System (PROMIS®), which can be administered and scored electronically (e.g., web, computer, voice response) or uploaded "paper and pencil" instruments [44]. PROMIS® is an NIH funded initiative, that aims to enhance and standardize measures of PROs through computer adaptive testing. Computer adaptive testing uses item response theory to minimize the number of survey items the patient is asked to complete in order to understand the status of a particular symptom or functionality (e.g., physical), without loss of scale precision or content validity [43, 44]; thus, minimizing patient burden, and increasing the likelihood the patient will complete the assessment. If patients report clinically elevated symptoms, patients can be triaged in "real time" to social work and/or clinical teams depending on the stated concerns, thus creating opportunities for interventions. Basch et al. evaluated the efficacy of an electronically integrated PRO system to a PRO monitoring method (the Symptom Tracking and Reporting – STAR) that was administered at the physician's discretion (usual care), among patients with advanced cancers undergoing chemotherapy ($n = 766$) [45]. At 6 months, the intervention group reported significantly less decline in HRQoL, less admissions to the ER, less hospitalizations, and remained on their chemotherapy for longer, compared to the usual care condition [45]. This finding is significant as it provides support for changing the health care delivery system to one where patients are engaged as active participants to improve the experience, efficiency, and outcomes of care.

mHealth for managing symptoms in cancer patients

The widespread availability of smart phones and other mobile technologies (e.g., wearables) created new opportunities to use mobile health (mHealth) technologies to assist communication and delivery of care. The World Health Organization defines mHealth as "medical and public health practice supported by mobile devices, such as mobile phones, patient monitoring devices, personal digital assistants, and other wireless devices" [46]. The benefits of mHealth are bidirectional, they can be used to collect context rich data from patients, as well as deliver health interventions regardless of patient's physical location (see Figure 8.2).

mHealth has been used to treat symptoms commonly experienced by people living with cancer, such as pain and psychological distress. Researchers at Duke University have adapted a Pain Coping Skills Training (PCST) protocol for patients with chronic disease [47] to an mHealth behavioral cancer pain intervention that relies on mobile technologies [48]. The intervention consisted of four 30–45-minute sessions delivered via videoconferencing (i.e., Skype) to the participants at home. Participants who completed the intervention experienced significant improvements in pain, physical symptoms, psychological distress, and pain catastrophizing [48]. In addition, the intervention was found to be a feasible and acceptable approach for reducing pain among cancer survivors. This intervention has demonstrated one way

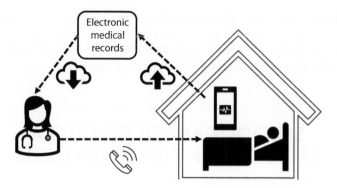

FIGURE 8.2 A representation of how patients and providers can be connected through digital technologies to increase reach of survivorship care.

to bridge intensive outpatient services and home settings, allowing for continuity of care and increased access to care for cancer survivors.

Reach of eHealth in remote communities for symptom management

Telemedicine is the use of information technology to provide remote personalized health care to patients, which allows for communication and exchange of data between patients and clinicians [49]. One example demonstrating the use of telehealth was focused on the administration of chemotherapy in a rural community under remote guidance from oncologists in Australia [50]. Chan and colleagues evaluated the safety of using tele-oncology in delivering chemotherapy to patients living in rural towns in Australia [50]. The study compared the dose intensity and corresponding toxicity profiles for patients undergoing chemotherapy in an urban tertiary cancer center in northern Queensland, with those for patients treated at a small rural hospital, supervised by the same medical oncologists. Outcomes included dose intensity (doses, number of cycles, and lines of treatment) and toxicity rates (rate of serious side effects, hospital admissions and mortality). Over the course of five years, a total of 89 patients received 626 cycles of chemotherapy in the small rural hospital, and 117 patients received 799 cycles at the cancer center. The authors reported no significant differences between the urban

---

CALL OUT BOX: EVIDENCE-BASED PRACTICE IN CANCER SURVIVORSHIP CARE

Implementation of evidence-based guidelines can be challenging due to differences observed between the environment in which the intervention was developed and the complex real-life nature of clinical practice settings. When organizations implement evidence-based therapies, they often do so inconsistently or in a manner that is different from the original study design and this may result in suboptimal results. Translational research [51] involves five phases that are listed below and serves to bridge the gap between conceptual design and implementation of novel interventions:

1T_0: Identification of opportunities and approaches to health problems
2T_1: Takes approaches identified in the first phase and applies them to a specific population or situation
3T_2: Evaluates the approach and results in an evidence-based guideline
4T_3: Moves evidence-based guidelines into practice
5T_4: Evaluates the outcomes in the clinical setting

and rural hospital in dose intensities, proportion of side-effects, and hospital admissions. Also, there were no toxicity-related deaths in either group. These findings suggest that tele-oncology can be used to safely administer chemotherapy in rural towns under the supervision of medical oncologists from larger centers, provided adequate conditions exist at the rural hospital.

SPECIFIC CANCER SYMPTOM MANAGEMENT INTERVENTIONS

In the following sections, we describe various examples of symptom management interventions designed for patients with specific tumor types.

Solid Tumors

Patients with head and neck cancers (HNC) report many unmet needs throughout their survivorship experience that affect their HRQoL and mood [52]. Treatment for HNC may involve changes to critical structures for speaking, eating, and breathing, which can result in impairments of functionality (e.g., dysphagia and breathing difficulties), and cosmetic burden (e.g., facial and neck disfigurement) [53]. Typical symptoms associated with HNC include pain, distress, dehydration, malnutrition, nausea, constipation, and sleep disturbance [52]. van der Meulen and colleagues showed that a nurse-led psychosocial intervention consisting of six bimonthly 45-minute counseling sessions focused on symptom management improved HRQoL and depressive symptoms and the effects were long-lasting [54, 55]. Participants in the intervention group showed significant improvements in emotional and physical functioning, pain, swallowing, social contact, mouth opening and depressive symptoms at 12-months. At 18-months, participants in the intervention group reported significantly better global HRQoL, role and emotional functioning, pain, swallowing, mouth opening, and depressive symptoms; and at 24-months reported significantly better ratings of emotional functioning and fatigue compared to the control group.

Reb and colleagues conducted a pilot study to evaluate the feasibility and acceptability of a Self-Management Survivorship Care Planning Intervention (SM-SCP) in colorectal and lung cancer survivors [56] Typical symptoms experienced by colorectal cancer survivors include bowel dysfunction, pain, fatigue, and sexual dysfunction that negatively affects their quality of life (QOL) [57–60]. Lung cancer survivors experience chronic pain, psychological distress, cough, fatigue, and impaired pulmonary function [56, 61, 62]. The intervention consisted of the design of an integrated survivorship care plan that included self-management skills coaching. Nurses leading the intervention used various behavioral approaches (e.g., goal setting, problem-solving skills, self-monitoring skills for late and long-term effects) to engage survivors and create the treatment summary care plan. The intervention was feasible and acceptable and showed significant improvements in depression, anxiety, self-efficacy, physical functioning, role limitations, physical pain, general health, health transition, physical health summary, and HRQoL from baseline to post-intervention (2-months) [56].

Hematologic Cancers

Patients treated for hematologic malignancies often experience fatigue/lack of energy, difficulty sleeping, drowsiness, dry mouth, pain, numbness of hands/feet, shortness of breath, difficulty concentrating, cough, lack of appetite and feeling nervous, irritable, sad, and worried [63]. A pilot randomized study evaluated the feasibility and efficacy of an application-based intervention to improve fatigue compared with a wait list control, among a group of patients with chronic myeloid leukemia treated with targeted therapies [64].

The intervention consisted of CBT for targeted therapy-related fatigue and was delivered via Facetime. Patients assigned to the intervention condition had significantly greater improvements in fatigue and overall QOL after treatment (18-weeks post baseline), compared to the control.

Chang and colleagues compared the effects of a three-week walking exercise program to reduce fatigue in patients with leukemia receiving chemotherapy [65]. The intervention consisted of 12 minutes of a walking exercise program per day, five days a week, for three consecutive weeks. Participants in the intervention group reported improved fitness, and lower levels of fatigue intensity and interference, symptom distress, anxiety, and depression compared to the control group [65].

CONTINUUM-BASED CANCER SYMPTOM MANAGEMENT INTERVENTIONS

Early Cancer Survivorship (<1 Year)

During the first year following a cancer diagnosis, patients often receive more intensive care, placing them at higher risk for symptom burden [66, 67]. Most of the behavioral and psychosocial interventions delivered in this time frame focus on managing symptoms associated with systemic therapies including chemotherapy (e.g., fatigue, pain, anorexia, nausea, and vomiting) [68–72]. For example, Given et al. (2004) examined the efficacy of a 20-week, nurse-administered cognitive-behavioral intervention for patients with several types of cancer undergoing a first course of chemotherapy. The intervention aimed to provide self-management knowledge and skills and assist patients to adopt self-management behaviors. The intervention was efficacious at reducing symptom severity among the patients with higher levels of symptom severity at baseline, compared with treatment as usual [69].

Short-Term or Transitional Survivorship (1–5 Years)

A quarter of all cancer survivors report high symptom burden 1-year post-diagnosis [67]. Among cancer survivors with high symptom burden, common symptoms include pain, fatigue, nausea and vomiting, bowel/bladder control problems, weight change, and respiratory symptoms [67]. Evidence suggests that patients in this phase may benefit from self-management interventions [72]. The Health Navigation program is a 12-week web-based educational program for cancer survivors who completed active treatment [73]. The intervention included five components: self-assessment and graphic reports; online educational modules; messaging service, caregiver support; and health professional monitoring. Compared to usual care, the intervention showed significant improvement in fatigue, anxiety, and overall QOL [73].

Long-Term Survivorship (5+ Years)

The most reported symptoms at this stage attributed to either the cancer or its treatment are pain, weakness, numbness, urinary incontinence, hair loss, and bowel incontinence [74]. For older long-term survivors, the presence of comorbidities may exacerbate their risk for poor HRQoL and physical functioning [75]. Self-management interventions may have a positive effect on the symptoms attributed to cancer or its treatment as well as on other co-occurring chronic diseases (e.g., diabetes, cardiac disease). The Stanford Chronic Disease Self-Management Program (CDSMP) is an evidence-based chronic disease self-management intervention [76] that was adapted to serve cancer patients. This program includes six peer-led weekly group sessions and was designed to improve patient's self-efficacy by promoting goal setting, skills mastery, problem solving, and decision making. Some of the topics covered in the CDSMP included the use of cognitive symptom management techniques, dealing with negative emotions, physical activity, and nutrition [77]. Two effectiveness trials found that this intervention significantly improved pain, depression, and sleep among cancer survivors [77, 78]. Also, being that this intervention is peer-led allows for a more affordable and scalable approach to long-term symptom management.

Advanced Stage Cancer

Patients with advanced stage cancer (stage III or IV) face unique challenges such as losing hope, dying-related anxiety, managing pain caused by the spread of cancer, non-curative treatment goals, feeling like a burden to others, social isolation, and financial toxicity [79]. Pain, fatigue, sleep disorders, depression, and cachexia are the most common symptoms in advanced cancer [80, 81]. Most of the interventions designed for patients with advanced cancer are either supportive, existential or cognitive-behavioral [79]. Supportive interventions focus on providing emotional support, encouraging emotional expression, and promoting adaptive coping strategies. Existential interventions focus on spiritual well-being, enhancing acceptance, hope, and value living. Cognitive-behavioral therapy interventions focus on reframing patients' thoughts and behaviors, promoting problem-solving skills, setting goals, and relaxation. A randomized control trial examined the efficacy of a brief cognitive-behavioral strategy intervention on reducing symptom cluster burden in patients with advanced cancer. The intervention included a single one-on-one training session with a nurse, an educational booklet; and an MP3 player with symptom-focused imagery, nature-focused imagery, relaxation exercises, and nature sounds [82]. Patients receiving the intervention reported less symptom cluster distress post-intervention when compared to the control condition. Mediators of the intervention effect were changes in stress, outcome expectancy and perceived control [82].

Palliative Care

Palliative care (PC) provides a valuable tool for reducing the symptom burden experienced by people living with cancer across the continuum of care. The American Society of Clinical Oncology (ASCO) recommends that any patient with advanced cancer should receive PC early in the disease course and concurrent with active treatment [83]. The integration of PC into oncology practice has improved patients' HRQOL and symptom control, patient-clinician communication, patient and caregiver satisfaction, and reduced healthcare costs [84, 85]. The ENABLE (Educate, Nurture, Advise, Before Life Ends) intervention is a telehealth early PC intervention for patients with advanced cancer and their family caregivers [86, 87]. The intervention includes an initial in-person PC consultation, six 45-minute weekly telephone coaching sessions led by an advanced practice nurse, and monthly follow-up. The sessions focus on enhancing problem solving, symptom management, self-care, decision making, advance care planning, and identifying personal growth opportunities. The patients assigned to the intervention reported improvements in HRQoL and lower depression when compared to those receiving usual care [88]. Subsequent analyses showed that participants assigned to the early PC intervention had a 15% statistically significant improvement in 1-year survival, compared to the usual care group [86].

SPECIFIC POPULATIONS

Despite overall improvements in cancer incidence and mortality, certain populations (e.g., older adults, racial/ethnic minorities) are at risk for higher symptom burden and worse overall health outcomes. In this section we describe symptom management interventions that have been tailored for older adults, individuals who identify as being in racial/ethnic minority groups and those living in rural communities.

Older Adults

Older adults with cancer have a higher prevalence of frailty, geriatric syndromes, lower self-rated health, limitations in activities of daily living (ADL), and limitations in instrumental ADL, compared to older adults without cancer [89]. Some of the most common symptoms among older adults with cancer include pain, fatigue, impaired cognition, anxiety, depression, cachexia, anorexia, and dyspnea. Comprehensive cancer rehabilitation, a multi-disciplinary approach designed to optimize HRQOL and functioning in physical, social, and vocational domains [90] is becoming more commonly applied to older cancer survivors. Among cancer survivors, rehabilitation has been linked to improvements in pain, function, and HRQOL, and has been shown to ameliorate physical and cognitive impairments at every stage of the treatment [91]. Furthermore, coordination of care across multiple providers to address multiple comorbidities, polypharmacy, and age-related functional declines remains challenging, yet it is essential for the restoration of wellbeing and functionality [90].

Comorbidities

In addition to the presence of cancer, patients may have underlying health problems that impact their QOL and ultimately exacerbate their current health status. However, patients can modify their lifestyle behaviors (e.g., diet, physical activity, stress-reduction exercises) to improve their health and wellbeing. Obesity is a modifiable risk-factor of breast cancer, and it places breast cancer survivors at greater risk for cancer recurrence and death [92]. An estimated 35% of cancer survivors in the United States are obese [93]. Interventions targeting weight loss and subsequent weight maintenance in breast cancer survivors may help reduce the risk of premature death from cancer recurrence as well as reduce overall mortality rates associated with obesity [94]. Research shows that higher dietary quality is associated with a reduced risk of death from non-cancer causes among breast cancer survivors [95], and this is important given that breast cancer survivors are more likely to die from comorbidities related to obesity than breast cancer [96, 97]. A recent study, conducted by Marchello and colleagues, examined changes in dietary quality after a 1-year weight maintenance intervention and assessed whether change in dietary quality differed in participants that varied in amount of weight regain (≤5% regain or >5% regain) [98]. They found that dietary quality can be maintained in breast cancer survivors after a weight loss intervention, and that higher dietary quality was associated with less weight regain.

Underrepresented Minorities

In the United States Black/African American men are disproportionately affected by prostate cancer, with 76% higher incidence compared to non-Hispanic White (NHW) men [99]. Also, Black/African American men with prostate cancer report lower HRQoL [100], and are 2.4 times more likely to die from prostate cancer [101], compared to NHW patients. Yanez et al. conducted a study which examined the acceptability, feasibility, and efficacy of a tablet-delivered psychosocial intervention for reducing disease-specific distress in older men with advanced prostate cancer, which also explored differences by race [102, 103]. Participants ($n = 74$) were randomized to either a 10-week Cognitive Behavioral Stress Management (CBSM) or an attention-control Health Promotion condition (control), both of which were delivered by tablets. The intervention was feasible given the good retention rates (>85%) and participants' ratings of acceptability (4/5 on weekly evaluations, and 3.6/4). At the 6-month timepoint, participants in the CBSM condition experienced significantly lower depressive symptoms, improved distress and functional wellbeing compared to those in the control condition. Secondary analyses showed that participants (Black/African American and NHW) in the CBSM group reported significant reductions in anxiety at 6 months that appeared to persist over time, thus providing preliminary evidence that racial/ethnic minorities can be effectively engaged in survivorship interventions with results indicating favorable outcomes. [102]

Rural Communities

Cancer survivors residing in rural areas experience unique challenges and barriers in survivorship care planning, adherence, and coordination [104, 105]. Rural cancer survivors report poorer mental health functioning, increased symptoms of anxiety, depression, distress, and more emotional problems, compared to urban cancer survivors [106]. Health disparities in rural communities may be due to a variety of reasons such as limited access to psychosocial or psycho-oncology services, social-isolation, fewer resources, and existing comorbidities.

CONCLUSION AND FUTURE DIRECTIONS

The available studies generally show that symptom management interventions can enable cancer survivors to achieve optimal physical and psychological well-being, and overall HRQOL. Various behavioral and psychosocial interventions have either improved patients' HRQoL, reduced symptom burden (e.g., psychological distress, fatigue, pain, etc.), and/or improved post-treatment adjustment. Symptom management interventions have ranged from educational programs, to supportive group therapy and individual treatments focused on providing a supportive environment where survivors can express concerns related to cancer survivorship. Interventions based on CBT models are common and use a variety of therapeutic techniques (e.g., cognitive restructuring, relaxation, problem solving skills, etc.) that have shown success in improving social support, self-esteem, emotional distress, physical function, and overall HRQoL among survivors. Other interventions include mindfulness-based stress reduction, health behavior change (e.g., The Stanford Chronic Disease Self-Management Program), and motivational interviewing have been found to improve health outcomes among cancer survivors. There are several ways participants can benefit from symptom management interventions including exchange of information, sharing experiences, reducing social isolation and skills training that facilitate self-efficacy and sense of control over the cancer experience. Interventions can be targeted to an individual or a dyad, depending on the goals of the therapy and targeted outcomes. Interventions can be administered at all phases of the cancer continuum, led by either healthcare providers or peers, and delivered via several modalities such as face-to-face, telephone, or technology-based (e.g., mHealth, telehealth).

Nonpharmacologic interventions using physical strategies with effects across two or more symptoms include: exercise, yoga, massage, cranial stimulation, ice/cooling of scalp and extremities, occupational therapy, physical therapy, tai chi, etc. Behavioral strategies include improving dietary quality, energy conservation, minimizing alcohol consumption, and sleep hygiene. Lastly, psychological strategies include, but are not limited to, psychoeducation, relaxation, cognitive behavioral strategies, guided imagery, mindfulness-based stress reduction, hypnosis, music therapy, coping strategies, psychosocial support, meditation, biofeedback, and motivational interviewing.

Ongoing research initiatives are now focused on the evaluation of dissemination and implementation models of evidence proven interventions, seeking to document the effectiveness of these programs in real-world settings. Several institutions have already integrated systematic PRO monitoring with health information technologies. With funding from the NCI, (the National Cancer Institute's IMPACT program, a newly formed consortium including Harvard University, The Mayo Clinic, and Northwestern University, is exploring mechanisms for integrating PRO data collected via patient portals (e.g., MyChart) into electronic health records (e.g., EPIC) and clinical workflow for cancer care (*link*: https://impactconsortium.org/). Given the complexity of possible interactions between personal, disease, and environmental characteristics, further research is needed to elucidate which type of symptom management intervention is most effective in improving health related QOL and reducing symptom burden among cancer survivors.

REFERENCES

1. National Cancer Institute, *NCI Dictionary of Cancer Terms*. 2020.
2. Sheikh-Wu, S.F., C.A. Downs, and D. Anglade, Interventions for managing a symptom cluster of pain, fatigue, and sleep disturbances during cancer survivorship: a systematic review. *Oncol Nurs Forum*, 2020. **47**(4): pp. e107–e119.
3. Burkett, V.S. and C.S. Cleeland, Symptom burden in cancer survivorship. *J Cancer Surviv*, 2007. **1**(2): pp. 167–175.
4. Henoch, I., et al., Symptom dimensions as outcomes in interventions for patients with cancer: a systematic review. *Oncol Nurs Forum*, 2018. **45**(2): pp. 237–249.
5. Wu, H.S. and J.K. Harden, Symptom burden and quality of life in survivorship: a review of the literature. *Cancer Nurs*, 2015. **38**(1): pp. e29–e54.
6. Ness, S., et al., Concerns across the survivorship trajectory: results from a survey of cancer survivors. *Oncol Nurs Forum*, 2013. **40**(1): pp. 35–42.
7. Ream, E., et al., Telephone interventions for symptom management in adults with cancer. *Cochrane Database Syst Rev*, 2020. **6**(6): p. Cd007568.
8. Henson, L.A., et al., Palliative care and the management of common distressing symptoms in advanced cancer: pain, breathlessness, nausea and vomiting, and fatigue. *J Clin Oncol*, 2020. **38**(9): pp. 905–914.
9. Guimond, A.J., H. Ivers, and J. Savard, Clusters of psychological symptoms in breast cancer: is there a common psychological mechanism? *Cancer Nurs*, 2020. **43**(5): pp. 343–353.
10. Collado-Hidalgo, A., et al., Inflammatory biomarkers for persistent fatigue in breast cancer survivors. *Clin Cancer Res*, 2006. **12**(9): pp. 2759–2766.
11. Kwekkeboom, K.L., et al., Mind-body treatments for the pain-fatigue-sleep disturbance symptom cluster in persons with cancer. *J Pain Symptom Manage*, 2010. **39**(1): pp. 126–138.
12. Miaskowski, C., et al., Advancing symptom science through symptom cluster research: expert panel proceedings and recommendations. *J Natl Cancer Inst*, 2017. **109**(4).
13. Lazarus, R.S. and S. Folkman, *Stress, appraisal, and coping*. 1984.
14. Bandura, A., Self-efficacy mechanism in human agency. *Am Psychol*, 1982. **37**(2): pp. 122–147.
15. McCorkle, R., et al., Self-management: enabling and empowering patients living with cancer as a chronic illness. *CA Cancer J Clin*, 2011. **61**(1): pp. 50–62.
16. Bandura, A., *Social foundations of thought and action*, 1986. Prentice-Hall: Englewood Cliffs, NJ. pp. 23–28.
17. Tallman, I., et al., A theory of problem-solving behavior. *Soc Psychol Q*, 1993. **56**(3): pp. 157–177.
18. Baumeister, R.F., B.J. Schmeichel, and K.D. Vohs, Self-regulation and the executive function: the self as controlling agent, in *Social Psychology: Handbook of Basic Principles, 2nd ed.* 2007. The Guilford Press: New York, NY. pp. 516–539.
19. Miller, W.R. and G.S. Rose, Toward a theory of motivational interviewing. *Am Psychol*, 2009. **64**(6): pp. 527–537.
20. Mishel, M.H., Uncertainty in illness. *Image: J Nurs Scholar*, 1988. **20**(4): pp. 225–232.
21. Parelkar, P., et al., Stress coping and changes in health behavior among cancer survivors: a report from the American Cancer Society's Study of Cancer Survivors-II (SCS-II). *J Psychosoc Oncol*, 2013. **31**(2): pp. 136–152.
22. Antoni, M.H., et al., The influence of bio-behavioural factors on tumour biology: pathways and mechanisms. *Nat Rev Cancer*, 2006. **6**(3): pp. 240–248.
23. Scherz, N., et al., Case management to increase quality of life after cancer treatment: a randomized controlled trial. *BMC Cancer*, 2017. **17**(1): p. 223.
24. Bower, J.E., et al., Mindfulness meditation for younger breast cancer survivors: a randomized controlled trial. *Cancer*, 2015. **121**(8): pp. 1231–1240.
25. Hwang, K.-H., O.-H. Cho, and Y.-S. Yoo, The effect of comprehensive care program for ovarian cancer survivors. *Clin Nurs Res*, 2016. **25**(2): pp. 192–208.
26. Boesen, E.H., et al., Psychoeducational intervention for patients with cutaneous malignant melanoma: a replication study. *J Clin Oncol*, 2005. **23**(6): pp. 1270–1277.
27. ORNISH, D., et al., Intensive lifestyle changes may affect the progression of prostate cancer. *J Urol*, 2005. **174**(3): pp. 1065–1070.
28. Baum, A. and B.L. Andersen, *Psychosocial Interventions for Cancer*. 2009.
29. Zhang, M.-F., et al., Effectiveness of mindfulness-based therapy for reducing anxiety and depression in patients with cancer: a meta-analysis. *Medicine*, 2015. **94**(45): p. e0897.
30. Hu, Y., T. Liu, and F. Li, Association between dyadic interventions and outcomes in cancer patients: a meta-analysis. *Support Care Cancer*, 2019. **27**(3): pp. 745–761.
31. Fujinami, R., et al., Family caregivers' distress levels related to quality of life, burden, and preparedness. *Psychooncology*, 2015. **24**(1): pp. 54–62.
32. Girgis, A., et al., Some things change, some things stay the same: a longitudinal analysis of cancer caregivers' unmet supportive care needs. *Psychooncology*, 2013. **22**(7): pp. 1557–1564.
33. Kim, Y., et al., Prevalence and predictors of depressive symptoms among cancer caregivers 5 years after the relative's cancer diagnosis. *J Consult Clin Psychol*, 2014. **82**(1): pp. 1–8.

34. Adashek, J.J. and I.M. Subbiah, Caring for the caregiver: a systematic review characterising the experience of caregivers of older adults with advanced cancers. *ESMO Open*, 2020. **5**(5).

35. Teixeira, R.J., et al., The impact of coping strategies of cancer caregivers on psychophysiological outcomes: an integrative review. *Psychol Res Behav Manag*, 2018. **11**: pp. 207–215.

36. Pasacreta, J.V., et al., Participant characteristics before and 4 months after attendance at a family caregiver cancer education program. *Cancer Nurs*, 2000. **23**(4): pp. 295–303.

37. Dalton, J.A., et al., Tailoring cognitive-behavioral treatment for cancer pain. *Pain Manag Nurs*, 2004. **5**(1): pp. 3–18.

38. Jarden, M., et al., The effect of a multimodal intervention on treatment-related symptoms in patients undergoing hemato-poietic stem cell transplantation: a randomized controlled trial. *J Pain Symptom Manage*, 2009. **38**(2): pp. 174–190.

39. Kwekkeboom, K.L., et al. Guideline-recommended symptom management strategies that cross over two or more cancer symptoms in oncology nursing forum. 2020. *Oncology Nursing Society*.

40. Wu, L.M., et al., Computerized cognitive training in prostate cancer patients on androgen deprivation therapy: a pilot study. *Support Care Cancer*, 2018. **26**(6): pp. 1917–1926.

41. Miriovsky, B.J., L.N. Shulman, and A.P. Abernethy, Importance of health information technology, electronic health records, and continuously aggregating data to comparative effectiveness research and learning health care. *J Clin Oncol*, 2012. **30**(34): pp. 4243–4248.

42. Wernhart, A., S. Gahbauer, and D. Haluza, eHealth and telemedicine: practices and beliefs among healthcare professionals and medical students at a medical university. *PLOS ONE*, 2019. **14**(2): p. e0213067.

43. Penedo, F.J., et al., The increasing value of eHealth in the delivery of patient-centred cancer care. *Lancet Oncol*, 2020. **21**(5): pp. e240–e251.

44. Cella, D., et al., The Patient-Reported Outcomes Measurement Information System (PROMIS): progress of an NIH Roadmap cooperative group during its first two years. *Medical Care*, 2007. **45**(5 Suppl 1): pp. S3–S11.

45. Basch, E., et al., Symptom monitoring with patient-reported outcomes during routine cancer treatment: a randomized controlled trial. *J Clin Oncol*, 2016. **34**(6): pp. 557–565.

46. World Health Organization, mHealth: new horizons for health through mobile technologies. mHealth: new horizons for health through mobile technologies, 2011.

47. Keefe, F.J., et al., Effects of spouse-assisted coping skills training and exercise training in patients with osteoarthritic knee pain: a randomized controlled study. *Pain*, 2004. **110**(3): pp. 539–549.

48. Somers, T.J., et al., A pilot study of a mobile health pain coping skills training protocol for patients with persistent cancer pain. *J Pain Symptom Manage*, 2015. **50**(4): pp. 553–558.

49. Cox, A., et al., Cancer survivors' experience with telehealth: a systematic review and thematic synthesis. *J Med Internet Res*, 2017. **19**(1): pp. e11–e11.

50. Chan, B.A., et al., Do teleoncology models of care enable safe delivery of chemotherapy in rural towns? *Med J Aust*, 2015. **203**(10): pp. 406–406.e6.

51. Wagner, J.A. and D.L. Kroetz, Transforming translation: impact of clinical and translational science. *Clin Transl Sci*, 2016. **9**(1): pp. 3–5.

52. Senchak, J.J., C.Y. Fang, and J.R. Bauman, Interventions to improve quality of life (QOL) and/or mood in patients with head and neck cancer (HNC): a review of the evidence. *Cancers Head Neck*, 2019. **4**: p. 2.

53. Devins, G.M., et al., The burden of stress in head and neck cancer. *Psychooncology*, 2013. **22**(3): pp. 668–676.

54. van der Meulen, I.C., et al., Long-term effect of a nurse-led psychosocial intervention on health-related quality of life in patients with head and neck cancer: a randomised controlled trial. *Br J Cancer*, 2014. **110**(3): pp. 593–601.

55. van der Meulen, I.C., et al., One-year effect of a nurse-led psychosocial intervention on depressive symptoms in patients with head and neck cancer: a randomized controlled trial. *Oncologist*, 2013. **18**(3): pp. 336–344.

56. Reb, A., et al., Empowering survivors after colorectal and lung cancer treatment: pilot study of a Self-Management Survivorship Care Planning intervention. *Eur J Oncol Nurs*, 2017. **29**: pp. 125–134.

57. Bours, M.J., et al., Candidate predictors of health-related quality of life of colorectal cancer survivors: a systematic review. *Oncologist*, 2016. **21**(4): pp. 433–452.

58. Gosselin, T.K., et al., The symptom experience in rectal cancer survivors. *J Pain Symptom Manage*, 2016. **52**(5): pp. 709–718.

59. Sun, V., et al., Surviving colorectal cancer: long-term, persistent ostomy-specific concerns and adaptations. *J Wound Ostomy Continence Nurs*, 2013. **40**(1): pp. 61–72.

60. Sun, V., et al., From diagnosis through survivorship: health-care experiences of colorectal cancer survivors with ostomies. *Support Care Cancer*, 2014. **22**(6): pp. 1563–1570.

61. Kenzik, K.M., et al., How much do cancer-related symptoms contribute to health-related quality of life in lung and colorec-tal cancer patients? A report from the Cancer Care Outcomes Research and Surveillance (CanCORS) Consortium. *Cancer*, 2015. **121**(16): pp. 2831–2839.

62. Kim, J.Y., et al., The impact of lung cancer surgery on quality of life trajectories in patients and family caregivers. *Lung Cancer*, 2016. **101**: pp. 35–39.

63. Manitta, V., et al., The symptom burden of patients with hematological malignancy: a cross-sectional observational study. *J Pain Symptom Manage*, 2011. **42**(3): pp. 432–442.

64. Jim, H.S.L., et al., Internet-assisted cognitive behavioral intervention for targeted therapy-related fatigue in chronic myeloid leukemia: Results from a pilot randomized trial. *Cancer*, 2020. **126**(1): pp. 174–180.

65. Chang, P.H., et al., Effects of a walking intervention on fatigue-related experiences of hospitalized acute myelogenous leukemia patients undergoing chemotherapy: a randomized controlled trial. *J Pain Symptom Manage*, 2008. **35**(5): pp. 524–534.

66. Bubis, L.D., et al., Symptom burden in the first year after cancer diagnosis: an analysis of patient-reported outcomes. *J Clin Oncol*, 2018. **36**(11): pp. 1103–1111.

67. Shi, Q., et al., Symptom burden in cancer survivors 1 year after diagnosis. *Cancer*, 2011. **117**(12): pp. 2779–2790.

68. Traeger, L., et al., Nursing intervention to enhance outpatient chemotherapy symptom management: patient-reported outcomes of a randomized controlled trial. *Cancer*, 2015. **121**(21): pp. 3905–3913.

69. Given, C., et al., Effect of a cognitive behavioral intervention on reducing symptom severity during chemotherapy. *J Clin Oncol*, 2004. **22**(3): pp. 507–516.

70. Ream, E., A. Richardson, and C. Alexander-Dann, Supportive intervention for fatigue in patients undergoing chemotherapy: a randomized controlled trial. *J Pain Symptom Manage*, 2006. **31**(2): pp. 148–161.

71. Williams, S.A. and A.M. Schreier, The role of education in managing fatigue, anxiety, and sleep disorders in women undergoing chemotherapy for breast cancer. *Appl Nurs Res*, 2005. **18**(3): pp. 138–147.

72. McCorkle, R., et al., Self-management: enabling and empowering patients living with cancer as a chronic illness. *CA Cancer J Clin*, 2011. **61**(1): pp. 50–62.

73. Yun, Y.H., et al., Web-based tailored education program for disease-free cancer survivors with cancer-related fatigue: a randomized controlled trial. *J Clin Oncol*, 2012. **30**(12): pp. 1296–1303.

74. Deimling, G.T., et al., The health of older-adult, long-term cancer survivors. *Cancer Nurs*, 2005. **28**(6).

75. Leach, C.R., et al., The complex health profile of long-term cancer survivors: prevalence and predictors of comorbid conditions. *J Cancer Surviv*, 2015. **9**(2): pp. 239–251.

76. Lorig, K.R., et al., Evidence suggesting that a chronic disease self-management program can improve health status while reducing hospitalization: a randomized trial. *Med Care*, 1999: pp. 5–14.

77. Salvatore, A.L., et al., National study of chronic disease self-management: 6-month and 12-month findings among cancer survivors and non-cancer survivors. *Psychooncology*, 2015. **24**(12): pp. 1714–1722.

78. Risendal, B.C., et al., Meeting the challenge of cancer survivorship in public health: results from the evaluation of the chronic disease self-management program for cancer survivors. *Front Public Health*, 2015. **2**: p. 214.

79. Taylor-Ford, M., Clinical considerations for working with patients with advanced cancer. *J Clin Psychol Med Settings*, 2014. **21**(3): pp. 201–213.

80. Teunissen, S.C.C.M., et al., Symptom prevalence in patients with incurable cancer: a systematic review. *J Pain Symptom Manage*, 2007. **34**(1): pp. 94–104.

81. Tsai, J.-S., et al., Significance of symptom clustering in palliative care of advanced cancer patients. *J Pain Symptom Manage*, 2010. **39**(4): pp. 655–662.

82. Kwekkeboom, K., et al., Randomized controlled trial of a brief cognitive-behavioral strategies intervention for the pain, fatigue, and sleep disturbance symptom cluster in advanced cancer. *Psychooncology*, 2018. **27**(12): pp. 2761–2769.

83. Ferrell, B.R., et al., Integration of palliative care into standard oncology care: American Society of Clinical Oncology Clinical Practice Guideline Update. *J Clin Oncol*, 2017. **35**(1): pp. 96–112.

84. Hui, D., et al., Improving patient and caregiver outcomes in oncology: team-based, timely, and targeted palliative care. *CA Cancer J Clin*, 2018. **68**(5): pp. 356–376.

85. Haun, M.W., et al., Early palliative care for adults with advanced cancer. *Cochrane Database Syst Rev*, 2017. **6**(6): p. Cd011129.

86. Bakitas, M.A., et al., Early versus delayed initiation of concurrent palliative oncology care: patient outcomes in the ENABLE III randomized controlled trial. *J Clin Oncol*, 2015. **33**(13): pp. 1438–1445.

87. Bakitas, M., et al., Project ENABLE: a palliative care demonstration project for advanced cancer patients in three settings. *J Palliat Med*, 2004. **7**(2): pp. 363–372.

88. Bakitas, M., et al., Effects of a palliative care intervention on clinical outcomes in patients with advanced cancer: the Project ENABLE II randomized controlled trial. *JAMA*, 2009. **302**(7): pp. 741–749.

89. Mohile, S.G., et al., Association of a cancer diagnosis with vulnerability and frailty in older Medicare beneficiaries. *J Natl Cancer Inst*, 2009. **101**(17): pp. 1206–1215.

90. Pergolotti, M., K.D. Lyons, and G.R. Williams, Moving beyond symptom management towards cancer rehabilitation for older adults: answering the 5W's. *J Geriatr Oncol*, 2018. **9**(6): pp. 543–549.

91. Silver, J.K., J. Baima, and R.S. Mayer, Impairment-driven cancer rehabilitation: an essential component of quality care and survivorship. *CA Cancer J Clin*, 2013. **63**(5): pp. 295–317.

92. Chlebowski, R.T., E. Aiello, and A. McTiernan, Weight loss in breast cancer patient management. *J Clin Oncol*, 2002. **20**(4): pp. 1128–1143.

93. National Cancer Institute (NCI), Obesity and Cancer: Pursuing Precision Public Health, in Cancer Trends Progress Report. 2020.

94. Playdon, M., et al., Weight loss intervention for breast cancer survivors: a systematic review. *Curr Breast Cancer Rep*, 2013. **5**(3): pp. 222–246.

95. George, S.M., et al., Better postdiagnosis diet quality is associated with reduced risk of death among postmenopausal women with invasive breast cancer in the women's health initiative. *Cancer Epidemiol Biomarkers Prev*, 2014. **23**(4): p. 575.

96. Demark-Wahnefried, W., et al., Riding the crest of the teachable moment: promoting long-term health after the diagnosis of cancer. *J Clin Oncol*, 2005. **23**(24): pp. 5814–5830.

97. Patnaik, J.L., et al., Cardiovascular disease competes with breast cancer as the leading cause of death for older females diagnosed with breast cancer: a retrospective cohort study. *Breast Cancer Res*, 2011. **13**(3): p. R64.

98. Marchello, N.J., et al., Rural breast cancer survivors are able to maintain diet quality improvements during a weight loss maintenance intervention. *J Cancer Surviv*, 2020.

99. American Cancer Society, *Cancer Facts & Figures for African Americans 2019–2021*.

100. Kinlock, B.L., et al., High levels of medical mistrust are associated with low quality of life among black and white men with prostate cancer. *Cancer Control*, 2017. **24**(1): pp. 72–77.

101. Mehnert, A., et al., Depression, anxiety, post-traumatic stress disorder and health-related quality of life and its association with social support in ambulatory prostate cancer patients. *Eur J Cancer Care (Engl)*, 2010. **19**(6): pp. 736–745.

102. Bouchard, L.C., et al., Brief report of a tablet-delivered psychosocial intervention for men with advanced prostate cancer: Acceptability and efficacy by race. *Transl Behav Med*, 2019. **9**(4): pp. 629–637.

103. Yanez, B., et al., Feasibility, acceptability, and preliminary efficacy of a technology-assisted psychosocial intervention for racially diverse men with advanced prostate cancer. *Cancer*, 2015. **121**(24): pp. 4407–4415.

104. Butow, P.N., et al., Psychosocial well-being and supportive care needs of cancer patients living in urban and rural/regional areas: a systematic review. *Support Care Cancer*, 2012. **20**(1): pp. 1–22.

105. Baseman, J., D. Revere, and L.M. Baldwin, A mobile breast cancer survivorship care app: pilot study. *JMIR Cancer*, 2017. **3**(2): p. e14.

106. Burris, J.L. and M. Andrykowski, Disparities in mental health between rural and nonrural cancer survivors: a preliminary study. *Psychooncology*, 2010. **19**(6): pp. 637–645.

Effects of Cancer Therapy on Cognition

9

Rebecca A. Harrison and Shelli R. Kesler

WHAT IS CANCER-RELATED COGNITIVE IMPAIRMENT (CRCI)?

Cancer and its therapies are associated with increased risk for neurotoxic injury resulting in acute, chronic, and/or progressive cognitive impairment. This condition is known colloquially as "chemobrain." However, radiation, surgery, and other therapies as well as the cancer itself have also been associated with cognitive decline and therefore, cancer-related cognitive impairment (CRCI), is a more accurate term. CRCI affects an estimated 60% or more of patients with cancer (1, 2). As of 2019, there were approximately 17 million cancer survivors in the United States (3), which translates into over 10 million individuals at high risk for CRCI, twice the number of Americans with Alzheimer's disease (4). Further, the median age of adult-onset cancer diagnosis is 66 years, making CRCI a condition that intersects disease, aging, and neurodegeneration (5, 6).

The severity of CRCI has been classified via neuropsychological tests as being "mild to moderate" (7). However, patient reported outcomes suggest much greater severity. Biomarker studies have suggested that chemotherapy is associated with two to four years of gray matter aging (8, 9) and over 14 years of cellular aging (10). The accelerated aging evidence has raised concern regarding increased risk for neurodegenerative disease. Some epidemiological studies have suggested that cancer and chemotherapy are associated with increased risk of Alzheimer's disease while other reports have not supported these findings (11). It seems more likely that there are shared risk factors that explain the overlap between cancer and neurodegeneration (12).

Most CRCI studies to date have focused on primary breast cancer although growing evidence indicates CRCI across cancer types (13). This may be surprising given that primary breast cancer originates outside the central nervous system (CNS) and has limited CNS-directed therapies. In fact, the existence of CRCI has been controversial as a result. Some of the main arguments presented against the existence of CRCI in non-CNS cancer have included (1) systemic chemotherapy does not cross the blood-brain barrier, (2) cognitive effects are simply due to the stress of having cancer, and (3) objective evaluation shows "normal" cognitive functioning in many patients.

DOI: 10.1201/9781003055426-9

Chemotherapy and the Blood-Brain Barrier

Most chemotherapies, especially those prescribed for non-CNS cancers, are administered systemically (e.g., intravenously, orally) and many of them have restricted direct access to the brain because they cannot actively cross the blood-brain barrier. However, chemotherapy treatment can disrupt blood-brain barrier function (14). Additionally, restricted direct access does not necessarily mean complete exclusion. Accordingly, there is evidence of measurable passive uptake of systemically administered chemotherapy in the CNS (15). The amount of passive uptake is very minimal, but in vitro and in vivo studies have shown that these same amounts cause significant neuronal death (16) and suppression of neural progenitor proliferation (17, 18). Therefore, even very small quantities of chemotherapy in the brain may be more than enough to result in significant brain injury.

In fact, neuroimaging studies have consistently demonstrated widespread, long-term structural and functional brain injury following cancer and its treatments, even in non-CNS origin cancers. These findings have demonstrated effects in all cortical lobes as well as several subcortical structures including hippocampus, thalamus, and cerebellum [Figure 9.1, see (19, 20) for reviews]. Notably, one neuroimaging study showed that anthracycline-based chemotherapies, which do not actively cross the blood-brain barrier, were significantly more toxic to functional brain networks and cognitive functioning in patients with primary breast cancer than non-anthracyclines, which actively cross the blood-brain barrier (21). Therefore, the argument that the blood-brain barrier would prevent CRCI does not seem to be supported by the evidence.

CRCI and Psychological Distress

Many patients with cancer have reported being told their cognitive complaints were "just stress" and not possibly due to cancer therapies. Patients with cancer do in fact have much higher incidences of depression and anxiety compared to the general population (22) and these symptoms are known to exacerbate cognitive problems (19, 23–25). However, multiple studies have demonstrated brain injury and associated cognitive impairment in patients with non-CNS cancer even after excluding those with significant psychological distress or fatigue, and/or simultaneously controlling for these factors in statistical models (26–32). Despite distress and fatigue levels being higher than that of controls, these studies have noted that symptoms are, on average, subclinical in patients and not highly correlated with objective cognitive testing (33). Furthermore, treatment-naive patients tend to show significantly better cognitive performance and neurobiologic status, frequently even indistinguishable from that of healthy controls, despite showing similar levels of distress and fatigue to treated patients (12, 34–37). Thus, the literature supports that CRCI can occur independently of distress. However, distress is often difficult to disentangle from CRCI and treating symptoms of anxiety, depression, and fatigue can result in improved cognitive function in some cases.

Evaluation of CRCI

Another argument against the existence of CRCI stems from frequent findings of normal cognitive performance on objective evaluation. Despite the significant and widespread brain changes observed in neuroimaging studies of CRCI, behavioral assessments show less consistent effects (19, 20, 38). Some studies indicate that patients show deficits on both objective and subjective measures of cognitive function (20, 39–42) while other studies show no effects (43–46). This inconsistency likely reflects variations in patient sampling, assessment selection, and statistical analysis, among others. However, a well-known issue in the CRCI literature is that patient reported outcome measures often indicate very significant cognitive dysfunction whereas objective measures tend to show average or normal functioning (41, 47, 48).

Clinically, CRCI is most often evaluated using standardized neuropsychological tests but many of these measures were developed to assess severe neuropathology and therefore may have ceiling effects

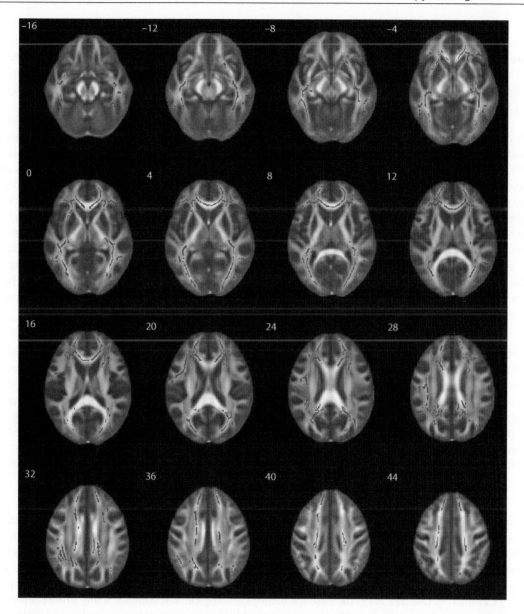

FIGURE 9.1   CRCI is associated with widespread brain injury. Multiple studies have indicated diffuse functional and structural brain deficits in patients with cancer, especially following chemotherapy treatment. In this example, red indicates areas of significantly lower white matter integrity in female breast cancer survivors compared to females with no cancer history. Cancer survivors were 6 years, on average, post-chemotherapy. (From Kesler SR, Watson CL, Blayney DW. Brain network alterations and vulnerability to simulated neurodegeneration in breast cancer. *Neurobiol Aging*. 2015;36(8):2429–42.)

for CRCI. Neuropsychological tests also assess very broad domains of cognitive function, summarizing multiple cognitive processes into one score. It may be that CRCI is associated with deficits in some but not all of these processes, requiring greater precision of measurement (49). Relatedly, there are currently no specific diagnostic criteria for CRCI and statistical thresholds used to distinguish impaired versus non-impaired patients remain arbitrary (43). Neuropsychological testing is limited in terms of sensitivity to CRCI but also lacks ecological validity for assessing cognitive function in general (41, 50). For example, one standardized test that has been recommended for assessing CRCI (51) requires the patient to connect numbered circles with a line as quickly as possible. In controlled assessment settings, this is believed to measure various aspects of visual tracking, attention, and processing speed, but the actions themselves have little if any transference to real-world skills. Patients reporting CRCI most often describe difficulties with daily tasks that are not well reflected in neuropsychological testing scores, such as taking notes during a work meeting, completing exams and schoolwork on time, or tracking conversations with friends and family (52).

"Normal" neuropsychological test scores may represent a decline from a previously higher level of performance. This decline would potentially be observed with serial evaluation, but pre-treatment neuropsychological surveillance is not currently standard of care for most patients, especially those with non-CNS origin cancer. Additionally, neuropsychological tests are highly susceptible to practice effects and standards for determining reliable change across repeated assessments have not been established. Further, like most biological processes, cognition exists on a continuum and research suggests that CRCI involves various subtypes characterized by different levels and combinations of symptoms (53). This suggests that the binary definition of CRCI that is typically employed (i.e., impaired vs. not impaired) excludes many patients who may have real-world deficits following cancer and its treatments. In other words, one level of impairment may be manageable for some patients but not for others. Accordingly, patients with higher educational and occupational achievement tend to endorse greater subjective cognitive impairment. These patients were likely above average cognitively before cancer treatment and then struggled to perform at their high-level jobs after declining to average cognitive ability.

Patient L.D., a 53 year old female breast cancer survivor, was an engineer prior to her diagnosis. She demonstrated average to above average neuropsychological performance after cancer treatment with the exception of memory encoding. However, in addition to memory problems, she reported multiple difficulties with attention, executive function, processing speed and language during her daily life and indicated that she "could not function at the same level as before cancer." She struggled with work performance and was eventually let go from her job as a result. She was denied disability even after several appeals and despite her neuropsychologist advocating on her behalf. She reported that her oncologist did not support her claims telling her that her cognitive symptoms could not be due to cancer treatment.

Patient reported outcome measures involve patient ratings of their own functioning so tend to be more ecologically valid. Patient reported outcomes assess cognitive functioning over a greater time period (e.g., past two weeks) compared to neuropsychological tests, which are based on a single time point. However, patient reported outcomes are also not without their flaws. Patient reported outcome measures are highly susceptible to the influence of response biases, transient situational factors, attitudes, and psychological distress (54, 55). As is the case for neuropsychological assessments, many different patient reported outcome measures exist. Their use has been highly inconsistent across studies of CRCI with no current consensus regarding which measure is best for this syndrome. Additionally, very few studies have used patient reported outcomes as a primary end point (48) making it difficult to determine the pattern of subjective cognitive function that characterizes CRCI. It is likely that subjective and objective cognitive function represent overlapping but separate phenotypes of CRCI and therefore it is critical to include both approaches when evaluating this syndrome.

REAL-WORLD IMPACT OF CRCI

CRCI impacts cancer patients during acute treatment and into the survivorship period. While the functional implications of CRCI are not well-studied, data does suggest it has a far-reaching impact on multiple dimensions of patient life. In addition to the financial incentives, returning to work can restore some normalcy to patients, improve quality of life, and provide a sense of meaningful contribution to society. However, as illustrated above, patients with CRCI often demonstrate difficulties with occupational functioning. With nearly half of all cancer patients being under the age of 65 years, the impact of cognition on vocational capabilities and return to work is a viable concern. Cancer is associated with significant economic burden including loss of productivity (56) and is the second leading cause of long-term disability applications (57), contributing to financial toxicity. A majority (approximately 64%) of patients with cancer return to work at some point following their diagnosis, however, they are at increased risk for negative employment outcomes (58). Long-term survivors are 1.4 times more likely to be unemployed than healthy controls, with a higher incidence of unemployment among those in the United States (59). Older, less educated, lower socioeconomic status patients are particularly vulnerable to negative employment outcomes (60).

Another area of potential impact, especially for younger patients, includes educational pursuits. Most research to date regarding educational impact of CRCI has involved survivors of pediatric cancers. Learning difficulties, increased special education placement and reduced educational attainment are commonly observed among these patients (61, 62). However, adult patients with and survivors of cancer are also at risk for academic difficulties.

> Six months after completing surgery and chemoradiation for nasopharyngeal carcinoma, patient Y.C., a 36 year old female, returned to nursing school and noted difficulty with her concentration and her retention of information. She reported that a three to four hour lecture would take her "a couple of days" to completely review. She was not able to follow lectures in the moment. She noted her grades had dropped, even though she was taking just as long or longer to prepare as she had prior to her diagnosis. She had recently failed an exam, because she was not able to complete the exam in time.

CRCI has been repeatedly associated with decreased quality of life and overall survival in multiple cancer types (63–65). This relationship is complex and is likely reflective of the overall reserve and health of the patient, the aggressiveness of the cancer, and the imparted treatments, among other variables. It does highlight CRCI as an early predictive factor for survival outcome that warrants clinical attention. In patients with newly diagnosed glioblastoma, the identification of cognitive impairment has been found as an independent predictor of overall survival (66), with the domains of executive function and attention being the most strongly associated with survival outcome. Cognitive impairment has also been shown to predict survival in patients with breast, prostate or colorectal cancer (67) demonstrating this relationship extends beyond CNS cancers. The reason for this is currently unclear though it may relate to shared genetic risk factors between cancer and cognitive decline and/or effects of tumor pathogenesis on the brain as described below and/or the significant relationship between CRCI and reduced adherence to cancer treatments (44, 64).

CRCI can have a deep personal impact on patient well-being. In a qualitative study of 74 breast cancer survivors, cognitive dysfunction was reported as the most distressing post-treatment symptom, resulting in reduced quality of life and level of daily functioning (68). CRCI has been shown to negatively impact patients' self-confidence and social relationships (69). Cognitive deficit is also associated with loss of autonomy (67). These findings support CRCI as having a far-reaching impact on patient quality of life, function, and survival, emphasizing the importance of a fundamental fluency in this area among those caring for and studying cancer patients and survivors.

WHAT CAUSES CRCI?

Although the precise pathophysiology of CRCI remains unclear, there are several candidate mechanisms including direct neurotoxicity, cancer pathogenesis, inflammation, oxidative stress, altered cerebral blood supply, DNA damage, mitochondrial dysfunction and hypothalamic-pituitary-adrenal (HPA) axis dysregulation, among others (Figure 9.2). The final common biologic pathway of these mechanisms

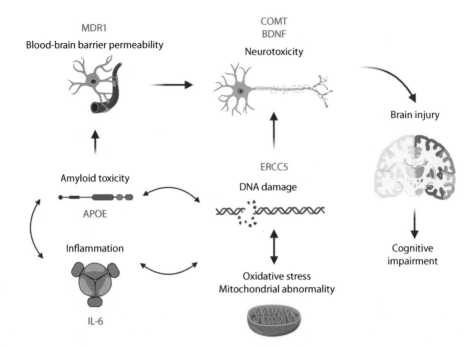

FIGURE 9.2 Candidate mechanisms of CRCI. Cancer-related cognitive impairment is believed to result from several possible biologic pathways including cancer pathogenesis, direct neurotoxicity of treatments, inflammatory response, DNA damage, oxidative stress, and mitochondrial dysfunction. These mechanisms interact to have both direct and indirect effects on the brain, not all of which are illustrated here. Several genes (shown in red text) may moderate certain mechanisms. The final common pathway of these mechanisms is altered brain structure and function (brain injury), which results in cognitive impairment. MDR1: multi-drug resistance 1, APOE: apolipoprotein, IL-6: interleukin-6, 5-HTTLPR: serotonin-transporter-linked polymorphic region, COMT: catechol-O-methyltransferase; BDNF: brain-derived neurotrophic factor, ERCC5: excision repair 5, endonuclease. (Figure created with BioRender.com.)

is diffuse brain injury as indicated by neuroimaging studies [see (19, 20) for reviews]. Notably, many of the candidate mechanisms for CRCI are closely associated with aging (70) and accordingly, older patients tend to have poorer cognitive outcome following chemotherapy (71).

Cancer Pathogenesis

Several studies have shown negative impact on brain function prior to treatment initiation, as well as a correlation between CRCI and disease severity, (72) suggesting a role of cancer pathogenesis in CRCI. A study of breast cancer patients showed that one third of patients had some evidence of cognitive impairment prior to the initiation of anticancer therapy (73). In a separate cohort of patients with breast cancer, mood and psychological distress were both significant predictors of pre-treatment self-reported cognitive dysfunction (74, 75), suggesting psychological distress from the diagnosis itself may be contributing to pretreatment changes. Another study demonstrated widespread though subtle differences in brain connectivity among pre-treatment patients with breast cancer compared to healthy controls (29). Tumor-induced inflammation and cytokine release are commonly hypothesized mechanisms of CRCI as well as other symptoms of cancer (fatigue, anorexia) (76, 77). Cytokines actively cross the blood-brain barrier (78) and also indirectly lead to impairment of blood-brain barrier integrity (79). Cytokines activate microglia and astrocytes, stimulate local inflammation and induce oxidative and nitrosative brain damage (80–82). Patel et al. noted that cognitive deficits were highly correlated with markers of peripheral inflammation in pre-treatment patients with breast cancer (83).

Malignant tumors and inflammatory responses are also associated with aberrant angiogenesis (84). One study observed elevated plasma vascular endothelial growth factor (VEGF), a common angiogenic factor, in patients with breast cancer following chemotherapy treatment, that was negatively correlated with cognition (85). VEGF is expressed in the brain and is believed to play an important role in neurodegeneration. However, the study did not evaluate baseline, pre-treatment VEGF levels. Long-term breast cancer survivors also have increased incidence of cerebral small vessel disease following cancer therapies (86) but it is currently unknown if these vascular effects exist prior to treatment initiation. Certain tumors also incite abnormal neurogenesis and nerve growth factor release (87–89), which may result in aberrant CNS activity via peripheral innervation. Tumor aggressiveness has been associated with tumor-related neurogenesis (87). The potential roles of tumor-related angiogenesis and neurogenesis in CRCI require further investigation.

Treatment-related Neurotoxicities

Surgery

The perioperative period can be associated with cognitive impairment, with anesthetic exposure, perioperative stress, and the surgery itself being potential contributors. This is often referred to as postoperative cognitive dysfunction (POCD) and tends to be more common in older patients (90). However, several studies suggest at least transient POCD in younger patients with cancer as well. For example, a study of middle-aged breast cancer patients found differences in functional brain activation patterns during visuospatial working memory tasks among early post-operative breast cancer patients prior to chemotherapy exposure (91). Since there was no pre-operative assessment, the effects of tumor pathogenesis could not be excluded from these findings. However, a longitudinal study of patients with breast cancer found that attentional function declined pre-surgery to 2 years after surgery (92). Risk factors for POCD include duration of surgery and anesthesia, hypoxia, hypercarbia, and hypotension (93). Proposed mechanisms of POCD include sustained impact of anesthetic exposure, intraoperative blood pressure fluctuations, perioperative infections, pain medications, and systemic inflammatory response (94). However, the contribution of surgery and anesthesia to persistent CRCI remains unclear.

Neurosurgery for CNS cancers is associated with additional risk factors and complications. Advanced surgical technology has resulted in improved tumor removal or resection. However, this tends to involve larger volumes of brain tissue being removed, which is potentially damaging to functioning brain regions (95). Accordingly, some patients show improvement in cognitive function following tumor resection while others show worsening of cognitive function (95, 96). The location and size of the tumor seem to significantly influence the patient's cognitive outcome following resection. Additionally, cognitive decline following tumor resection may be only temporary (95, 97) and in many cases, surgery tends to improve cognitive performance.

Chemotherapy

As noted above, chemotherapy is believed to have some direct neurotoxic effects on neurons, synapses and neural progenitor cells. Chemotherapy may also have indirect effects on the brain via inflammation, DNA damage, oxidative stress, and mitochondrial injury. Chemotherapy induces cytokine release and several studies have demonstrated elevated peripheral cytokine levels in patients with cancer, even several years post-chemotherapy (98, 99). Additionally, lower brain volumes and/or cognitive functioning have been shown to be correlated with increased peripheral inflammation in chemotherapy treated patients (100–102) and rodents (103).

Most chemotherapies exert their anti-cancer effects by disrupting various phases of the cell cycle to prevent cell division. The mechanism of action is direct or indirect DNA or RNA damage including double strand breaks, intercalation, and inhibition of enzymes, among others. Radiation therapy and certain hormone blockade therapies (e.g., Tamoxifen) have also been associated with significant DNA damage (104–106). These mechanisms affect normal cells as well as malignant ones, which can cause several side effects, including CRCI. Specifically, there are sites of ongoing neurogenesis in the brain including the hippocampus, olfactory areas, and subventricular zones. As noted above, several preclinical studies have demonstrated significantly suppressed neurogenesis following chemotherapy treatment (18, 107, 108). This impairs the neuroplasticity that supports new learning and brain network resilience.

Chemotherapy (and radiation treatments) produce massive free radicals including reactive oxygen species (ROS) that are toxic to many organs, including the brain. Oxidative stress can further damage DNA, which compounds the accumulated DNA damage and inefficient DNA repair mechanisms associated with the aging process (109). As noted below, patients with an apolipoprotein (APOE) e4 genotype may have increased risk for CRCI, potentially related to decreased amyloid-beta clearance. Some studies have observed increased levels of amyloid-beta in patients with cancer (110) as well as an association between amyloid-beta, tumor development, and metastatic potential (111). Amyloid-beta is believed to induce oxidative stress and oxidative DNA damage (112, 113). Several preclinical studies have related oxidative stress to brain injury and associated cognitive impairment in chemotherapy animal models (114, 115). Conroy and colleagues showed that oxidative DNA damage in patients with breast cancer was related to lower gray matter density, which was associated with poorer memory performance. These patients were 6 years post-chemotherapy on average yet had significantly higher levels of DNA damage compared to age-matched controls, suggesting that this is long-term effect (116).

Given its critical role in energy production, impairment of mitochondrial function has widespread effects on organ systems, especially the brain, which is the greatest consumer of metabolic resources. Mitochondria produce energy via oxidative phosphorylation, which inherently generates ROS as a by-product. Under normal conditions, these ROS levels seem to support certain cellular processes (113). However, chemotherapies, especially anthracyclines, have been shown to damage mitochondria via inflammation, oxidative stress, and impaired autophagy (117–119). Damaged mitochondria show reduced respiratory activity and paradoxically exacerbated production of ROS (120, 121). Mitochondrial DNA is even more susceptible to oxidative damage compared to nuclear DNA due to its proximity to ROS production and lack of repair mechanisms. Mitochondrial DNA thus has a higher mutation rate than nuclear DNA (122) and several of these mutations have been linked to cognitive impairment (123). Neuroimaging studies of CRCI provide indirect evidence of metabolic dysfunction including increased cerebral perfusion (which is coupled with metabolism) (124), increased cerebral glucose uptake (125), costly brain network over-integration (126) and metabolically greedy cortical hub vulnerability (2, 127). Additionally, mesenchymal stem cells, which are believed to donate their mitochondria to sites of injury, have been shown to ameliorate cognitive impairment and brain injury in chemotherapy-treated rodents (128, 129).

Radiation Therapy

Locoregional radiation

Breast cancer patients who receive upfront radiation therapy have increased rates of chronic fatigue, though not as high as those treated with chemotherapy in addition to radiation (130). To date, very few studies have focused on locoregional radiation and therefore the effects of this therapy on cognition remain largely unclear. One study found that breast cancer patients who received locoregional therapy had similar cognitive outcomes to those receiving systemic chemotherapy at 18-month follow up (131) but others have shown a negative impact of locoregional radiation on cognitive performance as well as brain functional activation (132, 133). It is also difficult to separate the potential effects of radiation and chemotherapy since many patients receive both treatments. While the mechanism by which locoregional radiation causes neurocognitive changes are not well defined, systemic inflammatory response, DNA damage, and oxidative stress are leading candidates.

CNS-directed radiation
Radiation therapy is a central component of the treatment for many primary and metastatic brain tumors. One of the main toxicities of CNS-directed radiation therapy is short- and long-term cognitive deficit. Preclinical study has identified several contributory biologic mechanisms that occur longitudinally after radiation exposure. These include impairment of neuronal stem cell proliferation and differentiation (134), and microglial activation with upregulation of CNS inflammatory pathways (135). Vascular mechanisms are also thought to contribute to the neurotoxicity of radiation, with capillary loss preceding radiation-induced neurocognitive changes (136).

In a longitudinal study of patients with low grade gliomas, patients who received upfront radiation therapy were compared to those that had deferred radiation to time of progression. While initial follow up at 6 years did not reveal significant cognitive differences between groups (137), the impact of early radiation therapy was significant at the 12-year follow up, where progressive neurocognitive decline in multiple cognitive domains was evident in the early-radiation therapy group (138). This supports a time-dependent impact of radiation therapy on brain health, which has been corroborated in other studies (139). In patients with brain metastases, attempts to reduce the cognitive toxicities of whole brain radiation therapy (WBRT) have resulted in new avenues of clinical research.

Efforts have been made to reduce the volume of radiation therapy administered, limit exposure of vulnerable structures, and impart neuroprotective strategies. In one study of oligometastatic disease, patients were randomized to receive stereotactic radiosurgery (SRS) versus a combination of SRS and WBRT. The administration of adjuvant WBRT was associated with worse cognitive outcomes, despite better control of CNS disease (140). As hippocampal dysfunction is a central feature of radiation-induced cognitive impairment, hippocampal avoidant radiation therapy has been evaluated as a method to improve the cognitive outcomes of WBRT. A single-arm phase II cooperative group trial (RTOG 0933) found a relative preservation of cognitive function in the hippocampal sparing group compared to historical controls (141). A phase III study to confirm these results is currently underway (NRG CC003).

Hormone blockade

Estrogen and androgen deprivation therapies are common in certain diagnoses including breast and prostate cancers. These sex hormones are well-known to be critical for cognitive function. Estrogen and androgen receptors are widely distributed throughout the brain and are critical for synaptic density and pruning as well as neurotransmitter signaling, particularly in the hippocampus and prefrontal cortex (142, 143), which are two highly commonly affected areas of the brain in patients with CRCI.

Research to date supports neurocognitive deterioration with selective estrogen receptor modulators (SERMs) (144–146), including decline in memory, visuospatial function, and processing speed being associated with tamoxifen therapy (144, 146). Patients who receive both chemotherapy and tamoxifen may be at the highest risk for CRCI (147). Also, many chemotherapy treated patients experience chemotherapy-induced amenorrhea (148) and this change in estrogen levels may mediate cognitive outcomes. Aromatase inhibitors, which prevent the conversion of androgen to estrogen, have been found to have less pronounced effects than SERMs on overall cognitive function when compared in longitudinal evaluation (149). However, studies have been very limited in this area with inconsistent results (150, 151).

Several studies have demonstrated both acute and chronic cognitive impairment in men treated with androgen deprivation therapy. Deficits have been noted in the domains of executive function, spatial processing, attention, and memory (152–155). A systematic review and meta-analysis from 2018 suggested inconclusive findings across studies (156) while a subsequent, large population-based study indicated 1.57 increased odds of mild cognitive impairment associated with androgen deprivation therapy (157).

The inconsistencies in CRCI study findings for both estrogen and androgen blockade therapies point to the need for further research in this area.

Genetic Predispositions

In recent years, germline genetic polymorphisms have been found to contribute a distinct vulnerability to CRCI. Carriers of the apolipoprotein E epsilon 4 allele (*APOE4*) have been found to have increased vulnerability to Alzheimer's disease (158), as well as increased cognitive impairment after stroke (159) and traumatic brain injury (160). In patients treated with chemotherapy, this has also been found to contribute to increased neurologic toxicity (161–163), suggesting it underlies a more generalized risk of cognitive change after brain insults. However, the effect of *APOE4* on CRCI is complex given that *APOE4* may also be a risk factor for development of certain cancers (164, 165).

The potential genetic and epigenetic changes influencing cognitive outcomes also encompass a broader network of genes that are thought to play important roles in brain health. For instance, the *Val* allele of the catechol-o-methyltransferase (*COMT*) gene, responsible for mediating enzymatic degradation of catecholamines, is proposed to increase the vulnerability of dopamine-dependent neural circuitry to cancer-related neurotoxicities (166). Polymorphisms in the human multidrug resistance gene (*MDR1*) have been hypothesized to be involved in CRCI given that they are associated with increased entry of cytotoxic agents into the nervous system (167), but to date, have not been formally studied in association with CRCI. Brain-derived neurotrophic factor (*BDNF*) is a neurotrophin that contributes to the development and maintenance of neural circuitry (168). While the role of *BDNF* in the development of CRCI continues to be elucidated, lower serum *BDNF* levels in long-term breast cancer survivors have been associated with greater subjective cognitive complaints, and *Met* allele carriers seemed relatively protected against cognitive complaints after chemotherapy treatment (169).

The Excision Repair Cross-Complementation group 5 (*ERCC5*) gene polymorphisms are associated with the capacity for DNA damage repair. The presence of certain polymorphisms in this gene has been associated with a vulnerability to cognitive impairment. For instance, in one study of post-menopausal breast cancer patients, polymorphisms in *ERCC5* were the most strongly associated of all genes studied with changes in global cognitive function prior to the initiation of adjuvant therapy (170). Further, patients with breast cancer who are carriers of the *ERCC5* rs873601 G minor allele have been shown to have increased odds of frequent cognitive problems (171). It is hypothesized that mutations in *ERCC5* may reduce a patient's ability to repair DNA damage and remove ROS, thus rendering the brain increasingly vulnerable to the toxicities of cancer and its therapies (116, 172).

Finally, genes that modulate systemic inflammation have also been proposed to influence the neuro-inflammation that can occur as a result of cancer therapy. In one study, polymorphisms in genes encoding for the pro-inflammatory cytokines tumor necrosis factor-alpha and interleukin 6 (*IL-6*) were analyzed for their impact on cognitive outcomes in breast cancer patients. *IL-6* mutation was associated with an increase in perceived cognitive impairment (173). At this time, further study is warranted to determine how an individual's baseline genetic profile may influence their vulnerability to CRCI.

WHAT CAN BE DONE ABOUT CRCI?

Diagnosing CRCI

Given the prevalence of CRCI, and its potential to appear months and years after treatment for cancer, it is important for all physicians to be aware of this syndrome and be able to communicate basic evidence about it to patients. Patients most often complain of cognitive decline in the survivorship phase after the stresses of cancer diagnosis and therapy have subsided and they begin to return to normal activities. Therefore, oncology and primary care clinicians who are conducting post-therapy clinical follow-ups should be prepared to discuss and evaluate CRCI. When patients present with subjective cognitive complaints, or these are raised by their family, one of the most important initial steps is to acknowledge that this is a real and established condition. Cognitive symptoms can appear before, during, and after a cancer diagnosis, highlighting the importance of educating patients and their family members about CRCI throughout the disease and treatment course. It is often very helpful to inform patients that there is a known, organic contributor to these symptoms.

The diagnosis of CRCI can occur at any time after a diagnosis of cancer has been made and should be considered whenever a patient presents with cognitive complaints and/or associated functional changes. CRCI should be listed as a potential side effect of cancer therapies prior to initiating therapy and should also be evaluated throughout the patient's treatment course within the framework of therapy-related adverse effects (e.g., "How are you tolerating your therapy? Any side effects such as fatigue, nausea, cognitive changes….").

As noted above, there are currently no standardized diagnostic criteria for this syndrome. Therefore, CRCI is a diagnosis of exclusion, made by eliminating other factors that could result in cognitive disorder such as medical comorbidities, secondary contributors (e.g., vitamin deficiencies and thyroid dysfunction) and overlapping clinical syndromes (e.g., fatigue or mood disorder). Inclusion of CRCI as an issue in the patient's medical record should occur once a clinician has rendered the diagnosis, ensuring it receives longitudinal attention and care along with other sequelae of cancer. Whether this diagnosis is made by an oncologist or primary care physician versus a neurologist or neuropsychologist should depend on the comfort level of the treating physician with their clinical assessment. However, patients with moderate to severe clinical syndrome should likely be referred to a neurologist and/or neuropsychologist given the potential personal, social, and vocational implications of the diagnosis.

These specialists can assist in characterizing cognitive change, evaluating its impact on function, delineating secondary contributors to the cognitive deficits, and ordering further paraclinical testing to support the diagnosis. Neuropsychologists specialize in the quantitative assessment and characterization of cognitive function. They can assist in delineating the specific cognitive domains that are affected and also help evaluate the potential role of patient history, mood, and fatigue. As noted above, standard neuropsychological testing often identifies a lower incidence of cognitive impairment than subjective inquiry suggesting it may not be perfectly sensitive in identifying impairment. Patients presenting with comorbid affective symptoms, such as depression and anxiety, may also benefit from the input and care of a psychiatrist.

Biologic Therapy

At this time, the identification of dedicated treatments for CRCI is limited by the challenges in its definition, lack of consensus for diagnosis, evolving biologic understanding of its underpinnings, and heterogeneous clinical manifestations (174). Despite these challenges, attempts to target the contributory cellular mechanisms are underway, and hold clinical promise in ameliorating symptoms and altering the trajectory of CRCI. Repurposing pharmacologic agents used for other indications is one proposed approach. For instance, agents such as lithium and fluoxetine have the potential to counteract the reduction in neuro- and gliogenesis observed in CRCI (175–177). Similarly, phosphodiesterase inhibitors used to treat hypertension and erectile dysfunction, have been found to ameliorate the loss of dendritic structure identified after chemotherapy exposure (178, 179). Reductions in neurotransmitter release have been targeted with drugs used for dementias, such as cholinesterase inhibitors and NMDA-receptor antagonists, and these have been explored in patients with CRCI with promise of benefit (180–182). Stimulant medications, through supplementing neurotransmitters such as dopamine and norepinephrine that are prominently involved in attention and motivation, may be particularly effective in those patients suffering from dysfunction in these domains, or cancer-related fatigue (183, 184). Nguyen and Ehrlich (2020) provided a comprehensive overview of drugs with strong repurposing potential for treating CRCI (174).

Patient Y.C. underwent formal neuropsychological testing to further characterize her cognitive symptoms after neurological exam. This revealed impairments in areas of attention and processing speed in comparison to other cognitive domains. Given these findings and the functional impact of her cognitive symptoms, she was started on amphetamine-dextroamphetamine. This was instituted 9 months after her completion of chemoradiation therapy. After two dose titrations, she reported considerable improvement in her cognitive function as well as her school performance. She has since successfully graduated from her Bachelor of Nursing program.

Several biologic treatments are currently in preclinical testing phase. Chiu et al. (2017) showed prevention of CRCI and associated brain injury by co-administration of chemotherapy with pifithrin-μ, which acts via the p53 pathway to protect mitochondria (118). A further study by this same research group demonstrated that nasally administered mesenchymal stem cells rescued white matter structure, connectome organization, memory, and problem-solving performance in chemotherapy treated mice (128). Mesenchymal stem cells can be derived from various tissue types and are believed to donate their mitochondria to sites of cellular injury and improve the microenvironment (185). Other drugs that have been successfully used to prevent or rescue CRCI in chemotherapy treated animals include levetiracetam, an FDA-approved anti-epileptic medication (16), Infliximab, a tumor necrosis factor-alpha inhibitor (186), KU-32, which is believed to repair mitochondrial damage (187), PAN-811, a ribonucleotide reductase inhibitor that reduces free radicals (188), astaxanthin, a carotenoid with antioxidant properties (189), and 2-Hydroxypropyl-β-cyclodextrin, a cyclodextrin that activates transcription factor EB (119). Further, Dietrich and colleagues (2018) demonstrated that bone marrow-derived granulocyte-colony stimulating factor-responsive cells enhanced functional brain repair after whole body radiation therapy (190).

Behavioral Interventions

Non-pharmacologic therapies should play a central role in the management of CRCI given that patients are often hesitant to add further medications to their treatment regimens. Some of the most robust data involves physical exercise for CRCI treatment. In a sample of women with breast cancer undergoing chemotherapy treatment, self-reported exercise behavior and cardiorespiratory fitness measures were positively correlated with cognitive performance (191). Another study found that moderate physical activity among breast cancer survivors was associated with both improved memory function as well as reduced white matter lesions (192). These findings have been replicated in murine models of CNS radiotherapy, where mice allowed to exercise during radiation therapy had greater information acquisition, behavioral control, and processing speed, as well as greater preservation of brain volume and connectome organization (193). A systematic review published in 2020 indicated a statistically significant effect of exercise on subjective cognitive function both during and after adjuvant treatment. Fewer studies noted change in neuropsychological outcomes (194), but this likely reflects the inadequacy of neuropsychological tests for CRCI measurement.

Potential mechanisms for the impact of aerobic exercise include the established impact of exercise on neurogenesis, particularly in the hippocampus, (195) allowing for greater neuroplasticity and recovery from the neurotoxic impact of cancer and its therapy. Exercise is also known to stimulate neurotrophic factors, such as BDNF, which may also contribute to its neurorestorative impact (196). Physical exercise may also modulate CRCI via epigenetic mechanisms including effects on DNA methylation (197). In addition to aerobic exercise, yoga has also been found to have a positive impact on CRCI (198–200). Yoga can reduce systemic markers of inflammation, as well as improve fatigue and mood (200).

Neuromodulation is an emerging intervention approach based on directly interfacing with brain function. Neurofeedback techniques involve non-invasively showing participants their own brain activity in real-time to train them how to control it (201). A case report of a female breast cancer survivor indicated that neuro-feedback alleviated her cognitive difficulties as well as other symptoms including fatigue, sleep disruption, pain and negative mood with improvements maintained at 6 month follow-up (202). A pilot study in breast cancer survivors showed improved self-reported cognitive function as well as fatigue after neurofeedback intervention, with participants serving as their own waitlist controls (203). A randomized controlled trial in chemotherapy treated breast cancer survivors demonstrated significant improvement in objective memory performance as well as quality of life in the neurofeedback group compared to the control group (204).

Non-invasive brain stimulation (NBS) is another neuromodulation technique that involves application of electrical stimulation to the scalp adjacent to target cortical regions. This can induce neuroplastic, neurotransmitter, and/or neuroreceptor changes underlying cognitive function (205). Significant improvements in sustained attention were observed in a small sample of breast cancer survivors randomized to NBS compared to those assigned to sham control (206).

Cognitive training involves programs aimed at improving brain function through a defined regimen of cognitive exercises and practices. These may take on varied forms, including some combination of education and self-awareness, compensatory strategies, cognitive-behavioral techniques, and mindfulness meditation (207–209). Both home-based and hospital/clinic-based programs have demonstrated similar effects on CRCI (210, 211), suggesting different settings and modes of administration may be efficacious. Endpoints used for clinical trials of cognitive training are varied, however studies have shown improved performance in multiple cognitive domains, including memory, executive function, attention, verbal fluency, and global cognitive function (207, 210, 212, 213). The availability of in-person cognitive training may vary depending on local resources and interests, however online programs allow for broader access.

The literature is currently unclear regarding optimal timing for CRCI interventions. Some patients enrolled in the clinical trials described above have been undergoing active cancer therapy while most have been long-term survivors who were several years post-primary therapy. This suggests that interventions may be useful at various stages of cancer treatment and recovery and that there is likely not a cutoff point after which no gains can be made. Optimal timing of intervention may depend on individual patient preferences, medical status, comorbidities and resources. For example, interventions during active treatment can be difficult for patients who are overwhelmed, frail or ill. Most studies implementing CRCI interventions have typically required that participants be at least 6 months post-primary therapy in order to allow for natural neurologic recovery and medical stability. This is based on research suggesting that CRCI appears to follow a course similar to traumatic brain injury where most deficits occur within the first 6 months after adjuvant therapies followed by a one to two year recovery/stabilization period (214). There is also some evidence suggesting that certain interventions, such as cognitive training, may not result in additional benefit when implemented prior to this period (209, 211). However, no studies have directly compared effects of early versus late intervention for CRCI and further research in this area is needed.

Approximately 3 years post-chemotherapy, patient L.D. was prescribed a 30 minute per day, five days per week, 12-week course of in-house computerized cognitive exercises focusing on executive functions. This was coupled with education regarding compensatory strategies (e.g., notetaking, smartphone use, self-talk, active listening) and stress management techniques (e.g., relaxation exercises). The patient was also encouraged to increase physical activity to at least 150 minutes of moderate intensity per week. Although neuropsychological testing did not reveal significant changes in her performance, the patient reported, "I have experienced tremendous improvements and successes. My flexibility in thinking and my problem solving have improved. I am better able to communicate with others, especially physicians. I am better able to hold more information in my head and work with it. My ability to drive has improved because now I am able to keep track of the constantly changing environment, anticipate, plan and execute efficiently. I am faster and more efficient at performing tasks. I am able to function at a higher level with more confidence."

SUMMARY AND CONCLUSIONS

CRCI is one of the most common adverse effects of cancer therapies characterized by various memory, thinking, and attention difficulties. These deficits can be acute and/or chronic, evident years and even decades post-adjuvant therapy. Research evidence supports that CRCI is a biologically induced, measurable syndrome that significantly reduces quality of life as well as overall survival. The specific pathophysiologic mechanisms of CRCI remain unclear, but the final common biologic pathway appears to be altered brain structure and function that results in cognitive decline. Objective assessment of CRCI can be difficult given that neuropsychological testing tends to lack sensitivity, specificity and ecological validity for these symptoms. The National Cancer Institute of the National Institutes of Health has called for improved, syndrome-specific, evidence-based assessments for CRCI (49). Until such tools are developed, all available sources of information should be considered including any neuropsychological or neurological evaluations, as well as patient and family reports, with the latter holding equal if not greater weight. Appropriate referrals to neurology, neuropsychology and psychiatry are often indicated to further evaluate CRCI and assist with treatment planning.

Currently, there are no standardized, evidence-based interventions for CRCI, likely in part due to the lack of clarity regarding its mechanistic underpinnings. However, there are several safe, available treatments that can potentially be helpful for certain patients, including physical activity, a short course of psychostimulant and/or cognitive training. Neuromodulation shows some promising results for improving cognitive function, but further study is required. Disadvantages of these techniques include their limited availability for most participants and the requirement of multiple in-person sessions (although telehealth applications are growing). Cognitive training also shows potential for addressing CRCI symptoms and is available broadly via online programs but is notoriously lacking in real-world transfer effects. Some data suggest that the true benefits of cognitive training may be the protective increase in neural reserve (215) and/or associated positive psychological aspects including improved internal locus of control, self-efficacy, and distraction from real-world problems, which may be difficult to measure or realize. Biologically, several efforts are underway to test repurposed or novel drugs in preclinical trials that may hold promise for treating and even preventing CRCI.

Physical activity remains one of the best interventions for brain and overall health but compliance with physical activity recommendations is challenging for many patients especially those with pain, frailty, and other physical limitations. However, even very mild, non-aerobic activities such as gentle yoga or simple stretching exercises can help improve cognitive function as well as other symptoms such as psychological distress, fatigue, and sleep disruption. Validation-based communication can enhance shared decision making by accepting the patient's experience as understandable, even if one does not necessarily agree with it. This includes validating the existence of CRCI by discussing the research evidence demonstrating that (1) neuropsychological testing does not always reflect patient experience and (2) there have been measurable brain changes associated with this syndrome. Such a discussion can be an intervention in itself by providing an evidence-based explanation for patients who are confused and frustrated regarding their symptoms.

REFERENCES

1. Janelsins MC, Kesler SR, Ahles TA, Morrow GR. Prevalence, mechanisms, and management of cancer-related cognitive impairment. *Int Rev Psychiatry.* 2014;26(1):102–13.
2. Kesler SR, Rao A, Blayney DW, Oakley-Girvan IA, Karuturi M, Palesh O. Predicting long-term cognitive outcome following breast cancer with pre-treatment resting state fMRI and random forest machine learning. *Front Hum Neurosci.* 2017; 11:555.

3. Institute NC. Statistics, Graphs and Definitions 2020. Available from: https://cancercontrol.cancer.gov/ocs/statistics/index.html.
4. Association As. Facts and Figures 2020. Available from: https://www.alz.org/alzheimers-dementia/facts-figures.
5. Guida JL, Ahles TA, Belsky D, Campisi J, Cohen HJ, DeGregori J, et al. Measuring aging and identifying aging phenotypes in cancer survivors. *J Natl Cancer Inst*. 2019;111(12):1245–54.
6. van der Willik KD, Schagen SB, Ikram MA. Cancer and dementia: two sides of the same coin? *Eur J Clin Invest*. 2018;48(11):e13019.
7. Wefel JS, Kesler SR, Noll KR, Schagen SB. Clinical characteristics, pathophysiology, and management of noncentral nervous system cancer-related cognitive impairment in adults. *CA: Cancer J Clin*. 2015;65(2):123–38.
8. Henneghan A, Rao V, Harrison RA, Karuturi M, Blayney DW, Palesh O, et al. Cortical brain age from pre-treatment to post-chemotherapy in patients with breast cancer. *Neurotox Res*. 2020;37(4):788–99.
9. Koppelmans V, de Ruiter MB, van der Lijn F, Boogerd W, Seynaeve C, van der Lugt A, et al. Global and focal brain volume in long-term breast cancer survivors exposed to adjuvant chemotherapy. *Breast Cancer Res Treat*. 2012;132(3):1099–106.
10. Sanoff HK, Deal AM, Krishnamurthy J, Torrice C, Dillon P, Sorrentino J, et al. Effect of cytotoxic chemotherapy on markers of molecular age in patients with breast cancer. *J Natl Cancer Inst*. 2014;106(4):dju057.
11. Koppelmans V, Breteler MM, Boogerd W, Seynaeve C, Schagen SB. Late effects of adjuvant chemotherapy for adult onset non-CNS cancer; cognitive impairment, brain structure and risk of dementia. *Crit Rev Oncol Hematol*. 2013;88(1):87–101.
12. Kesler SR, Rao V, Ray WJ, Rao A, Alzheimer's Disease Neuroimaging Initiative. Probability of Alzheimer's disease in breast cancer survivors based on gray-matter structural network efficiency. *Alzheimers Dement (Amst)*. 2017;9:67–75.
13. McDonald BC. Editorial: Cognitive and neuroimaging effects of chemotherapy: evidence across cancer types and treatment regimens. *J Natl Cancer Inst*. 2017;109(12):1–3.
14. Bernatz S, Ilina EI, Devraj K, Harter PN, Mueller K, Kleber S, et al. Impact of Docetaxel on blood-brain barrier function and formation of breast cancer brain metastases. *J Exp Clin Cancer Res*. 2019;38(1):434.
15. Rousselle C, Clair P, Lefauconnier J-M, Kaczorek M, Scherrmann J-M, Temsamani J. New advances in the transport of doxorubicin through the blood-brain barrier by a peptide vector-mediated strategy. *Mol Pharmacol*. 2000;57(4):679–86.
16. Manchon JF, Dabaghian Y, Uzor NE, Kesler SR, Wefel JS, Tsvetkov AS. Levetiracetam mitigates doxorubicin-induced DNA and synaptic damage in neurons. *Sci Rep*. 2016;6:25705.
17. Dietrich J, Han R, Yang Y, Mayer-Proschel M, Noble M. CNS progenitor cells and oligodendrocytes are targets of chemotherapeutic agents in vitro and in vivo. *J Biol*. 2006;5(7):22.
18. Dietrich J, Kesari S. Effect of cancer treatment on neural stem and progenitor cells. *Cancer Treat Res*. 2009;150:81–95.
19. Feng Y, Zhang XD, Zheng G, Zhang LJ. Chemotherapy-induced brain changes in breast cancer survivors: evaluation with multimodality magnetic resonance imaging. *Brain Imaging Behav*. 2019;13(6):1799–814.
20. Li M, Caeyenberghs K. Longitudinal assessment of chemotherapy-induced changes in brain and cognitive functioning: a systematic review. *Neurosci Biobehav Rev*. 2018;92:304–17.
21. Kesler SR, Blayney DW. Neurotoxic effects of anthracycline- vs nonanthracycline-based chemotherapy on cognition in breast cancer survivors. *JAMA Oncol*. 2016;2(2):185–92.
22. Niedzwiedz CL, Knifton L, Robb KA, Katikireddi SV, Smith DJ. Depression and anxiety among people living with and beyond cancer: a growing clinical and research priority. *BMC Cancer*. 2019;19(1):943.
23. Yang Y, Hendrix CC. Cancer-related cognitive impairment in breast cancer patients: influences of psychological variables. *Asia Pac J Oncol Nurs*. 2018;5(3):296–306.
24. Tager FA, McKinley PS, Schnabel FR, El-Tamer M, Cheung YK, Fang Y, et al. The cognitive effects of chemotherapy in post-menopausal breast cancer patients: a controlled longitudinal study. *Breast Cancer Res Treat*. 2010;123(1):25–34.
25. Perrier J, Viard A, Levy C, Morel N, Allouache D, Noal S, et al. Longitudinal investigation of cognitive deficits in breast cancer patients and their gray matter correlates: impact of education level. *Brain Imaging Behav*. 2020;14(1):226–41.
26. Bruno J, Hosseini SM, Kesler S. Altered resting state functional brain network topology in chemotherapy-treated breast cancer survivors. *Neurobiol Dis*. 2012;48(3):329–38.
27. McDonald BC, Conroy SK, Ahles TA, West JD, Saykin AJ. Alterations in brain activation during working memory processing associated with breast cancer and treatment: a prospective functional magnetic resonance imaging study. *J Clin Oncol: Official J Am Soc Clin Oncol*. 2012;30(20):2500–8.
28. Tao L, Lin H, Yan Y, Xu X, Wang L, Zhang J, et al. Impairment of the executive function in breast cancer patients receiving chemotherapy treatment: a functional MRI study. *Eur J Cancer Care (Engl)*. 2017;26(6).
29. Kesler SR, Adams M, Packer M, Rao V, Henneghan AM, Blayney DW, et al. Disrupted brain network functional dynamics and hyper-correlation of structural and functional connectome topology in patients with breast cancer prior to treatment. *Brain Behav*. 2017;7(3):e00643.
30. Cheng H, Li W, Gong L, Xuan H, Huang Z, Zhao H, et al. Altered resting-state hippocampal functional networks associated with chemotherapy-induced prospective memory impairment in breast cancer survivors. *Sci Rep*. 2017;7:45135.
31. Chen X, He X, Tao L, Li J, Wu J, Zhu C, et al. The working memory and dorsolateral prefrontal-hippocampal functional connectivity changes in long-term survival breast cancer patients treated with tamoxifen. *Int J Neuropsychopharmacol*. 2017;20(5):374–82.
32. Miao H, Chen X, Yan Y, He X, Hu S, Kong J, et al. Functional connectivity change of brain default mode network in breast cancer patients after chemotherapy. *Neuroradiology*. 2016;58(9):921–8.

33. Kaiser J, Dietrich J, Amiri M, Ruschel I, Akbaba H, Hantke N, et al. Cognitive performance and psychological distress in breast cancer patients at disease onset. *Front Psychol.* 2019;10:2584.
34. Kesler SR, Waffel JS, Hosseini SM, Cheung M, Watson CL, Hoeft F. Default mode network connectivity distinguishes chemotherapy-treated breast cancer survivors from controls. *Proc Natl Acad Sci U S A.* 2013;110(28):11600–5.
35. Sales MVC, Suemoto CK, Apolinario D, Serrao V, Andrade CS, Conceicao DM, et al. Effects of adjuvant chemotherapy on cognitive function of patients with early-stage colorectal cancer. *Clin Colorectal Cancer.* 2019;18(1):19–27.
36. Stouten-Kemperman MM, de Ruiter MB, Caan MW, Boogerd W, Kerst MJ, Reneman L, et al. Lower cognitive performance and white matter changes in testicular cancer survivors 10 years after chemotherapy. *Hum Brain Mapp.* 2015;36(11):4638–47.
37. Menning S, de Ruiter MB, Veltman DJ, Boogerd W, Oldenburg HS, Reneman L, et al. Changes in brain activation in breast cancer patients depend on cognitive domain and treatment type. *PLOS ONE.* 2017;12(3):e0171724.
38. Kesler SR. Default mode network as a potential biomarker of chemotherapy-related brain injury. *Neurobiol Aging.* 2014;35(Suppl 2):S11–9.
39. Park J-H, Bae SH, Jung Y-S, Jung Y-M. Prevalence and characteristics of chemotherapy-related cognitive impairment in patients with breast cancer. *J Korean Acad Nurs.* 2015;45(1):118–28.
40. Kesler SR, Kent JS, O'Hara R. Prefrontal cortex and executive function impairments in primary breast cancer. *Arch Neurol.* 2011;68(11):1447–53.
41. Hutchinson AD, Hosking JR, Kichenadasse G, Mattiske JK, Wilson C. Objective and subjective cognitive impairment following chemotherapy for cancer: a systematic review. *Cancer Treat Rev.* 2012;38(7):926–34.
42. Pullens MJJ, De Vries J, Roukema JA. Subjective cognitive dysfunction in breast cancer patients: a systematic review. *Psychooncology.* 2010;19(11):1127–38.
43. Bernstein LJ, McCreath GA, Komeylian Z, Rich JB. Cognitive impairment in breast cancer survivors treated with chemotherapy depends on control group type and cognitive domains assessed: a multilevel meta-analysis. *Neurosci Biobehav Rev.* 2017;83:417–28.
44. Rick O, Reuß-Borst M, Dauelsberg T, Hass HG, König V, Caspari R, et al. NeuroCog FX study: a multicenter cohort study on cognitive dysfunction in patients with early breast cancer. *Psychooncology.* 2018;27(8):2016–22.
45. Kitahata R, Nakajima S, Uchida H, Hayashida T, Takahashi M, Nio S, et al. Self-rated cognitive functions following chemotherapy in patients with breast cancer: a 6-month prospective study. *Neuropsychiatr Dis Treat.* 2017;13:2489–96.
46. Amidi A, Christensen S, Mehlsen M, Jensen AB, Pedersen AD, Zachariae R. Long-term subjective cognitive functioning following adjuvant systemic treatment: 7–9 years follow-up of a nationaie cohort of women treated for primary breast cancer. *Br J Cancer.* 2015;113(5):794–801.
47. Savard J, Ganz PA. Subjective or objective measures of cognitive functioning—what's more important? *JAMA Oncol.* 2016;2(10):1263–4.
48. Bray VJ, Dhillon HM, Vardy JL. Systematic review of self-reported cognitive function in cancer patients following chemotherapy treatment. *J Cancer Surviv.* 2018;12(4):537–59.
49. Horowitz TS, Suls J, Treviño M. A call for a neuroscience approach to cancer-related cognitive impairment. *Trends Neurosci.* 2018;41(8):493–6.
50. Howieson D. Current limitations of neuropsychological tests and assessment procedures. *Clin Neuropsychol.* 2019;33(2):200–8.
51. Wefel JS, Vardy J, Ahles T, Schagen SB. International Cognition and Cancer Task Force recommendations to harmonise studies of cognitive function in patients with cancer. *Lancet Oncol.* 2011;12(7):703–8.
52. Henderson FM, Cross AJ, Baraniak AR. 'A new normal with chemobrain': experiences of the impact of chemotherapy-related cognitive deficits in long-term breast cancer survivors. *Health Psychol Open.* 2019;6(1). doi: 10.1177/2055102919832234.
53. Kesler SR, Petersen ML, Rao V, Harrison RA, Palesh O. Functional connectome biotypes of chemotherapy-related cognitive impairment. *J Cancer Surviv.* 2020;14(4):483–93.
54. O'Leary TE, Diller L, Recklitis CJ. The effects of response bias on self-reported quality of life among childhood cancer survivors. *Qual Life Res.* 2007;16(7):1211–20.
55. Harila MJ, Salo J, Lanning M, Vilkkumaa I, Harila-Saari AH. High health-related quality of life among long-term survivors of childhood acute lymphoblastic leukemia. *Pediatr Blood Cancer.* 2010;55(2):331–6.
56. Yabroff KR, Lund J, Kepka D, Mariotto A. Economic burden of cancer in the United States: estimates, projections, and future research. *Cancer Epidemiol Biomarkers Prev.* 2011;20(10):2006–14.
57. Health and Productivity Benchmarking [Internet]. 2016. Available from: https://www.ibiweb.org/benchmarking/.
58. Mehnert A. Employment and work-related issues in cancer survivors. *Crit Rev Oncol Hematol.* 2011;77(2):109–30.
59. de Boer AG, Taskila T, Ojajarvi A, van Dijk FJ, Verbeek JH. Cancer survivors and unemployment: a meta-analysis and meta-regression. *JAMA.* 2009;301(7):753–62.
60. van Muijen P, Weevers NL, Snels IA, Duijts SF, Bruinvels DJ, Schellart AJ, et al. Predictors of return to work and employment in cancer survivors: a systematic review. *Eur J Cancer Care (Engl).* 2013;22(2):144–60.
61. Krull KR, Brinkman TM, Li C, Armstrong GT, Ness KK, Srivastava DK, et al. Neurocognitive outcomes decades after treatment for childhood acute lymphoblastic leukemia: a report from the St Jude lifetime cohort study. *J Clin Oncol: Official J Am Soc Clin Oncol.* 2013;31(35):4407–15.
62. Zheng DJ, Krull KR, Chen Y, Diller L, Yasui Y, Leisenring W, et al. Long-term psychological and educational outcomes for survivors of neuroblastoma: a report from the Childhood Cancer Survivor Study. *Cancer.* 2018;124(15):3220–30.

63. Robb C, Boulware D, Overcash J, Extermann M. Patterns of care and survival in cancer patients with cognitive impairment. *Crit Rev Oncol Hematol.* 2010;74(3):218–24.

64. Stilley CS, Bender CM, Dunbar-Jacob J, Sereika S, Ryan CM. The impact of cognitive function on medication management: three studies. *Health Psychol.* 2010;29(1):50–5.

65. Krull KR, Hardy KK, Kahalley LS, Schuitema I, Kesler SR. Neurocognitive outcomes and interventions in long-term survivors of childhood cancer. *J Clin Oncol: Official J Am Soc Clin Oncol.* 2018;36(21):2181–9.

66. Peters KB, Woodring S, Healy P, Herndon JE, Lipp ES, Minchew J, et al. Baseline cognitive function to predict survival in patients with glioblastoma. *J Clin Oncol.* 2016;34(15_suppl):10125.

67. Libert Y, Dubruille S, Borghgraef C, Etienne AM, Merckaert I, Paesmans M, et al. Vulnerabilities in older patients when cancer treatment is initiated: does a cognitive impairment impact the two-year survival? *PLOS ONE.* 2016;11(8):e0159734.

68. Boykoff N, Moieni M, Subramanian SK. Confronting chemobrain: an in-depth look at survivors' reports of impact on work, social networks, and health care response. *J Cancer Surviv.* 2009;3(4):223–32.

69. Von Ah D, Habermann B, Carpenter JS, Schneider BL. Impact of perceived cognitive impairment in breast cancer survivors. *Eur J Oncol Nurs.* 2013;17(2):236–41.

70. Mandelblatt JS, Hurria A, McDonald BC, Saykin AJ, Stern RA, VanMeter JW, et al. Cognitive effects of cancer and its treatments at the intersection of aging: what do we know; what do we need to know? *Semin Oncol.* 2013;40(6):709–25.

71. Ahles TA, Saykin AJ, McDonald BC, Li Y, Furstenberg CT, Hanscom BS, et al. Longitudinal assessment of cognitive changes associated with adjuvant treatment for breast cancer: impact of age and cognitive reserve. *J Clin Oncol.* 2010;28(29):4434–40.

72. Ahles TA, Saykin AJ, McDonald BC, Furstenberg CT, Cole BF, Hanscom BS, et al. Cognitive function in breast cancer patients prior to adjuvant treatment. *Breast Cancer Res Treat.* 2008;110(1):143–52.

73. Wefel JS, Lenzi R, Theriault RL, Davis RN, Meyers CA. The cognitive sequelae of standard-dose adjuvant chemotherapy in women with breast carcinoma. *Cancer.* 2004;100(11):2292–9.

74. Cimprich B, So H, Ronis DL, Trask C. Pre-treatment factors related to cognitive functioning in women newly diagnosed with breast cancer. *Psychooncology.* 2005;14(1):70–8.

75. Pullens MJ, De Vries J, Van Warmerdam LJ, Van De Wal MA, Roukema JA. Chemotherapy and cognitive complaints in women with breast cancer. *Psychooncology.* 2013;22(8):1783–9.

76. Cleeland CS, Bennett GJ, Dantzer R, Dougherty PM, Dunn AJ, Meyers CA, et al. Are the symptoms of cancer and cancer treatment due to a shared biologic mechanism? A cytokine-immunologic model of cancer symptoms. *Cancer.* 2003;97(11):2919–25.

77. Lee BN, Dantzer R, Langley KE, Bennett GJ, Dougherty PM, Dunn AJ, et al. A cytokine-based neuroimmunologic mechanism of cancer-related symptoms. *Neuroimmunomodulation.* 2004;11(5):279–92.

78. Wilson CJ, Finch CE, Cohen HJ. Cytokines and cognition–the case for a head-to-toe inflammatory paradigm. *J Am Geriatr Soc.* 2002;50(12):2041–56.

79. Konsman JP, Vigues S, Mackerlova L, Bristow A, Blomqvist A. Rat brain vascular distribution of interleukin-1 type-1 receptor immunoreactivity: relationship to patterns of inducible cyclooxygenase expression by peripheral inflammatory stimuli. *J Comp Neurol.* 2004;472(1):113–29.

80. Lynch MA. Age-related neuroinflammatory changes negatively impact on neuronal function. *Front Aging Neurosci.* 2010;1:6.

81. Aluise CD, Miriyala S, Noel T, Sultana R, Jungsuwadee P, Taylor TJ, et al. 2-Mercaptoethane sulfonate prevents doxorubicin-induced plasma protein oxidation and TNF-alpha release: implications for the reactive oxygen species-mediated mechanisms of chemobrain. *Free Radical Biol Med.* 2011;50(11):1630–8.

82. Joshi G, Aluise CD, Cole MP, Sultana R, Pierce WM, Vore M, et al. Alterations in brain antioxidant enzymes and redox proteomic identification of oxidized brain proteins induced by the anti-cancer drug adriamycin: implications for oxidative stress-mediated chemobrain. *Neuroscience.* 2010;166(3):796–807.

83. Patel SK, Wong AL, Wong FL, Breen EC, Hurria A, Smith M, et al. Inflammatory biomarkers, comorbidity, and neurocognition in women with newly diagnosed breast cancer. *J Natl Cancer Inst.* 2015;107(8):1–7.

84. Farnsworth RH, Lackmann M, Achen MG, Stacker SA. Vascular remodeling in cancer. *Oncogene.* 2014;33(27):3496–505.

85. Ng T, Cheung YT, Ham Guo MS, Kee YC, Ho HK, Fan G, et al. Plasma vascular endothelial growth factor level and cognitive changes in breast cancer patients. *J Clin Oncol (Meeting Abstracts).* 2013;31(15_suppl):e20566.

86. Koppelmans V, Vernooij MW, Boogerd W, Seynaeve C, Ikram MA, Breteler MM, et al. Prevalence of cerebral small-vessel disease in long-term breast cancer survivors exposed to both adjuvant radiotherapy and chemotherapy. *J Clin Oncol: Official J Am Soc Clin Oncol.* 2015;33(6):588–93.

87. Zhao Q, Yang Y, Liang X, Du G, Liu L, Lu L, et al. The clinicopathological significance of neurogenesis in breast cancer. *BMC Cancer.* 2014;14(1):1–6.

88. Pundavela J, Roselli S, Faulkner S, Attia J, Scott RJ, Thorne RF, et al. Nerve fibers infiltrate the tumor microenvironment and are associated with nerve growth factor production and lymph node invasion in breast cancer. *Mol Oncol.* 2015;9(8):1626–35.

89. Cole SW, Nagaraja AS, Lutgendorf SK, Green PA, Sood AK. Sympathetic nervous system regulation of the tumour microenvironment. *Nat Rev Cancer.* 2015;15(9):563–72.

90. Zhang J, Liu G, Zhang F, Fang H, Zhang D, Liu S, et al. Analysis of postoperative cognitive dysfunction and influencing factors of dexmedetomidine anesthesia in elderly patients with colorectal cancer. *Oncol Lett.* 2019;18(3):3058–64.

91. Scherling C, Collins B, Mackenzie J, Bielajew C, Smith A. Pre-chemotherapy differences in visuospatial working memory in breast cancer patients compared to controls: an FMRI study. *Front Hum Neurosci.* 2011;5:122.

92. Chen ML, Miaskowski C, Liu LN, Chen SC. Changes in perceived attentional function in women following breast cancer surgery. *Breast Cancer Res Treat.* 2012;131(2):599–606.

93. Rundshagen I. Postoperative cognitive dysfunction. *Dtsch Arztebl Int.* 2014;111(8):119–25.

94. Almahozi A, Radhi M, Alzayer S, Kamal A. Effects of memantine in a mouse model of postoperative cognitive dysfunction. *Behav Sci (Basel).* 2019;9(3).

95. Talacchi A, Santini B, Savazzi S, Gerosa M. Cognitive effects of tumour and surgical treatment in glioma patients. *J Neurooncol.* 2011;103(3):541–9.

96. Satoer D, Vork J, Visch-Brink E, Smits M, Dirven C, Vincent A. Cognitive functioning early after surgery of gliomas in eloquent areas. *J Neurosurg.* 2012;117(5):831–8.

97. Teixidor P, Gatignol P, Leroy M, Masuet-Aumatell C, Capelle L, Duffau H. Assessment of verbal working memory before and after surgery for low-grade glioma. *J Neurooncol.* 2007;81(3):305–13.

98. Janelsins MC, Mustian KM, Palesh OG, Mohile SG, Peppone LJ, Sprod LK, et al. Differential expression of cytokines in breast cancer patients receiving different chemotherapies: implications for cognitive impairment research. *Support Care Cancer.* 2012;20(4):831–9.

99. Vardy JL, Dhillon HM, Pond GR, Rourke SB, Bekele T, Renton C, et al. Cognitive function in patients with colorectal cancer who do and do not receive chemotherapy: a prospective, longitudinal, controlled study. *J Clin Oncol: Official J Am Soc Clin Oncol.* 2015;33(34):4085–92.

100. Kesler S, Janelsins M, Koovakkattu D, Palesh O, Mustian K, Morrow G, et al. Reduced hippocampal volume and verbal memory performance associated with interleukin-6 and tumor necrosis factor-alpha levels in chemotherapy-treated breast cancer survivors. *Brain Behav Immun.* 2013;30 Suppl:S109–16.

101. Apple AC, Schroeder MP, Ryals AJ, Wagner LI, Cella D, Shih PA, et al. Hippocampal functional connectivity is related to self-reported cognitive concerns in breast cancer patients undergoing adjuvant therapy. *Neuroimage Clin.* 2018;20:110–8.

102. Williams AM, Shah R, Shayne M, Huston AJ, Krebs M, Murray N, et al. Associations between inflammatory markers and cognitive function in breast cancer patients receiving chemotherapy. *J Neuroimmunol.* 2018;314:17–23.

103. Yang M, Kim J-S, Kim J, Jang S, Kim S-H, Kim J-C, et al. Acute treatment with methotrexate induces hippocampal dysfunction in a mouse model of breast cancer. *Brain Res Bull.* 2012;89(1–2):50–56.

104. Wozniak K, Kolacinska A, Blasinska-Morawiec M, Morawiec-Bajda A, Morawiec Z, Zadrozny M, et al. The DNA-damaging potential of tamoxifen in breast cancer and normal cells. *Arch Toxicol.* 2007;81(7):519–27.

105. Borrego-Soto G, Ortiz-Lopez R, Rojas-Martinez A. Ionizing radiation-induced DNA injury and damage detection in patients with breast cancer. *Genet Mol Biol.* 2015;38(4):420–32.

106. Hu R, Hilakivi-Clarke L, Clarke R. Molecular mechanisms of tamoxifen-associated endometrial cancer (review). *Oncol Lett.* 2015;9(4):1495–501.

107. El-Agamy SE, Abdel-Aziz AK, Esmat A, Azab SS. Chemotherapy and cognition: comprehensive review on doxorubicin-induced chemobrain. *Cancer Chemother Pharmacol.* 2019;84(1):1–14.

108. Dietrich J, Prust M, Kaiser J. Chemotherapy, cognitive impairment and hippocampal toxicity. *Neuroscience.* 2015;309:224–32.

109. Maynard S, Fang EF, Scheibye-Knudsen M, Croteau DL, Bohr VA. DNA damage, DNA repair, aging, and neurodegeneration. *Cold Spring Harb Perspect Med.* 2015;5(10):a025130.

110. Jin WS, Bu XL, Liu YH, Shen LL, Zhuang ZQ, Jiao SS, et al. Plasma amyloid-beta levels in patients with different types of cancer. *Neurotox Res.* 2017;31(2):283–8.

111. Lim S, Yoo BK, Kim H-S, Gilmore HL, Lee Y, Lee H-p, et al. Amyloid-β precursor protein promotes cell proliferation and motility of advanced breast cancer. *BMC Cancer.* 2014;14(1):928.

112. Butterfield DA, Swomley AM, Sultana R. Amyloid beta-peptide (1-42)-induced oxidative stress in Alzheimer disease: importance in disease pathogenesis and progression. *Antioxid Redox Signal.* 2013;19(8):823–35.

113. Mao P, Reddy PH. Aging and amyloid beta-induced oxidative DNA damage and mitochondrial dysfunction in Alzheimer's disease: implications for early intervention and therapeutics. *Biochim Biophys Acta.* 2011;1812(11):1359–70.

114. Keeney JTR, Ren X, Warrier G, Noel T, Powell DK, Brelsfoard JM, et al. Doxorubicin-induced elevated oxidative stress and neurochemical alterations in brain and cognitive decline: protection by MESNA and insights into mechanisms of chemotherapy-induced cognitive impairment ("chemobrain"). *Oncotarget.* 2018;9(54).

115. Bagnall-Moreau C, Chaudhry S, Salas-Ramirez K, Ahles T, Hubbard K. Chemotherapy-induced cognitive impairment is associated with increased inflammation and oxidative damage in the hippocampus. *Mol Neurobiol.* 2019;56(10):7159–72.

116. Conroy SK, McDonald BC, Smith DJ, Moser LR, West JD, Kamendulis LM, et al. Alterations in brain structure and function in breast cancer survivors: effect of post-chemotherapy interval and relation to oxidative DNA damage. *Breast Cancer Res Treat.* 2013;137(2):493–502.

117. Ren X, Keeney JTR, Miriyala S, Noel T, Powell DK, Chaiswing L, et al. The triangle of death of neurons: oxidative damage, mitochondrial dysfunction, and loss of choline-containing biomolecules in brains of mice treated with doxorubicin. Advanced insights into mechanisms of chemotherapy induced cognitive impairment ("chemobrain") involving TNF-alpha. *Free Radical Biol Med.* 2018;134:1–8.

118. Chiu GS, Maj MA, Rizvi S, Dantzer R, Vichaya EG, Laumet G, et al. Pifithrin-mu prevents cisplatin-induced chemobrain by preserving neuronal mitochondrial function. *Cancer Res.* 2017;77(3):742–52.

119. Manchon J, Uzor N, Kesler S, Wefel J, Townley A, Pradeep S, et al. TFEB ameliorates the impairment of the autophagy-lysosome pathway in neurons induced by doxorubicin. *Aging.* 2016;8(12):3507–19.

120. Guo C, Sun L, Chen X, Zhang D. Oxidative stress, mitochondrial damage and neurodegenerative diseases. *Neural Regen Res.* 2013;8(21):2003–14.

121. Zorov DB, Juhaszova M, Sollott SJ. Mitochondrial reactive oxygen species (ROS) and ROS-induced ROS release. *Physiol Rev.* 2014;94(3):909–50.

122. Nguyen NNY, Kim SS, Jo YH. Deregulated mitochondrial DNA in diseases. *DNA Cell Biol.* 2020;39(8):1385–400.

123. Inczedy-Farkas G, Trampush JW, Perczel Forintos D, Beech D, Andrejkovics M, Varga Z, et al. Mitochondrial DNA mutations and cognition: a case-series report. *Arch Clin Neuropsychol.* 2014;29(4):315–21.

124. Nudelman KN, Wang Y, McDonald BC, Conroy SK, Smith DJ, West JD, et al. Altered cerebral blood flow one month after systemic chemotherapy for breast cancer: a prospective study using pulsed arterial spin labeling MRI perfusion. *PLOS ONE.* 2014;9(5):e96713.

125. Tang TT, Zawaski JA, Kesler SR, Beamish CA, Reddick WE, Glass JO, et al. A comprehensive preclinical assessment of late-term imaging markers of radiation-induced brain injury. *Neurooncol Adv.* 2019;1(1):vdz012.

126. Xuan H, Gan C, Li W, Huang Z, Wang L, Jia Q, et al. Altered network efficiency of functional brain networks in patients with breast cancer after chemotherapy. *Oncotarget.* 2017;8(62):105648.

127. Kesler SR, Noll K, Cahill DP, Rao G, Wefel JS. The effect of IDH1 mutation on the structural connectome in malignant astrocytoma. *J Neurooncol.* 2017;131(3):565–74.

128. Chiu GS, Boukelmoune N, Chiang ACA, Peng B, Rao V, Kingsley C, et al. Nasal administration of mesenchymal stem cells restores cisplatin-induced cognitive impairment and brain damage in mice. *Oncotarget.* 2018;9(85):35581–97.

129. Brown WR, Blair RM, Moody DM, Thore CR, Ahmed S, Robbins ME, et al. Capillary loss precedes the cognitive impairment induced by fractionated whole-brain irradiation: a potential rat model of vascular dementia. *J Neurol Sci.* 2007;257(1):67–71.

130. Bower JE, Ganz PA, Desmond KA, Bernaards C, Rowland JH, Meyerowitz BE, et al. Fatigue in long-term breast carcinoma survivors: a longitudinal investigation. *Cancer.* 2006;106(4):751–8.

131. Ehrenstein JK, van Zon SKR, Duijts SFA, van Dijk BAC, Dorland HF, Schagen SB, et al. Type of cancer treatment and cognitive symptoms in working cancer survivors: an 18-month follow-up study. *J Cancer Surviv.* 2020;14(2):158–67.

132. Stouten-Kemperman MM, de Ruiter MB, Boogerd W, Veltman DJ, Reneman L, Schagen SB. Very late treatment-related alterations in brain function of breast cancer survivors. *J Int Neuropsychol Soc.* 2014;21:1–12.

133. Stouten-Kemperman MM, de Ruiter MB, Koppelmans V, Boogerd W, Reneman L, Schagen SB. Neurotoxicity in breast cancer survivors ≥10 years post-treatment is dependent on treatment type. *Brain Imaging Behav.* 2015;9(2):275–84.

134. Monje ML, Mizumatsu S, Fike JR, Palmer TD. Irradiation induces neural precursor-cell dysfunction. *Nat Med.* 2002;8(9):955–62.

135. Lee WH, Sonntag WE, Mitschelen M, Yan H, Lee YW. Irradiation induces regionally specific alterations in pro-inflammatory environments in rat brain. *Int J Radiat Biol.* 2010;86(2):132–44.

136. Coderre JA, Morris GM, Micca PL, Hopewell JW, Verhagen I, Kleiboer BJ, et al. Late effects of radiation on the central nervous system: role of vascular endothelial damage and glial stem cell survival. *Radiat Res.* 2006;166(3):495–503.

137. Klein M, Heimans JJ, Aaronson NK, van der Ploeg HM, Grit J, Muller M, et al. Effect of radiotherapy and other treatment-related factors on mid-term to long-term cognitive sequelae in low-grade gliomas: a comparative study. *Lancet.* 2002;360(9343):1361–8.

138. Douw L, Klein M, Fagel SS, van den Heuvel J, Taphoorn MJ, Aaronson NK, et al. Cognitive and radiological effects of radiotherapy in patients with low-grade glioma: long-term follow-up. *Lancet Neurol.* 2009;8(9):810–8.

139. Surma-aho O, Niemelä M, Vilkki J, Kouri M, Brander A, Salonen O, et al. Adverse long-term effects of brain radiotherapy in adult low-grade glioma patients. *Neurology.* 2001;56(10):1285–90.

140. Brown PD, Jaeckle K, Ballman KV, Farace E, Cerhan JH, Anderson SK, et al. Effect of radiosurgery alone vs radiosurgery with whole brain radiation therapy on cognitive function in patients with 1 to 3 brain metastases: a randomized clinical trial. *JAMA.* 2016;316(4):401–9.

141. Gondi V, Pugh SL, Tome WA, Caine C, Corn B, Kanner A, et al. Preservation of memory with conformal avoidance of the hippocampal neural stem-cell compartment during whole-brain radiotherapy for brain metastases (RTOG 0933): a phase II multi-institutional trial. *J Clin Oncol: Official J Am Soc Clin Oncol.* 2014;32(34):3810–6.

142. Hara Y, Waters EM, McEwen BS, Morrison JH. Estrogen effects on cognitive and synaptic health over the lifecourse. *Physiol Rev.* 2015;95(3):785–807.

143. Hajszan T, MacLusky NJ, Leranth C. Role of androgens and the androgen receptor in remodeling of spine synapses in limbic brain areas. *Horm Behav.* 2008;53(5):638–46.

144. Castellon SA, Ganz PA, Bower JE, Petersen L, Abraham L, Greendale GA. Neurocognitive performance in breast cancer survivors exposed to adjuvant chemotherapy and tamoxifen. *J Clin Exp Neuropsychol.* 2004;26(7):955–69.

145. Shilling V, Jenkins V, Fallowfield L, Howell T. The effects of hormone therapy on cognition in breast cancer. *J Steroid Biochem Mol Biol.* 2003;86(3–5):405–12.

146. Palmer JL, Trotter T, Joy AA, Carlson LE. Cognitive effects of Tamoxifen in pre-menopausal women with breast cancer compared to healthy controls. *J Cancer Surviv.* 2008;2(4):275–82.

147. Bender CM, Sereika SM, Berga SL, Vogel VG, Brufsky AM, Paraska KK, et al. Cognitive impairment associated with adjuvant therapy in breast cancer. *Psychooncology.* 2006;15(5):422–30.

148. Mar Fan H, Houédé-Tchen N, Chemerynsky I, Yi Q-L, Xu W, Harvey B. Menopausal symptoms in women undergoing chemotherapy-induced and natural menopause: a prospective controlled study. *Ann Oncol.* 2010;21(5):983–7.

149. Phillips KA, Ribi K, Sun Z, Stephens A, Thompson A, Harvey V, et al. Cognitive function in postmenopausal women receiving adjuvant letrozole or tamoxifen for breast cancer in the BIG 1-98 randomized trial. *Breast.* 2010;19(5):388–95.

150. Jenkins V, Shilling V, Fallowfield L, Howell A, Hutton S. Does hormone therapy for the treatment of breast cancer have a detrimental effect on memory and cognition? A pilot study. *Psychooncology.* 2004;13(1):61–6.

151. Jenkins VA, Ambroisine LM, Atkins L, Cuzick J, Howell A, Fallowfield LJ. Effects of anastrozole on cognitive performance in postmenopausal women: a randomised, double-blind chemoprevention trial (IBIS II). *Lancet Oncol.* 2008;9(10):953–61.

152. Gonzalez BD, Jim HSL, Booth-Jones M, Small BJ, Sutton SK, Lin H-Y, et al. Course and predictors of cognitive function in patients with prostate cancer receiving androgen-deprivation therapy: a controlled comparison. *J Clin Oncol: Official J Am Soc Clin Oncol.* 2015;33(18):2021–7.

153. Mohile SG, Lacy M, Rodin M, Bylow K, Dale W, Meager MR, et al. Cognitive effects of androgen deprivation therapy in an older cohort of men with prostate cancer. *Crit Rev Oncol/Hematol.* 2010;75(2):152–9.

154. Cherrier MM, Rose AL, Higano C. The effects of combined androgen blockade on cognitive function during the first cycle of intermittent androgen suppression in patients with prostate cancer. *J Urol.* 2003;170(5):1808–11.

155. Green HJ, Pakenham KI, Headley BC, Yaxley J, Nicol DL, Mactaggart PN, et al. Altered cognitive function in men treated for prostate cancer with luteinizing hormone-releasing hormone analogues and cyproterone acetate: a randomized controlled trial. *BJU Int.* 2002;90(4):427–32.

156. Sun M, Cole AP, Hanna N, Mucci LA, Berry DL, Basaria S, et al. Cognitive impairment in men with prostate cancer treated with androgen deprivation therapy: a systematic review and meta-analysis. *J Urol.* 2018;199(6):1417–25.

157. Alonso Quiñones HJ, Stish BJ, Hagen C, Petersen RC, Mielke MM. Prostate cancer, use of androgen deprivation therapy, and cognitive impairment: a population-based study. *Alzheimer Dis Assoc Disord.* 2020;34(2): 118–121.

158. Belloy ME, Napolioni V, Greicius MD. A quarter century of APOE and Alzheimer's disease: progress to date and the path forward. *Neuron.* 2019;101(5):820–38.

159. Montagne A, Nation DA, Zlokovic BV. *APOE4* accelerates development of dementia after stroke. *Stroke.* 2020;51(3):699–700.

160. Ben-Moshe H, Luz I, Liraz O, Boehm-Cagan A, Salomon-Zimri S, Michaelson D. ApoE4 exacerbates hippocampal pathology following acute brain penetration injury in female mice. *J Mol Neurosci.* 2020;70(1):32–44.

161. Ahles TA, Saykin AJ, Noll WW, Furstenberg CT, Guerin S, Cole B, et al. The relationship of APOE genotype to neuropsychological performance in long-term cancer survivors treated with standard dose chemotherapy. *Psychooncology.* 2003;12(6):612–9.

162. Koleck TA, Bender CM, Sereika SM, Ahrendt G, Jankowitz RC, McGuire KP, et al. Apolipoprotein E genotype and cognitive function in postmenopausal women with early-stage breast cancer. *Oncol Nurs Forum.* 2014;41(6):E313–25.

163. Mandelblatt JS, Small BJ, Luta G, Hurria A, Jim H, McDonald BC, et al. Cancer-related cognitive outcomes among older breast cancer survivors in the thinking and living with cancer study. *J Clin Oncol: Official J Am Soc Clin Oncol.* 2018;36(32):3211–22.

164. Saadat M. Apolipoprotein E (APOE) polymorphisms and susceptibility to breast cancer: a meta-analysis. *Cancer Res Treat.* 2012;44(2):121–6.

165. Porrata-Doria T, Matta JL, Acevedo SF. Apolipoprotein E allelic frequency altered in women with early-onset breast cancer. *Breast Cancer (Auckl).* 2010;4:43–8.

166. Small BJ, Rawson KS, Walsh E, Jim HS, Hughes TF, Iser L, et al. Catechol-O-methyltransferase genotype modulates cancer treatment-related cognitive deficits in breast cancer survivors. *Cancer.* 2011;117(7):1369–76.

167. Ren X, Boriero D, Chaiswing L, Bondada S, St Clair DK, Butterfield DA. Plausible biochemical mechanisms of chemotherapy-induced cognitive impairment ("chemobrain"), a condition that significantly impairs the quality of life of many cancer survivors. *Biochim Biophys Acta Mol Basis Dis.* 2019;1865(6):1088–97.

168. Phillips C. Brain-derived neurotrophic factor, depression, and physical activity: making the neuroplastic connection. *Neural Plast.* 2017;2017:7260130.

169. Yap NY, Tan NYT, Tan CJ, Loh KW-J, Ng RCH, Ho HK, et al. Associations of plasma brain-derived neurotrophic factor (BDNF) and Val66Met polymorphism (rs6265) with long-term cancer-related cognitive impairment in survivors of breast cancer. *Breast Cancer Res Treat.* 2020;183(3):683–96.

170. Koleck TA, Bender CM, Sereika SM, Brufsky AM, Lembersky BC, McAuliffe PF, et al. Polymorphisms in DNA repair and oxidative stress genes associated with pre-treatment cognitive function in breast cancer survivors: an exploratory study. *Springerplus.* 2016;5:422.

171. Merriman JD, Sereika SM, Conley YP, Koleck TA, Zhu Y, Phillips ML, et al. Exploratory study of associations between DNA repair and oxidative stress gene polymorphisms and cognitive problems reported by postmenopausal women with and without breast cancer. *Biol Res Nurs.* 2019;21(1):50–60.

172. Walker CH, Drew BA, Antoon JW, Kalueff AV, Beckman BS. Neurocognitive effects of chemotherapy and endocrine therapies in the treatment of breast cancer: recent perspectives. *Cancer Invest.* 2012;30(2):135–48.

173. Chae JW, Ng T, Yeo HL, Shwe M, Gan YX, Ho HK, et al. Impact of TNF-α (rs1800629) and IL-6 (rs1800795) polymorphisms on cognitive impairment in Asian breast cancer patients. *PLOS ONE.* 2016;11(10):e0164204.

174. Nguyen LD, Ehrlich BE. Cellular mechanisms and treatments for chemobrain: insight from aging and neurodegenerative diseases. *EMBO Mol Med.* 2020;12(6):e12075.

175. Huehnchen P, Boehmerle W, Springer A, Freyer D, Endres M. A novel preventive therapy for paclitaxel-induced cognitive deficits: preclinical evidence from C57BL/6 mice. *Transl Psychiatry.* 2017;7(8):e1185.

176. Lyons L, ElBeltagy M, Umka J, Markwick R, Startin C, Bennett G, et al. Fluoxetine reverses the memory impairment and reduction in proliferation and survival of hippocampal cells caused by methotrexate chemotherapy. *Psychopharmacology (Berl).* 2011;215(1):105–15.

177. Lyons L, ElBeltagy M, Bennett G, Wigmore P. Fluoxetine counteracts the cognitive and cellular effects of 5-fluorouracil in the rat hippocampus by a mechanism of prevention rather than recovery. *PLOS ONE.* 2012;7(1):e30010.

178. Callaghan CK, O'Mara SM. Long-term cognitive dysfunction in the rat following docetaxel treatment is ameliorated by the phosphodiesterase-4 inhibitor, rolipram. *Behav Brain Res.* 2015;290:84–9.

179. Johnston IN, Tan M, Cao J, Matsos A, Forrest DRL, Si E, et al. Ibudilast reduces oxaliplatin-induced tactile allodynia and cognitive impairments in rats. *Behav Brain Res.* 2017;334:109–18.

180. Winocur G, Binns MA, Tannock I. Donepezil reduces cognitive impairment associated with anti-cancer drugs in a mouse model. *Neuropharmacology.* 2011;61(8):1222–8.

181. Wartena R, Brandsma D, Belderbos J. Are memantine, methylphenidate and donepezil effective in sparing cognitive functioning after brain irradiation? *J Cancer Metastasis Treat.* 2018;4:59.

182. Lim I, Joung H-Y, Yu AR, Shim I, Kim JS. PET evidence of the effect of donepezil on cognitive performance in an animal model of chemobrain. *BioMed Res Int.* 2016;2016:6945415.

183. Gong S, Sheng P, Jin H, He H, Qi E, Chen W, et al. Effect of methylphenidate in patients with cancer-related fatigue: a systematic review and meta-analysis. *PLOS ONE.* 2014;9(1):e84391.

184. Vega JN, Dumas J, Newhouse PA. Cognitive effects of chemotherapy and cancer-related treatments in older adults. *Am J Geriatr Psychiatry.* 2017;25(12):1415–26.

185. Li C, Cheung MKH, Han S, Zhang Z, Chen L, Chen J, et al. Mesenchymal stem cells and their mitochondrial transfer: a double-edged sword. *Biosci Rep.* 2019;39(5):BSR20182417.

186. Wahdan SA, El-Derany MO, Abdel-Maged AE, Azab SS. Abrogating doxorubicin-induced chemobrain by immunomodulators IFN-beta 1a or infliximab: insights to neuroimmune mechanistic hallmarks. *Neurochem Int.* 2020;138:104777.

187. Sofis MJ, Jarmolowicz DP, Kaplan SV, Gehringer RC, Lemley SM, Garg G, et al. KU32 prevents 5-fluorouracil induced cognitive impairment. *Behav Brain Res.* 2017;329:186–90.

188. Jiang Z-G, Winocur G, Wojtowicz JM, Shevtsova O, Fuller S, Ghanbari HA. PAN-811 prevents chemotherapy-induced cognitive impairment and preserves neurogenesis in the hippocampus of adult rats. *PLOS ONE.* 2018;13(1):e0191866.

189. El-Agamy SE, Abdel-Aziz AK, Wahdan S, Esmat A, Azab SS. Astaxanthin ameliorates doxorubicin-induced cognitive impairment (chemobrain) in experimental rat model: impact on oxidative, inflammatory, and apoptotic machineries. *Mol Neurobiol.* 2018;55(7):5727–40.

190. Dietrich J, Baryawno N, Nayyar N, Valtis YK, Yang B, Ly I, et al. Bone marrow drives central nervous system regeneration after radiation injury. *J Clin Invest.* 2018;128(1):281–93.

191. Crowgey T, Peters KB, Hornsby WE, Lane A, McSherry F, Herndon JE, 2nd, et al. Relationship between exercise behavior, cardiorespiratory fitness, and cognitive function in early breast cancer patients treated with doxorubicin-containing chemotherapy: a pilot study. *Appl Physiol Nutr Metab [Physiologie appliquee, nutrition et metabolisme].* 2014;39(6):724–9.

192. Cooke GE, Wetter NC, Banducci SE, Mackenzie MJ, Zuniga KE, Awick EA, et al. Moderate physical activity mediates the association between white matter lesion volume and memory recall in breast cancer survivors. *PLOS ONE.* 2016;11(2):e0149552.

193. Sahnoune I, Inoue T, Kesler SR, Rodgers SP, Sabek OM, Pedersen SE, et al. Exercise ameliorates neurocognitive impairments in a translational model of pediatric radiotherapy. *Neuro Oncol.* 2018;20(5):695–704.

194. Campbell KL, Zadravec K, Bland KA, Chesley E, Wolf F, Janelsins MC. The effect of exercise on cancer-related cognitive impairment and applications for physical therapy: systematic review of randomized controlled trials. *Phys Therapy.* 2020;100(3):523–42.

195. Kempermann G, Fabel K, Ehninger D, Babu H, Leal-Galicia P, Garthe A, et al. Why and how physical activity promotes experience-induced brain plasticity. *Front Neurosci.* 2010;4:189.

196. Ferris LT, Williams JS, Shen CL. The effect of acute exercise on serum brain-derived neurotrophic factor levels and cognitive function. *Med Sci Sports Exerc.* 2007;39(4):728–34.

197. Wagner MA, Erickson KI, Bender CM, Conley YP. The influence of physical activity and epigenomics on cognitive function and brain health in breast cancer. *Front Aging Neurosci.* 2020;12:123.

198. Galantino ML, Greene L, Daniels L, Dooley B, Muscatello L, O'Donnell L. Longitudinal impact of yoga on chemotherapy-related cognitive impairment and quality of life in women with early stage breast cancer: a case series. *Explore (NY).* 2012;8(2):127–35.

199. Derry HM, Jaremka LM, Bennett JM, Peng J, Andridge R, Shapiro C, et al. Yoga and self-reported cognitive problems in breast cancer survivors: a randomized controlled trial. *Psychooncology.* 2015;24(8):958–66.

200. Kiecolt-Glaser JK, Bennett JM, Andridge R, Peng J, Shapiro CL, Malarkey WB, et al. Yoga's impact on inflammation, mood, and fatigue in breast cancer survivors: a randomized controlled trial. *J Clin Oncol: Official J Am Soc Clin Oncol.* 2014;32(10):1040–9.

201. Sulzer J, Haller S, Scharnowski F, Weiskopf N, Birbaumer N, Blefari ML, et al. Real-time fMRI neurofeedback: progress and challenges. *NeuroImage.* 2013;76:386–99.

202. Nelson DV, Esty ML. Neurotherapy as a catalyst in the treatment of fatigue in breast cancer survivorship. *EXPLORE.* 2016;12(4):246–9.

203. Alvarez J, Meyer FL, Granoff DL, Lundy A. The effect of EEG biofeedback on reducing postcancer cognitive impairment. *Integr Cancer Ther.* 2013;12(6):475–87.

204. Sarvghadi P, Ghaffari A, Rostami HR. The effects of neurofeedback training on short-term memory and quality of life in women with breast cancer. *Int J Therapy Rehab.* 2019;26(11):1–8.

205. Zimerman M, Hummel F. Non-invasive brain stimulation: enhancing motor and cognitive functions in healthy old subjects. *Front Aging Neurosci.* 2010;2: 149.

206. Gaynor AM, Pergolizzi D, Alici Y, Ryan E, McNeal K, Ahles TA, et al. Impact of transcranial direct current stimulation on sustained attention in breast cancer survivors: evidence for feasibility, tolerability, and initial efficacy. *Brain Stimul.* 2020;13(4):1108–16.

207. Ferguson RJ, Ahles TA, Saykin AJ, McDonald BC, Furstenberg CT, Cole BF, et al. Cognitive-behavioral management of chemotherapy-related cognitive change. *Psychooncology.* 2007;16(8):772–7.

208. McDougall GJ, Becker H, Acee TW, Vaughan PW, Delville CL. Symptom management of affective and cognitive disturbance with a group of cancer survivors. *Arch Psychiatr Nurs.* 2011;25(1):24–35.

209. Poppelreuter M, Weis J, Bartsch HH. Effects of specific neuropsychological training programs for breast cancer patients after adjuvant chemotherapy. *J Psychosoc Oncol.* 2009;27(2):274–96.

210. Von Ah D, Carpenter JS, Saykin A, Monahan P, Wu J, Yu M, et al. Advanced cognitive training for breast cancer survivors: a randomized controlled trial. *Breast Cancer Res Treat.* 2012;135(3):799–809.

211. Kesler S, Hadi Hosseini SM, Heckler C, Janelsins M, Palesh O, Mustian K, et al. Cognitive training for improving executive function in chemotherapy-treated breast cancer survivors. *Clin Breast Cancer.* 2013;13(4):299–306.

212. Schuurs A, Green HJ. A feasibility study of group cognitive rehabilitation for cancer survivors: enhancing cognitive function and quality of life. *Psychooncology.* 2013;22(5):1043–9.

213. Ferguson RJ, McDonald BC, Rocque MA, Furstenberg CT, Horrigan S, Ahles TA, et al. Development of CBT for chemotherapy-related cognitive change: results of a waitlist control trial. *Psychooncology.* 2012;21(2):176–86.

214. Correa DD, Ahles TA. Neurocognitive changes in cancer survivors. *Cancer J.* 2008;14(6):396–400.

215. Brem AK, Sensi SL. Towards combinatorial approaches for preserving cognitive fitness in aging. *Trends Neurosci.* 2018;41(12):885–97.

216. Kesler SR, Watson CL, Blayney DW. Brain network alterations and vulnerability to simulated neurodegeneration in breast cancer. *Neurobiol Aging.* 2015;36(8):2429–42.

Treating Tobacco Use in Cancer Survivors

10

Kathleen Gali and Judith J. Prochaska

INTRODUCTION

In 2019, 2.5 million cancer deaths globally were due to the use of tobacco (1). In the US, one in three cancer deaths are attributed to smoking tobacco (2), with considerable variation across US states and by sex. About one-quarter of US cancer deaths in women and one-third of cancer deaths in men can be explained by smoking. Smoking-attributable cancer death is highest in the southern states, where 40% of cancer deaths in men is attributable to smoking (3). Smoking raises the risk of at least 20 different types or subtypes of cancers in the body including lung, mouth, kidney, and colon cancer (4). Lung cancer is the most common cancer and the leading cause of cancer death. The risk of lung cancer diagnosis and lung cancer death increases by 80% with active cigarette smoking (5). The longer one smokes, and the more packs smoked per day, the greater the risk. Quitting smoking as early as possible can reduce the risk. Yet, smoking in cancer persists, with up to 50% of patients who smoke before a cancer diagnosis continuing to smoke during treatment (6).

Most patients who smoke want to quit and try to quit, but face challenges (7). Barriers to quitting include concerns about managing nicotine withdrawal symptoms, poor knowledge of or access to effective cessation therapies, and feelings of defeat or low self-efficacy (i.e., belief in one's ability to quit) due to prior failed quit attempts. When diagnosed with cancer, an additional barrier to care can be stigma in relation to the cancer diagnosis and tobacco addiction. Without medication and support, those who make a quit attempt are likely to relapse to smoking (8).

Tobacco smoking can complicate cancer treatments by interacting with medications (e.g., erlotinib, irinotecan) reducing serum concentrations, increasing cancer treatment side-effects, and slowing post-surgery recovery and wound healing (9–12). Smoking also can increase the risk of disease recurrence, second primary tumors, and other serious illnesses such as heart or lung disease or stroke (13). Quitting smoking as early as possible after a cancer diagnosis reduces the risk of complications and can increase survival and well-being (14).

Treating tobacco dependence means treating an addiction. When quitting tobacco, one has to deal with the physical addiction to nicotine and the psychological and social cues connected to smoking. Nicotine affects the dopamine reward system and upregulates nicotinic receptors in the brain (15). Stopping smoking decreases nicotine levels and causes a craving for nicotine and experiences of

DOI: 10.1201/9781003055426-10

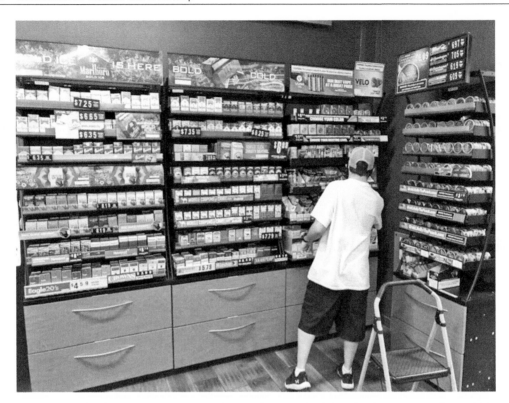

FIGURE 10.1 Tobacco display "power-wall" at a convenience store in Oregon. Image shows the variety of tobacco products sold from combustible cigarettes and cigars, to e-cigarettes, dip and chew products, and newer tobacco-free nicotine pouches. (Photo credit: Mark Martini, image taken October 23, 2020.)

withdrawal (15). Smoking cigarettes itself is habit forming with the constant hand-to-mouth motion, each hit from a cigarette bringing nicotine, with its stimulating and rewarding affects, to the brain. Various environmental and social cues can trigger smoking urges such as advertising and pack-displays at point-of-sale in retail stores (see Figure 10.1), smoking shown in the movies and on television, and being around friends and/or family members who smoke. To address both the addiction and conditioned habit of smoking, combination treatment of cessation medication and behavioral therapy is recommended.

The Continuous Update Project, supported by World Cancer Research Fund (WCRF) International, provides up-to-date analysis and information on cancer prevention and survival research (16). Their expert guided lifestyle recommendations identify smoking, other forms of tobacco, and secondhand smoke as the most important risk factors. To reduce the global burden of cancer, they recommend avoiding tobacco in any form plus maintaining a healthy diet and weight and being physically active.

The benefits of quitting tobacco have been well documented; yet barriers may prevent patients from accessing treatment. In this chapter, we review evidence-based treatments for quitting tobacco with a focus on the oncology setting and adult cigarette smoking. Most of the evidence to date has focused on treatments for quitting cigarettes; few studies have demonstrated success with treating smoking in adolescents. No studies to date have examined treatments for quitting electronic cigarettes (i.e., e-cigarettes or vapes). The latter part of the chapter considers system coordination to integrate treatment of tobacco within cancer care. Highlighted are a variety of population-based quality improvement (QI) models that are being implemented to treat tobacco use in cancer survivors funded by the National Cancer Institute's (NCI) Moonshot Initiative.

SMOKING CESSATION TREATMENT IN CANCER SURVIVORS

The National Comprehensive Cancer Network's (NCCN) guidelines recommend, regardless of cancer stage or prognosis, smoking cessation for the improvement in treatment outcomes. Recommendations are for the creation of a quit plan for all cancer patients who smoke, use of FDA-approved cessation medications, providing evidence-based motivational strategies and behavioral therapy (which can be brief), and continuous follow-up (17).

Pharmacotherapies to Aid Smoking Cessation

FDA-approved cessation medications are nicotine replacement therapy (NRT) in the form of gum, patches, lozenge, nasal spray, and inhaler; varenicline; and bupropion. Given their superior efficacy, varenicline and combination NRT (i.e., the combined use of nicotine patch plus nicotine gum or lozenge) are first-line options. In the inpatient setting, combined NRT is preferred as therapeutic effects are immediate; whereas for varenicline, the quit date is typically set 7 days out to build up the medication to therapeutic levels (17). Bupropion and single form NRT also are efficacious and FDA-approved. In the US, nicotine gums, lozenges, and patches can be purchased over the counter by adults 18 years and older, while prescriptions are needed for the nicotine nasal spray, nicotine inhaler, varenicline, and bupropion.

A minimum of 12 weeks of cessation medication treatment is recommended, although use for 6 months or longer may be necessary to prevent relapse or brief slips, which is common and can be managed. A medication guide for cessation medications that lists dosing and recommended treatment duration, precautions, advantages/disadvantages, adverse effects, and costs is shown in Table 10.1.

Varenicline

Varenicline is a partial nicotine receptor agonist binding with high affinity and selectivity at the $\alpha_4\beta_2$ neuronal nicotinic acetylcholine receptors, stimulating low-level agonist activity and competitively inhibiting binding of nicotine. Clinically this is experienced as reduced symptoms of nicotine withdrawal and lower reinforcement and reward associated with smoking. In head-to-head trials and concluded from meta-analyses, varenicline is the most effective single pharmacotherapy option in promoting smoking cessation and is comparably effective to combined NRT (18).

Tested in patients with cancer, varenicline showed a 84% retention rate, 40% abstinence at 12 weeks, and with no reports of expected side effects (e.g., nausea, sleep problems) (19). A second study of varenicline use in patients with cancer found no difference between 12 weeks versus 24 weeks of treatment (20).

Common side effects of varenicline are nausea, insomnia, and abnormal dreams. Varenicline safety has been extensively examined, especially in regard to cardiovascular events and neuropsychiatric changes. Studies have found varenicline to be safe and well tolerated. It should be noted, that while rare, patients with brain metastases with a history or elevated risk of seizure, should use varenicline with caution (17).

Nicotine replacement therapy

NRT facilitates smoking cessation by reducing withdrawal symptoms and by providing an alternative source of nicotine with less pleasurable (i.e., less dependence-producing) effects (15). The combination of a slow-acting (nicotine patch) with a fast-acting (nicotine gums, lozenges, sprays, and inhalers) form of

TABLE 10.1 FDA-approved medications for smoking cessation

	NICOTINE REPLACEMENT THERAPY (NRT) FORMULATIONS					BUPROPION SR	VARENICLINE
	GUM	LOZENGE	TRANSDERMAL PATCH	NASAL SPRAY	ORAL INHALER		
PRODUCT	**NICORETTE[1], GENERIC** OTC 2 mg, 4 mg original, cinnamon, fruit, mint (various)	**Nicorette[1], Generic Nicorette[1] Mini** OTC 2 mg, 4 mg; cinnamon, cherry, mint	**Habitrol[2], NicoDerm CQ[1], Generic** OTC 7 mg, 14 mg, 21 mg (24-hr release)	**Nicotrol NS[3]** Rx Metered spray 10 mg/mL nicotine solution	**Nicotrol Inhaler[3]** Rx 10 mg cartridge delivers 4 mg inhaled vapor	**Generic** (formerly Zyban) Rx 150 mg sustained-release tablet	**Chantix[3]** Rx 0.5 mg, 1 mg tablet
PRECAUTIONS	• Recent (≤2 weeks) myocardial infarction • Serious underlying arrhythmias • Serious or worsening angina pectoris • Temporomandibular joint disease • Pregnancy[4] and breastfeeding • Adolescents (<18 years)	• Recent (≤2 weeks) myocardial infarction • Serious underlying arrhythmias • Serious or worsening angina pectoris • Pregnancy[4] and breastfeeding • Adolescents (<18 years)	• Recent (≤2 weeks) myocardial infarction • Serious underlying arrhythmias • Serious or worsening angina pectoris • Pregnancy[4] and breastfeeding • Adolescents (<18 years)	• Recent (≤2 weeks) myocardial infarction • Serious underlying arrhythmias • Serious or worsening angina pectoris • Underlying chronic nasal disorders (rhinitis, nasal polyps, sinusitis) • Severe reactive airway disease • Pregnancy[4] and breastfeeding • Adolescents (<18 years)	• Recent (≤2 weeks) myocardial infarction • Serious underlying arrhythmias • Serious or worsening angina pectoris • Bronchospastic disease • Pregnancy[4] and breastfeeding • Adolescents (<18 years)	• Concomitant therapy with medications/conditions known to lower the seizure threshold • Hepatic impairment • Pregnancy[4] and breastfeeding • Adolescents (<18 years) • Treatment-emergent neuropsychiatric symptoms[5] **Contraindications:** • Seizure disorder • Concomitant bupropion (e.g., Wellbutrin) therapy • Current or prior diagnosis of bulimia or anorexia nervosa • Simultaneous abrupt discontinuation of alcohol or sedatives/benzodiazepines • MAO inhibitors in preceding 14 days; concurrent use of reversible MAO inhibitors	• Severe renal impairment (dosage adjustment is necessary) • Pregnancy[4] and breastfeeding • Adolescents (<18 years) • Treatment-emergent neuropsychiatric symptoms[5]

DOSING

1st cigarette ≤30 minutes after waking: 4 mg 1st cigarette >30 minutes after waking: 2 mg Weeks 1–6: 1 piece q 1–2 hours* Weeks 7–9: 1 piece q 2–4 hours* Weeks 10–12: 1 piece q 4–8 hours* • Maximum, 24 pieces/day • During initial 6 weeks of treatment, use at least 9 pieces/day • Chew each piece slowly • Park between cheek and gum when peppery or tingling sensation appears (~15–30 chews) • Resume chewing when tingle fades • Repeat chew/park steps until most of the nicotine is gone (tingle does not return; generally 30 min) • Park in different areas of mouth • No food or beverages 15 minutes before or during use • Duration: up to 12 weeks	1st cigarette ≤30 minutes after waking: 4 mg 1st cigarette >30 minutes after waking: 2 mg Weeks 1–6: 1 lozenge q 1–2 hours* Weeks 7–9: 1 lozenge q 2–4 hours* Weeks 10–12: 1 lozenge q 4–8 hours* • Maximum, 20 lozenges/day • During initial 6 weeks of treatment, use at least 9 lozenges/day • Allow to dissolve slowly (20–30 minutes) • Nicotine release may cause a warm, tingling sensation • Do not chew or swallow • Occasionally rotate to different areas of the mouth • No food or beverages 15 minutes before or during use • Duration: up to 12 weeks	_≥10 cigarettes/day:_ 21 mg/day x 4–6 weeks 14 mg/day x 2 weeks 7 mg/day x 2 weeks _≤10 cigarettes/day:_ 14 mg/day x 6 weeks 7 mg/day x 2 weeks • Rotate patch application site daily; do not apply a new patch to the same skin site for at least one week • May wear patch for 16 hours if patient experiences sleep disturbances (remove at bedtime); rule out other factors first, e.g., caffeine/tobacco smoke drug interaction, other medications, and lifestyle factors • Duration: 8–10 weeks	1–2 doses/hour* (8–40 doses/day) One dose = 2 sprays (one in **each** nostril); each spray delivers 0.5 mg of nicotine to the nasal mucosa • Maximum -5 doses/hour or -40 doses/day • During initial 6–8 weeks of treatment, use at least 8 doses/day • Gradually reduce daily dosage over an additional 4–6 weeks Do not sniff, swallow, or inhale through the nose as the spray is being administered • Duration: 12 weeks	6–16 cartridges/day Individualize dosing; initially use 1 cartridge q 1–2 hours* • Best effects with continuous puffing for 20 minutes • During initial 6 weeks of treatment use at least 6 cartridges/day • Gradually reduce daily dosage over the following 6–12 weeks • Nicotine in cartridge is depleted after 20 minutes of active puffing • Inhale into back of throat or puff in short breaths • Do NOT inhale into the lungs (like a cigarette) but "puff" as if lighting a pipe • Open cartridge retains potency for 24 hours • No food or beverages 15 minutes before or during use • Duration: 3–6 months	150 mg po q AM x 3 days, then 150 mg po bid • Do not exceed 300 mg/day • Begin therapy 1–2 weeks **prior** to quit date • Allow at least 8 hours between doses • Avoid bedtime dosing to minimize insomnia • Dose tapering is not necessary • Duration: 7–12 weeks, with maintenance up to 6 months in selected patients	Days 1–3: 0.5 mg po q AM Days 4–7: 0.5 mg po bid Weeks 2–12: 1 mg po bid • Begin therapy 1 week **prior** to quit date • Take dose after eating and with a full glass of water • Dose tapering is not necessary • Dosing adjustment is necessary for patients with severe renal impairment • Duration: 12 weeks; an additional 12-week course may be used in selected patients • May initiate up to 35 days before target quit date OR may reduce smoking over a 12-week period of treatment prior to quitting and continue treatment for an additional 12 weeks

(Continued)

TABLE 10.1 (Continued)　FDA-approved medications for smoking cessation

	NICOTINE REPLACEMENT THERAPY (NRT) FORMULATIONS					BUPROPION SR	VARENICLINE
	GUM	LOZENGE	TRANSDERMAL PATCH	NASAL SPRAY	ORAL INHALER		
ADVERSE EFFECTS	• Mouth and throat irritation • Jaw muscle soreness • Hiccups • GI complaints (dyspepsia, nausea) • May stick to dental work • Adverse effects more commonly experienced when chewing the lozenge or using incorrect gum chewing technique (due to rapid nicotine release): 　• *Lightheadedness/dizziness* 　• *Nausea/vomiting* 　• *Hiccups* 　• *Mouth and throat irritation*	• Mouth and throat irritation • Hiccups • GI complaints (dyspepsia, nausea)	• Local skin reactions (erythema, pruritus, burning) • Sleep disturbances (abnormal or vivid dreams, insomnia); associated with nocturnal nicotine absorption	• Nasal and/or throat irritation (hot, peppery, or burning sensation) • Ocular irritation/tearing • Sneezing • Cough	• *Mouth and/or throat irritation* • Cough • Hiccups • GI complaints (dyspepsia, nausea)	• *Insomnia* • Dry mouth • Nausea • Anxiety/difficulty concentrating • Constipation • Tremor • Rash • Seizures (risk is 0.15%) • Neuropsychiatric symptoms (rare; see PRECAUTIONS)	• *Nausea* • Sleep disturbances (insomnia, abnormal/ vivid dreams) • Headache • Flatulence • Constipation • Taste alteration • Neuropsychiatric symptoms (rare; see PRECAUTIONS)
ADVANTAGES	• Might serve as an oral substitute for tobacco • Might delay weight gain • Can be titrated to manage withdrawal symptoms • Can be used in combination with other agents to manage situational urges • Relatively inexpensive	• *Might serve as an oral substitute for tobacco* • Might delay weight gain • Can be titrated to manage withdrawal symptoms • Can be used in combination with other agents to manage situational urges • Relatively inexpensive	• Once-daily dosing associated with fewer adherence problems • Of all NRT products, its use is least obvious to others • Can be used in combination with other agents; delivers consistent nicotine levels over 24 hours • Relatively inexpensive	Can be titrated to rapidly manage withdrawal symptoms Can be used in combination with other agents to manage situational urges	Might serve as an oral substitute for tobacco Can be titrated to manage withdrawal symptoms • Mimics hand-to-mouth ritual of smoking • Can be used in combination with other agents to manage situational urges	• Twice-daily oral dosing is simple and associated with fewer adherence problems • Might delay weight gain • Might be beneficial in patients with depression • Can be used in combination with NRT agents • Relatively inexpensive (generic formulations)	• Twice-daily oral dosing is simple and associated with fewer adherence problems • Offers a different mechanism of action for patients who have failed other agents • Most effective cessation agent when used as monotherapy

	Nicotine gum[1]	Nicotine lozenge[2]	Nicotine patch	Nicotine nasal spray	Nicotine inhaler	Bupropion SR	Varenicline[3]
DISADVANTAGES	• Need for frequent dosing can compromise adherence • Might be problematic for patients with significant dental work • Proper chewing technique is necessary for effectiveness and to minimize adverse effects • Gum chewing might not be acceptable or desirable for some patients	• Need for frequent dosing can compromise adherence • Gastrointestinal side effects (nausea, hiccups, heartburn) might be bothersome	• When used as monotherapy, cannot be titrated to acutely manage withdrawal symptoms • Not recommended for use by patients with dermatologic conditions (e.g., psoriasis, eczema, atopic dermatitis)	• Need for frequent dosing can compromise adherence • Nasal administration might not be acceptable or desirable for some patients; nasal irritation often problematic • Not recommended for use by patients with chronic nasal disorders or severe reactive airway disease • Cost of treatment	• Need for frequent dosing can compromise adherence • Cartridges might be less effective in cold environments (≤60°F) • Cost of treatment	• Seizure risk is increased • Several contraindications and precautions preclude use in some patients (see PRECAUTIONS) • Patients should be monitored for potential neuropsychiatric symptoms[4] (see PRECAUTIONS)	• Patients should be monitored for potential neuropsychiatric symptoms[4] (see PRECAUTIONS) • Cost of treatment
Cost/day[5]	2 mg or 4 mg: $1.90–$5.49 (9 pieces)	2 mg or 4 mg: $2.97–$4.23 (9 pieces)	$1.52–$3.49 (1 patch)	$9.64 (8 doses)	$16.38 (6 cartridges)	$0.72 (2 tablets)	$17.20 (2 tablets)

1 Marketed by GlaxoSmithKline.

2 Marketed by Dr. Reddy's.

3 Marketed by Pfizer.

4 The U.S. Clinical Practice Guideline states that pregnant smokers should be encouraged to quit without medication based on insufficient evidence of effectiveness and theoretical concerns with safety. Pregnant smokers should be offered behavioral counseling interventions that exceed minimal advice to quit.

In July 2009, the FDA mandated that the prescribing information for all bupropion- and varenicline-containing products include a black-boxed warning highlighting the risk of serious neuropsychiatric symptoms, including changes in behavior, hostility, agitation, depressed mood, suicidal thoughts and behavior, and attempted suicide. Clinicians should advise patients to stop taking varenicline or bupropion SR and contact a health care provider immediately if they experience agitation, depressed mood, or any changes in behavior that are not typical of nicotine withdrawal, or if they experience suicidal thoughts or behavior. If treatment is stopped due to neuropsychiatric symptoms, patients should be monitored until the symptoms resolve. Based on results of a mandated clinical trial, the FDA removed this boxed warning in December 2016.

6 Approximate cost based on the recommended initial dosing for each agent and the wholesale acquisition cost from Red Book Online. Thomson Reuters, January 2021.

Note: For complete prescribing information and a comprehensive listing of warnings and precautions, please refer to the manufacturers' package inserts.

Abbreviations: MAO, monoamine oxidase; NRT, nicotine replacement therapy; OTC, over-the-counter (nonprescription product); Rx, prescription product.

*while awake

NRT is recommended as a first-line therapy providing comparable benefit to varenicline (17). The slow delivery of the nicotine patches helps ameliorate nicotine withdrawal symptoms, while the gum, lozenge, spray, or inhaler provide some acute nicotine relief. Combination NRT outperforms single form NRT (18); however, if combination NRT is not affordable or tolerated, single form NRT also is efficacious.

Dosing of NRT is guided by markers of nicotine dependence including time to first cigarette upon wakening and the number of cigarettes smoked per day. Nicotine patches are placed on the skin in the morning and deliver nicotine over 16–24 hours. Nicotine gum, lozenge, and inhaler are absorbed in relatively low doses of nicotine over 15–30 minutes and can be used every 1–2 hours.

Side effects from the nicotine patch include insomnia and/or abnormal dreams. Sleep disturbance can be avoided by removing the patch before bedtime. Side effects of the nicotine patch and gum include gastrointestinal symptoms, which can be reduced with instruction to "park" the products. The idea is to facilitate transfer of the nicotine through the oral mucosa into the blood stream, rather than creating nicotine-enriched saliva that is swallowed bringing nicotine into the stomach and gut. Burning and irritation effects of the nicotine nasal spray often decline with continued use. Overall, NRT products are well tolerated with benefits of use outweighing potential risks from continued smoking (21).

Additionally, randomized clinical trials have demonstrated nicotine mouth spray to be safe, efficacious, and acceptable for quitting smoking (22, 23). In 2019, an independent expert panel to the FDA recommended approval for over-the counter use (24). Nicotine mouth spray is sold in 45 countries, but is unavailable still in the US.

Bupropion

Bupropion, a stimulant drug that was originally marketed as an antidepressant, has been successfully used as a cessation aid, and received approval from the FDA for this indication. Bupropion's efficacy is comparable to single form NRT. Bupropion can be combined with NRT, with some trials showing increased benefit. Bupropion reduces the seizure threshold and should not be used in smokers who are at risk for seizures (e.g., patients with brain metastases with a history of seizures) (25).

Other medications with evidence, but not FDA-approved

Two additional medications in the US, nortriptyline and clonidine, have demonstrated efficacy for treating smoking, but are not FDA-approved for this indication (off-label), and tend to be used only by specialized tobacco treatment providers (17). Cytisine, considered one of the oldest medications for smoking cessation, is widely used in Central and Eastern Europe. The recommended treatment course is shorter (25 days versus 12 weeks), and cytisine is less costly (15, 26) than other cessation aids. Though not currently available in the US, clinical trials of cytisine are underway, and FDA approval is being sought (27).

E-cigarettes

To date, e-cigarettes have not been reviewed and approved by the FDA as a therapeutic aid for quitting smoking. In the US, e-cigarettes are regulated as a tobacco product, and there is insufficient evidence on the safety and efficacy to help in quitting smoking. No studies of e-cigarette use for quitting smoking have been published with a focus on cancer survivors (17).

Behavioral Support to Aid Smoking Cessation

Pharmacotherapy plus behavioral support increases quit attempts, and more intensive counseling can increase the success of quitting by 10%–20% (28). Compared to behavioral therapy or medication alone, combination medication and behavioral therapy is most effective (29). A number of behavioral treatments delivered via different channels (e.g., print, in-person, telephonic, digital health) have demonstrated evidence. Below we review different treatment forms with attention to feasibility of integration into oncology settings. At a minimum, all patients should be asked about their use of tobacco, and those who use tobacco should be advised to quit. A more comprehensive approach offers assistance and arranges follow-up, either in-person or via telephone or telemedicine. We detail quitline and digital health referral resources when in-house programs are not available.

5 "A"s

NCI's 5 "A"s (Ask-Advise-Assess-Assist-Arrange) is a framework for treating tobacco in health settings (30). The U.S. Preventive Services Task Force's Clinical Practice Guidelines recommends that clinicians: (i) **A**sk about tobacco use; (ii) **A**dvise patients who use tobacco to quit; (iii) **A**ssess readiness to quit; (iv) **A**ssist in the quit attempt by offering and providing counseling, medications, and referrals; and (v) **A**rrange for follow-up (31). The 5 "A"s framework guides providers on how to communicate to patients about tobacco use and treatments. In a survey of oncology patients, most reported being asked about their tobacco use and advised to quit, but less so were assisted with cessation medication (43%) or provided counseling (54.8%) or follow-up (30.7%) (32). When the 5 "A"s are incorporated, engagement in tobacco treatment and the likelihood of quitting and staying quit increases (33). Assessments should occur frequently, possibly at every clinic visit, to capture any changes in tobacco status. Relapse is a hallmark of nicotine addiction and if not assessed repeatedly an opportunity to help patients into a treatment program could be missed. A flowchart of the 5 "A"s tobacco cessation counseling framework is shown in Figure 10.2.

STEP One: ASK about Tobacco Use

↪ Suggested Dialogue

✓ Do you ever smoke or use any type of tobacco?
  – I take time to talk with all of my patients about tobacco use—because it's important.
✓ Condition X often is caused or worsened by exposure to tobacco smoke. Do you, or does someone in your household smoke?
✓ Medication X often is used for conditions linked with or caused by smoking. Do you, or does someone in your household smoke?

STEP Two: ADVISE to Quit

↪ Suggested Dialogue

  – Quitting is the most important thing you can do to protect your health now and in the future. I have training to help my patients quit, and when you are ready I would be more than happy to work with you to design a treatment plan.
  – What are your thoughts about quitting? Might you consider quitting sometime in the next month?
  – Prior to imparting advice, consider asking the patient for permission to do so – e.g., "May I tell you why this concerns me?" [then elaborate on patient-specific concerns]

STEP Three: Assess Readiness to Quit

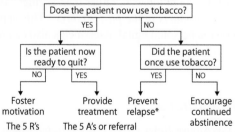

Foster motivation — The 5 R's

Provide treatment — The 5 A's or referral

Prevent relapse*

Encourage continued abstinence

* Relapse prevention interventions are not necessary if patient has not used tobacco for many years and is not at risk for re-initiation.

Fiore MC, Jaén CR, Baker TB, et al. *Treating Tobacco Use and Dependence: 2008 update.* Clinical Practice Guideline, Rockville, MD: U.S. Department of Health and Human Services. Public Health Service. May 2008.

STEP Four: ASSIST with Quitting

✓ **Assess Tobacco Use History**
  • Current use: type(s) of tobacco used, amount
  • Past use:
    – Duration of tobacco use
    – Changes in levels of use recently
  • Past quit attempts:
    – Number of attempts, date of most recent attempt, duration
    – Methods used previously—What did or didn't work? Why or why not?
    – Prior medication administration, dose, compliance, duration of treatment
    – Reasons for relapse
✓ **Discuss Key Issues** (for the upcoming or current quit attempt)
  • Reasons/motivation for wanting to quit (or avoid relapse)
  • Confidence in ability to quit (or avoid relapse)
  • Triggers for tobacco use
  • Routines and situations associated with tobacco use
  • Stress-related tobacco use
  • Concerns about weight gain
  • Concerns about withdrawal symptoms
✓ **Facilitate Quitting Process**
  • Discuss methods for quitting: pros and cons of the different methods
  • Set a quit date: ideally, less than 2 weeks away
  • Recommend Tobacco Use Log
  • Discuss coping strategies (cognitive, behavioral)
  • Discuss withdrawal symptoms
  • Discuss concept of "slip" versus relapse
  • Provide medication counseling: compliance, proper use, with demonstration
  • Offer to assist throughout the quit attempt
✓ **Evaluate the Quit Attempt** (at follow-up)
  • Status of attempt
  • "Slips" and relapse
  • Medication compliance and plans for discontinuation

STEP Five: ARRANGE Follow-up Counseling

✓ Monitor patients' progress throughout the quit attempt. Follow-up contact should occur during the first week after quitting. A second follow-up contact is recommended in the first month. Additional contacts should be scheduled as needed. Counseling contacts can occur face-to-face, by telephone, or by e-mail. Keep patient progress notes.
✓ Address temptations and triggers; discuss strategies to prevent relapse.
✓ Congratulate patients for continued success.

FIGURE 10.2 Tobacco cessation counseling 5 "A"s: Ask, Advise, Assess, Assist, and Arrange Follow-up. (Courtesy of The Regents of the University of California. Copyright © 1999–2021. All rights reserved. Updated January 15, 2021.)

Cancer centers are exploring innovative ways to incorporate the 5 "A"s into their practice. For example, at the Lurie Comprehensive Cancer Center of Northwestern University, patients are asked to report their tobacco use via a 5-item online assessment incorporated into their system's electronic health record (EHR) (34). Online patient assessments reduce stigma and staff burden and assist in efficient identification and documentation of smoking status. The items include questions on smoking history and current status, number of cigarettes smoked, and degree of tobacco dependence. If not completed online in the patient portal, patients can complete the assessment during a clinic visit. Once a positive tobacco screen is identified, a message is sent directly to a tobacco treatment specialist who contacts the patient and offers treatment options for quitting. In a quality improvement pilot, of the 164 patients with a positive tobacco screen, 87% were reached, and about 50% engaged in treatment.

In addition to cigarette smoking, given greater diversification in the tobacco product market, it is important to screen for current use of other forms of nicotine and tobacco use, such as cigars and cigarillos, hookah, smokeless oral tobacco products (dip, chew, snus), e-cigarettes or nicotine vapes, and tobacco-free nicotine pouches (e.g., Zyn, Velo, on!). Exposure to smoke in the home by family or friends also should be assessed and addressed. Secondhand smoke is a risk factor for cancer, heart disease, and stroke and should be avoided (35). Among patients with cancer not traditionally perceived as tobacco-related, secondhand smoke in the home was found to be a barrier to quitting smoking after diagnosis (36). Helping patients make a smoke-free home environment removes potential triggers, decreases further health risks through secondhand smoke exposure, and can increase the likelihood of quitting (37). If feasible, family members should be offered smoking cessation services or referred to treatment to aid in their quitting and to provide support to cancer survivors. Integrating family members into patients' tobacco treatment has been found feasible (38).

Once patients are identified as using tobacco, the next step is engaging them in tobacco treatment. Direct outreach achieves higher utilization rates than traditional referral by a provider or alert from the EHR. However, the direct approach has a higher time burden requiring staff to contact patients via phone and/or electronic message, possibly multiple times. The Duke Cancer Center Smoking Cessation Program reported 60 hours a month spent making outreach calls (39). For some programs, direct outreach may be too costly and burdensome.

When assessing tobacco use, clinicians are encouraged to consider potential stigma experienced by patients with cancer who smoke. There are tendencies, mostly by individuals who do not smoke, to place blame on patients who continue to smoke, and to fault their lack of intrinsic motivation to quit. Uninformed beliefs include that people should be able to quit and those who do not are foolish (40). This can affect patients' health outcomes, wellbeing, and ability to seek treatment for their tobacco use. Supportive approaches such as the use of non-judgmental language can help decrease the stigma felt by patients with cancer who smoke. For example, when asking about tobacco, rather than asking: *"are you a smoker;"* ask: *"have you used tobacco or other nicotine products in the past 30 days."* This approach puts emphasis on the behavior of smoking rather than on the person. Digital assessments also can reduce stigma.

Referrals to quitlines and digital health solutions

If limited in time for the full 5 "A"s, providers can Ask-Advise-Refer (AAR), where *refer* would be to an outside entity such as the toll-free national quitline (1-800-QUIT-NOW); NCI comprehensive website (www.smokefree.gov) with interactive programs, smartphone apps, and text messaging (see Figure 10.3); or to a local tobacco treatment program. In a study of utilization of the Michigan Tobacco Quitline among patients with cancer referred for treatment, 79% completed one or more counseling calls and 26% were tobacco-free at 6-months follow-up (41). Information about quitting and other support programs also can be found on various agency websites such as the Centers for Disease Control, American Cancer Society, American Lung Association, and state and county public health departments.

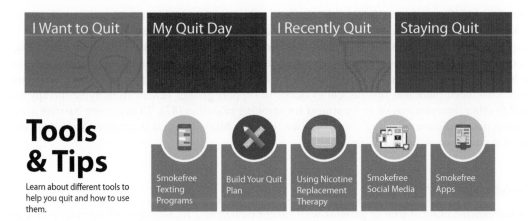

FIGURE 10.3   Welcome page of the National Cancer Institute's Smokefree.gov tobacco treatment resource which provides programs for the general public, veterans, women, teens, Spanish-speakers, and adults age 60 years and older. (Courtesy of National Cancer Institute.)

Smartphone technology

Patients are likely to differ in their preferences for treatment. Mobile technologies enable patients to receive support and learn techniques to deal with cravings at a self-directed pace. Researchers developed and are testing Quit2Heal, a smartphone app designed for patients with cancer who smoke that helps users cope with smoking urges. The app's tobacco treatment guide focuses on teaching skills to deal with cancer-related shame, stigma, depression, anxiety, and common triggers to smoke. A pilot study of the Quit2Heal app showed acceptability and potential effectiveness in helping patients with cancer quit smoking (42).

Within-system tobacco treatment counseling services

Ideally, for coordination of care and engagement in treatment, tobacco cessation services are integrated within an oncology clinic, overarching cancer center, or entire health system. Such services may be provided in-clinic during an existing patient visit, arranged for separate in-person appointments, or provided via phone counseling or telemedicine.

Intensive counseling goes beyond the brief, often one-time intervention, and involves multiple therapy sessions over an extended amount of time, and even extended medication support to help reduce the risk of relapse. Research found an intensive smoking counseling intervention that lasted up to 6 months improved quit rates among cancer survivors (37).

Cessation counseling orientations tend to be cognitive behavioral and motivational, although, increasingly, other clinical approaches (e.g., mindfulness, acceptance and commitment therapy) are being incorporated. Cognitive behavioral components focus on replacing negative thinking with more positive thinking and addressing the behaviors that may promote smoking toward healthier and protective behaviors against urges (43). Motivational techniques (e.g., open questions, affirmation, reflective listening, summary reflections) use an interview format by asking questions and listening for "change talk." A collaborative process with empathy can alleviate ambivalence about quitting smoking and support those who smoke make a commitment to quit (44). Mindfulness approaches can include guided meditation, incorporating mindful eating habits and yoga movements. A mindfulness group intervention was found to be feasible and acceptable as a treatment option for smoking cessation among cancer survivors (45). The acceptance-commitment therapy (ACT) approach has been shown to be a potential alternative to the predominant cognitive behavioral approach to smoking cessation counseling. ACT uses a mindfulness approach to help navigate the journey to quitting. Those who smoke are taught to acknowledge and accept their cravings to smoke, emotions, or thoughts, and take committed actions toward their quit goals. Research comparing ACT based interventions to cognitive behavioral have been found to be comparable in helping people quit smoking (46). Hypnotherapy has been used as a therapeutic tool to help people quit smoking. While a popular choice, a Cochrane review concluded there was insufficient evidence to support greater benefit from hypnotherapy compared to other interventions or no treatment for smoking cessation (47). To overcome barriers accessing care, due to distance, lack of transportation, or immobility, tobacco treatment counseling can be provided via phone or telemedicine.

Phone counseling

In a randomized clinical trial of patients with cancer treated at 2 NCI-designated comprehensive cancer centers, patients who received sustained telephone counseling plus free FDA-approved smoking cessation medication compared with short-term telephone counseling were more likely to be tobacco-free at 6-months follow-up (37). Telephone counseling was delivered by a certified tobacco treatment counselor in a motivational interviewing style with a focus on cognitive behavioral and stress management and resiliency strategies. The sustained intensive treatment group received 12 sessions: 4 weekly, 4 biweekly over 2 months, and then 3 booster sessions monthly. In contrast, the standard treatment group was only offered 4 weekly sessions. Besides intensive treatment, factors associated with quit status were increases in motivation to quit, self-efficacy, establishment of home smoking rules, and decreases in anxiety.

Telemedicine

The rise of sophisticated technology systems, as well as the surge in demand with the need for physical distancing during the COVID-19 pandemic (48), has led to exponential growth in the use of telemedicine. While telemedicine cannot offer physical hands-on exams or lab work that could be done during an in-person visit, it is a viable option for delivering tobacco cessation treatment. Rather than just a phone call, video allows the patient and counselor to see one another making the interaction more personal. To support the rise in the use of telemedicine, the American Academy of Family Physicians developed the Tobacco Cessation Telehealth Guide for providers, which includes information on billing codes (49). At Memorial Sloan Kettering, their tobacco cessation program made a rapid change from in-person to telehealth sessions during the beginning of the pandemic (50). They saw high patient attendance at the virtual sessions, and when compared to in-person visits, the virtual sessions had higher rates of completion. While their program was successful, and shown to be feasible and acceptable, the authors do note the barriers to implementation. These included getting set up with the technology for the telehealth sessions on both the clinician and patient sides, and issues dealing with insurance coverage for telehealth services. Once the technology is set up and the workflow has been established these barriers subside.

SYSTEM-BASED APPROACHES

Despite recommendations from various leading health organizations, tobacco treatment programs are not widely available at cancer centers and referral rates tend to be low. The 5 "A's are not always done fully by providers. Most ask, asses, and advise on quitting tobacco (72%–90%), but less discuss and provide cessation (30%–55%), and even a lower percentage address tobacco use at follow up (32, 51). Thus, rates of engagement in tobacco treatment are not as high as it could be (52). Barriers to implementation include lack of institutional buy-in, need for staff training, perceptions that patients are not interested in quitting, and availability of resources (51, 53, 54).

NCI Moonshot Cancer Center Cessation Initiative (C3I)

To address the need for cancer centers to implement evidence-based and sustainable tobacco treatment programs, the NCI Moonshot Initiative launched the Cancer Center Cessation Initiative (C3I). Since 2017, 3 cohorts (2017–2019, 2018–2020, and 2020–2022) for a total of 52 cancer centers, have received funding and support via the C3I Coordinating Center at the University of Wisconsin (55) (see Figure 10.4). C3I centers were expected to develop tobacco treatment programs through the enhancement of workflows to improve identification and documentation of tobacco use in EHRs, identify barriers to treatment and assist patients in overcoming them, achieve institutional buy-in, and develop a mechanism for sustainability after the funding period (56).

After 1 year of funding, the first cohort of C3I funded centers were able to integrate various tobacco treatment services into their existing clinical workflows. Availability of in-person counseling programs, cessation medication, and text- or web-based programs grew, as well as an increase in capacity to deliver the programs through hiring of skilled tobacco treatment specialists (57).

Moving from opt-in to opt-out

A major shift in addressing tobacco use in healthcare settings is the move away from the traditional "opt-in" approach, whereby the burden is put on the patient who has to request or follow through on a referral from their oncology provider. Alternatively, "opt-out" models automatically refer patients for

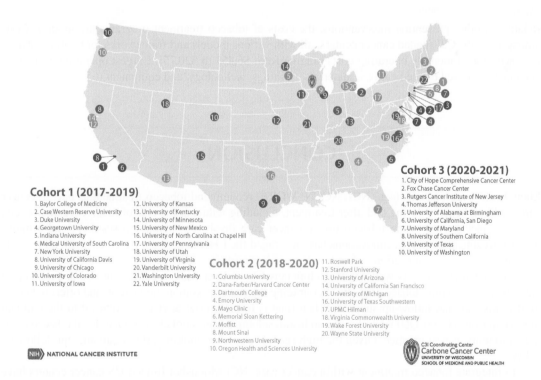

FIGURE 10.4 Map of the National Cancer Institute's Moonshot Cancer Center Cessation Initiative (C3I) funded programs. (Courtesy of National Cancer Institute.)

evidence-based tobacco cessation treatment. If patients are not interested, they have the option to opt-out from engaging in care. There have been ethical concerns raised due to the presumed consent within an opt-out model. Though after weighing the consequences, goods, and the rights of moral agents, and considering the preservation of autonomy with the principle of beneficence, the opt-out approach is deemed ethical and encouraged for health systems treating cancer survivors (58). The opt-out model for tobacco treatment has proven feasible in inpatient and cancer care settings (59, 60), with increased patient reach and engagement (61) and quit rates (62).

Stanford Cancer Center Tobacco Treatment Services

With C3I funding, the Stanford Cancer Center developed an opt-out model for tobacco treatment (63). Prior to integrating the tobacco treatment program, partnerships with pilot clinics were established, shadowing and observations in clinic occurred to determine how the program could fit within existing workflows, and strong relationships with clinic staff were developed to ensure the prioritization and sustainability of tobacco treatment integration. During this pre-implementation phase it was noticed that one of the major barriers to engagement in tobacco treatment was the reliance on clinician referrals in the EHR. Implementing an automated opt-out model was preferred to ensure all patients were screened for tobacco use and provided opportunities to engage in tobacco treatment. Once patients were identified as a tobacco user through the EHR, they were contacted by a tobacco treatment specialist and offered a menu of services that included individual counseling, group therapy, and same-day delivery of medication. Through this process, reach and engagement increased. Within a year, 33% of 273 patients reached had engaged in either one or two tobacco treatment services (63). Of those who completed a 6 months follow-up, 30% reported being tobacco-free. When asked about the program, 70% would refer the program to others, and 69% were satisfied with the program (64).

Costs

Relative to other prevention interventions, the costs of tobacco treatment programs are modest. Costs among 15 of the C3I funded cancer centers, all with various models and frameworks for treating tobacco in cancer, found monthly operating costs ranging from $6,453 to $20,751. Largest operating costs were personnel, followed by medications, materials, trainings, technology, and equipment (65).

CONCLUSION

Many health organizations (e.g., NCI, NCCN, WCRF) recommend tobacco treatment as part of cancer care, yielding benefits during and after treatment, including reducing the risk of recurrence and second primary cancers. Addressing tobacco use in cancer care involves systematic assessment and a multi-pronged treatment approach. Innovations have leveraged the EHR to assess tobacco use with all patients and trigger treatment connections when tobacco use is reported.

The oncology team, as well as other clinicians who deliver care to cancer survivors, can support patients with becoming tobacco-free by encouraging the use of cessation medication and offering behavioral counseling and follow-up support. When time is limited, brief advice and referral to the national tobacco quitline (1-800-QUIT-NOW), digital health solutions (e.g., smokefree.gov), or local tobacco treatment programs is best practice. Given the high risk of relapse to smoking after a quit attempt, follow-up is key.

To integrate tobacco treatment within cancer care, NCI Moonshot funded US cancer centers have been testing different system-level models (e.g., opt-out) and treatment delivery channels (e.g., telemedicine) within clinic workflows. Findings from these innovative tobacco treatment quality improvement programs are indicating great potential. Programs have increased patient engagement at a reasonable cost per quit. Ultimately, supporting cancer survivors in quitting tobacco can improve treatment outcomes and optimize patient quality of life.

REFERENCES

1. Global Burden of Disease Collaborative Network. Global Burden of Disease Study 2019 (GBD 2019) Results. 2021. http://ghdx.healthdata.org/gbd-results-tool. Accessed 19 Jan 2021.
2. Jacobs EJ, Newton CC, Carter BD, et al. What proportion of cancer deaths in the contemporary United States is attributable to cigarette smoking? *Ann Epidemiol.* 2015;25(3):179–82.e1.
3. Lortet-Tieulent J, Goding Sauer A, Siegel RL, et al. State-level cancer mortality attributable to cigarette smoking in the United States. *JAMA Intern Med.* 2016;176(12):1792–8.
4. Wild CP, Weiderpass E, Stewart BW. World Cancer Report: Cancer Research for Cancer Prevention. Lyon, France: International Agency for Research on Cancer [Internet]. 2020. http://publications.iarc.fr/586. Accessed 20 Jan 2021.
5. The Health Consequences of Smoking: A Report of the Surgeon General. Atlanta (GA): Dept. of Health and Human Services, Centers for Disease Control and Prevention, National Center for Chronic Disease Prevention and Health Promotion, Office on Smoking and Health. 2004.
6. Burke L, Miller L-A, Saad A, et al. Smoking behaviors among cancer survivors: an observational clinical study. *J Oncol Pract.* 2009;5(1):6–9.
7. Paul CL, Tzelepis F, Boyes AW, et al. Continued smoking after a cancer diagnosis: a longitudinal study of intentions and attempts to quit. *J Cancer Surviv.* 2019;13(5):687–94.
8. Ostroff JS, Jacobsen PB, Moadel AB, et al. Prevalence and predictors of continued tobacco use after treatment of patients with head and neck cancer. *Cancer.* 1995;75(2):569–76.
9. Marin VP, Pytynia KB, Langstein HN, et al. Serum cotinine concentration and wound complications in head and neck reconstruction. *Plast Reconstr Surg.* 2008;121(2):451–7.
10. Gajdos C, Hawn MT, Campagna EJ, et al. Adverse effects of smoking on postoperative outcomes in cancer patients. *Ann Surg Oncol.* 2012;19(5):1430–8.
11. O'Malley M, King AN, Conte M, et al. Effects of cigarette smoking on metabolism and effectiveness of systemic therapy for lung cancer. *J Thorac Oncol.* 2014;9(7):917–26.
12. Peppone LJ, Mustian KM, Morrow GR, et al. The effect of cigarette smoking on cancer treatment-related side effects. *Oncologist.* 2011;16(12):1784–92.
13. Parsons A, Daley A, Begh R, et al. Influence of smoking cessation after diagnosis of early stage lung cancer on prognosis: systematic review of observational studies with meta-analysis. *BMJ.* 2010;340:b5569.
14. Garces YI, Yang P, Parkinson J, et al. The relationship between cigarette smoking and quality of life after lung cancer diagnosis. *Chest.* 2004;126(6):1733–41.
15. Prochaska JJ, Benowitz NL. Current advances in research in treatment and recovery: nicotine addiction. *Sci Adv.* 2019;5(10):eaay9763.
16. World Cancer Research Fund/American Institute for Cancer Research. Continuous Update Project Expert Report. Recommendations and public health and policy implications. 2018. Available at dietandcancerreport.org. Accessed 22 Jan 2021.
17. Shields PG, Bierut L, Herbst RS, et al. NCCN Clinical Practice Guidelines in Oncology (NCCN Guidelines): Smoking Cessation. 2020. https://www.nccn.org/professionals/physician_gls/pdf/smoking.pdf. Accessed 22 Jan 2021. A UCSF Smoking Cessation Leadership Center, https://smokingcessationleadership.ucsf.edu/curricula/rx-change. Accessed 21 Apr 2021
18. Cahill K, Stevens S, Perera R, et al. Pharmacological interventions for smoking cessation: an overview and network meta-analysis. *Cochrane Database Syst Rev.* 2013(5):Cd009329.
19. Price S, Hitsman B, Veluz-Wilkins A, et al. The use of varenicline to treat nicotine dependence among patients with cancer. *Psychooncology.* 2017;26(10):1526–34.
20. Schnoll R, Leone F, Veluz-Wilkins A, et al. A randomized controlled trial of 24 weeks of varenicline for tobacco use among cancer patients: efficacy, safety, and adherence. *Psychooncology.* 2019;28(3):561–9.
21. Fiore MC, Jaén CR, Baker TB, et al. *Treating tobacco use and dependence: 2008 update.* Rockville, MD: US Department of Health and Human Services. 2008.
22. Nides M, Danielsson T, Saunders F, et al. Efficacy and safety of a nicotine mouth spray for smoking cessation: a randomized, multicenter, controlled study in a naturalistic setting. *Nicotine Tob Res.* 2018;22(3):339–45.
23. Tønnesen P, Lauri H, Perfekt R, et al. Efficacy of a nicotine mouth spray in smoking cessation: a randomised, double-blind trial. *Eur Respir J.* 2012;40(3):548–54.

24. Joseph S, Mishra M. GSK's over-the-counter nicotine oral spray gets FDA panel backing. 2019. https://www.reuters.com/article/us-gsk-fda-idUSKBN1W32V2. Accessed 16 Feb 2021.

25. Hughes JR, Stead LF, Hartmann-Boyce J, et al. Antidepressants for smoking cessation. *Cochrane Database Syst Rev.* 2014(1).

26. Tutka P, Vinnikov D, Courtney RJ, et al. Cytisine for nicotine addiction treatment: a review of pharmacology, therapeutics and an update of clinical trial evidence for smoking cessation. *Addiction.* 2019;114(11):1951–69.

27. ClinicalTrials.gov. https://clinicaltrials.gov/ct2/show/NCT03709823. Accessed 16 Feb 2021.

28. Hartmann-Boyce J, Hong B, Livingstone-Banks J, et al. Additional behavioural support as an adjunct to pharmacotherapy for smoking cessation. *Cochrane Database Syst Rev.* 2019(6).

29. U.S. Department of Health and Human Services. Smoking Cessation: A Report of the Surgeon General. Atlanta, GA: U.S. Department of Health and Human Services, Centers for Disease Control and Prevention, National Center for Chronic Disease Prevention and Health Promotion, Office on Smoking and Health. 2020.

30. Clinical Practice Guideline Treating Tobacco Use and Dependence 2008 Update Panel Liaisons and Staff. A clinical practice guideline for treating tobacco use and dependence: 2008 update. A U.S. Public Health Service report. *Am J Prev Med.* 2008;35(2):158–76.

31. U.S. Preventive Services Task Force. Final Recommendation Statement: Interventions for Tobacco Smoking Cessation in Adults, Including Pregnant Persons. 2021. https://www.uspreventiveservicestaskforce.org/uspstf/recommendation/tobacco-use-in-adults-and-pregnant-women-counseling-and-interventions. Accessed 23 Jan 2021.

32. Neil JM, Price SN, Friedman ER, et al. Patient-level factors associated with oncology provider-delivered brief tobacco treatment among recently diagnosed cancer patients. *Tob Use Insights.* 2020;13:1179173X20949270.

33. Quinn VP, Hollis JF, Smith KS, et al. Effectiveness of the 5-As tobacco cessation treatments in nine HMOs. *J Gen Intern Med.* 2009;24(2):149–54.

34. May JR, Klass E, Davis K, et al. Leveraging patient reported outcomes measurement via the electronic health record to connect patients with cancer to smoking cessation treatment. *Int J Environ Res Public Health.* 2020;17(14):5034.

35. Brennan P, Buffler PA, Reynolds P, et al. Secondhand smoke exposure in adulthood and risk of lung cancer among never smokers: a pooled analysis of two large studies. *Int J Cancer.* 2004;109(1):125–31.

36. Eng L, Qiu X, Su J, et al. The role of second-hand smoke exposure on smoking cessation in non-tobacco-related cancers. *Cancer.* 2015;121(15):2655–63.

37. Park ER, Perez GK, Regan S, et al. Effect of sustained smoking cessation counseling and provision of medication vs shorter-term counseling and medication advice on smoking abstinence in patients recently diagnosed with cancer: a randomized clinical trial. *JAMA.* 2020;324(14):1406–18.

38. Ruebush E, Mitra S, Meyer C, et al. Using a family systems approach to treat tobacco use among cancer patients. *Int J Environ Res Public Health.* 2020;17(6):2050.

39. Davis JM, Thomas LC, Dirkes JEH, et al. Strategies for referring cancer patients in a smoking cessation program. *Int J Environ Res Public Health.* 2020;17(17).

40. Luberto CM, Hyland KA, Streck JM, et al. Stigmatic and sympathetic attitudes toward cancer patients who smoke: a qualitative analysis of an online discussion board forum. *Nicotine Tob Res.* 2016;18(12):2194–201.

41. Notier AE, Hager P, Brown KS, et al. Using a quitline to deliver opt-out smoking cessation for cancer patients. *JCO Oncol Pract.* 2020;16(6):e549–56.

42. Bricker JB, Watson NL, Heffner JL, et al. A smartphone app designed to help cancer patients stop smoking: results from a pilot randomized trial on feasibility, acceptability, and effectiveness. *JMIR Form Res.* 2020;4(1):e16652.

43. Perkins KA, Conklin CA, Levine MD. *Cognitive-behavioral therapy for smoking cessation: a practical guidebook to the most effective treatments.* London: Taylor & Francis. 2008.

44. Miller WR, Rollnick S. *Motivational interviewing: Helping people change.* New York, NY: Guilford Press. 2012. [Database]

45. Charlot M, D'Amico S, Luo M, et al. Feasibility and acceptability of mindfulness-based group visits for smoking cessation in low-socioeconomic status and minority smokers with cancer. *J Altern Complement Med.* 2019;25(7):762–9.

46. McClure Jennifer B, Bricker J, Mull K, et al. Comparative effectiveness of group-delivered acceptance and commitment therapy versus cognitive behavioral therapy for smoking cessation: a randomized controlled trial. *Nicotine Tob Res.* 2020;22(3):354–62.

47. Barnes J, McRobbie H, Dong CY, et al. Hypnotherapy for smoking cessation. *Cochrane Database Syst Rev.* 2019(6).

48. Koonin LM, Hoots B, Tsang CA, et al. Trends in the use of telehealth during the emergence of the COVID-19 pandemic—United States, January–March 2020. *Morb Mortal Wkly Rep.* 2020;69(43):1595.

49. American Academy of Family Physicians (AAFP). Tobacco Cessation Telehealth Guide. 2020.

50. Kotsen C, Dilip D, Carter-Harris L, et al. Rapid scaling up of telehealth treatment for tobacco-dependent cancer patients during the COVID-19 outbreak in New York City. *Telemed e-Health.* 2020;27(1):20–9.

51. Warren GW, Marshall JR, Cummings KM, et al. Practice patterns and perceptions of thoracic oncology providers on tobacco use and cessation in cancer patients. *J Thorac Oncol.* 2013;8(5):543–8.

52. Goldstein AO, Ripley-Moffitt CE, Pathman DE, et al. Tobacco use treatment at the US National Cancer Institute's Designated Cancer Centers. *Nicotine Tob Res.* 2013;15(1): 52–58.

53. Adsit R, Wisinski K, Mattison R, et al. A survey of baseline tobacco cessation clinical practices and receptivity to academic detailing. *WMJ.* 2016;115(3):143–6.

54. Warren GW, Marshall JR, Cummings KM, et al. Addressing tobacco use in patients with cancer: a survey of American Society of Clinical Oncology members. *J Oncol Pract*. 2013;9(5):258–62.

55. University of Wisconsin-Madison Center for Tobacco Research and Intervention. C3I Expands Consortium to Help Cancer Patients Quit Smoking. 2020. https://ctri.wisc.edu/2020/12/11/c3i-expands-consortium-to-help-cancer-patients-quit-smoking/. Accessed 22 Jan 2021.

56. National Cancer Institute. Cancer Center Cessation Initiative. 2020. https://cancercontrol.cancer.gov/brp/tcrb/cancer-center-cessation-initiative. Accessed 22 Jan 2021.

57. D'Angelo H, Rolland B, Adsit R, et al. Tobacco treatment program implementation at NCI Cancer Centers: progress of the NCI Cancer Moonshot-Funded Cancer Center Cessation Initiative. *Cancer Prev Res*. 2019;12(11):735–40.

58. Ohde JW, Master Z, Tilburt JC, et al. Presumed consent with opt-out: an ethical consent approach to automatically refer patients with cancer to tobacco treatment services. *J Clin Oncol*. 2021;39(8):876–80.

59. Nahhas GJ, Wilson D, Talbot V, et al. Feasibility of implementing a hospital-based "opt-out" tobacco-cessation service. *Nicotine Tob Re*. 2017;19(8):937–43.

60. Nolan M, Ridgeway JL, Ghosh K, et al. Design, implementation, and evaluation of an intervention to improve referral to smoking cessation services in breast cancer patients. *Support Care Cancer*. 2019;27(6):2153–8.

61. Richter KP, Ellerbeck EF. It's time to change the default for tobacco treatment. *Addiction*. 2015;110(3):381–6.

62. Amato KA, Reid ME, Ochs-Balcom HM, et al. Evaluation of a dedicated tobacco cessation support service for thoracic cancer center patients. *J Public Health Manag Pract*. 2018;24(5):E12.

63. Gali K, Pike B, Kendra MS, et al. Integration of tobacco treatment services into cancer care at Stanford. *Int J Environ Res Public Health*. 2020;17(6):2101.

64. Chieng A, Tran, C, Chandler, M, Gali, K, Pike, B, Kendra, M, Prochaska, JJ, editor. 6-Mo Tobacco Usage Among Cancer Patients Engaged in a Tobacco Treatment Program – Learning to Improve Engagement. Society for Research on Nicotine and Tobacco Conference. 2021; Virtual.

65. Salloum R, D'Angelo H, Theis R, et al. Mixed-methods Economic Evaluation of the Implementation of Tobacco Treatment Programs in National Cancer Institute-designated Cancer Centers. Research Square. 2021.

Special Considerations in Older Cancer Survivors

11

Juan Pablo Negrete-Najar, Andrea Perez-de-Acha, Ana Patricia Navarrete-Reyes, and Enrique Soto-Perez-de-Celis

Approximately 64% of cancer survivors in the US are aged ≥65 years, and one in five older adults is a cancer survivor. This number is expected to increase given the demographic and epidemiologic transitions and the increasingly better survival rates in older adults with cancer (1). In addition, the interaction between cancer treatment toxicity and age-related physiological changes makes older cancer survivors more likely to suffer from one or more systemic and/or psychological (depression, anxiety, and adjustment disorders) chronic conditions (2).

Older cancer survivors have a higher prevalence of geriatric syndromes, such as functional impairment and frailty, compared with their counterparts without cancer (3), ranging from those that minimally impact activities of daily living to those that impair major organ systems. Effects such as decreased general functioning and reduced energy level may persist for up to 20 years after a cancer diagnosis (4). Aging is a heterogenous process, which combined with the effects of cancer and cancer therapies, leads to wide variations in the needs of older survivors, requiring individualized assessment, treatment, and follow up. Therefore, physicians taking care of older survivors need a greater understanding of how to identify and manage age-related health issues (5).

In most high-income countries, old age is defined as being ≥65 years. However, older adults are a highly heterogeneous group, and chronological age alone provides limited information regarding the fitness of an individual (3). Therefore, knowledge of an older individual's functional and physiological age allows for a better understanding of their vulnerabilities and could lead to higher quality survivorship care (5).

GERIATRIC SYNDROMES AND OLDER CANCER SURVIVORS

"Geriatric syndrome" refers to multifactorial clinical conditions in older persons that don't fit into a discrete disease category, and include functional disability, incontinence, falls, frailty, pressure ulcers, malnutrition, and delirium, among others. They occur when the accumulated effects of impairments

DOI: 10.1201/9781003055426-11

in multiple systems render an older person vulnerable to situational challenges (6, 7). Although their clinical presentations are heterogeneous, they share many common features, including having multiple underlying etiologies, shared risk factors, causing considerable impact on quality of life (QoL), and disability.

The relationship between cancer survivorship and geriatric syndromes is not thoroughly understood. A few studies have addressed functionality/disability in older adults with a new cancer diagnosis. A study of over 900 patients aged ≥65 years with newly diagnosed breast, colon, lung, and prostate cancer found that physical functioning improved (8) while depressive symptoms decreased (9) over one year of follow up. On the contrary, in a cohort of older adults with breast cancer (BC), physical functioning and mental health declined over a follow up period of 15 months (10). Nevertheless, both studies showed that the number of comorbid conditions predicted changes in physical and mental health.

Studies comparing younger and older cancer survivors have consistently found greater psychologic impact among younger survivors (11–15). However, older adults consistently report worse physical functioning (11, 14, 16). When compared with the general population, age correlates with better emotional and social functioning among survivors, but also with worse physical function (11).

Studies comparing long-term BC survivors according to age at diagnosis, show that survivors diagnosed at an older age (≥65 years) report significantly worse QoL in the physical domain, whereas those diagnosed at younger ages report worse social QoL (17). Among the most significant problems cited by survivors are sexual issues, fatigue, and family-related conflict surrounding disease recurrence. Importantly QoL varies by cancer site, with head and neck, and bladder cancer survivors reporting the worst QoL (18, 19).

Additionally, older cancer survivors have higher rates of specific comorbidities, are less likely to report being in excellent health, and have more mobility and activity limitations when compared to the general population (20–22). Importantly, functional decline seems to be correlated with other comorbidities rather than with the cancer itself.

Long-term cancer survivors have more geriatric syndromes than age-matched individuals without a history of cancer, and the number of geriatric syndromes correlates with mortality. In women who were long-term cancer survivors, the presence of ≥3 geriatric syndromes was associated with a 4-fold increased risk of 10-year mortality (23). While cancer survivors without geriatric syndromes had a 1.3–1.4-fold increased risk of death when compared with age matched cancer-free controls, the highest mortality risk occurred among women with deficits in physical functioning (HR 2.0). Other geriatric syndromes, including functional disability, severe comorbidity, malnutrition, polypharmacy, and cognitive impairment also increase 5-year mortality in colorectal cancer survivors (24); while poor mental health, functional disability, comorbidities, and inability to manage finances increase the risk of mortality in surgically treated older patients with BC (25).

There is extensive evidence to support the use of a comprehensive geriatric assessment (CGA) early in the cancer care continuum, as it can assist with care planning and is associated with improved health-related outcomes in various settings (26). CGA is a multidisciplinary diagnostic and treatment process that identifies medical, psychosocial, and functional problems of an older person that can be used to develop a coordinated plan aimed at maximizing overall health and to understand an individual's functional and physiologic age, going beyond chronological age alone (26). Identifying geriatric conditions can prevent or delay complications through the use of targeted interventions to address impairments (5). Information gained from the CGA can identify unique patient needs and aid in planning individualized survivorship care.

Conducting a CGA may facilitate cancer surveillance practices and help in the prevention and management of common chronic health conditions (27). A CGA generally includes validated tools that assess several domains important in determining physiologic age (Table 11.1). The choice of specific tools for the assessment of each domain is driven by local expertise since there is no gold standard (28). CGA can be performed in a variety of settings and should lead to interventions aimed at decreasing the risk of morbidity and mortality among older cancer survivors (29).

TABLE 11.1 Frequently used tools for each domain of the CGA

DOMAIN	SELECTED TOOLS	COMMENTS
Functional status	Activities of Daily Living (Katz index)	6 skills needed to live independently at home
	Instrumental Activities of Daily Living (Lawton and Brody index)	8 tasks needed to live independently in the community
Performance-based measures	Timed Up and Go test	Quick, requires no training. Cut-off score 14 seconds
	Short Physical Performance Battery	Evaluates lower extremity function and mobility
	Gait speed	Gait speed at comfortable pace. Cut-off score <0.8 m/s
Cognitive function	Mini-Mental State Examination	Requires 5–10 minutes to apply. Cut-off score: 24 points
	Montreal Cognitive Assessment	Greater sensitivity to detect mild levels of cognitive impairment
	Mini-Cog	Simple 3-item screening tool
Nutrition	Mini Nutritional Assessment	Identifies older adults at risk for malnutrition
Psychological status	Geriatric Depression Scale	High sensitivity when compared to DSM-V criteria
	Patient Health Questionnaire-9	Brief, sensitive screening tool for depression

COMPREHENSIVE GERIATRIC ASSESSMENT

Functional Status

Functional status refers to the ability to perform routine daily tasks, self-care, and physical activities. Functional status has been shown to predict survival, identify mobility impairments, and postoperative morbidity and mortality (30). Functional assessment includes a review of the patient's ability to complete activities of daily living (ADLs) and instrumental activities of daily living (IADLs). ADLs are basic self-care skills needed to maintain independence at home, such as bathe, dress, toilet, feed one-self, maintain continence, and transfer from a bed or chair without assistance (Katz Index) (31). IADLs are those required to maintain independence in the community, such as using the telephone, taking transportation, shopping, housekeeping, preparing meals, managing finances, and taking medications (Lawton Index) (32). It is fundamental to inquire about the reason behind functional decline, since this will inform the type of intervention needed. For example, options for the treatment of pain-associated disability diverge from those of disability caused by cognitive impairment or weakness.

Objective Performance-Based Measures

Commonly used performance-based measures include gait speed, balance, and upper and lower extremity strength, which are associated with clinical outcomes (33). Commonly used tests include the Timed Up and Go test (TUG), the Short Physical Performance Battery and the hand grip test. Gait speed is an important indicator in older persons, since it is an independent predictor of mortality (34). Gait speeds ≥1.0 m/s suggest healthier aging, while gait speeds <0.8 m/s are related to poor health and functional status. TUG is a brief and simple test performed by measuring the time it takes for a patient to rise from a chair, walk a fixed distance across the room (10 feet), turn around, walk back to the chair, and sit down, with a cut-off score of 14 seconds (Figure 11.1) (35). Observation of the different TUG components may help identify deficits in balance, strength, and gait.

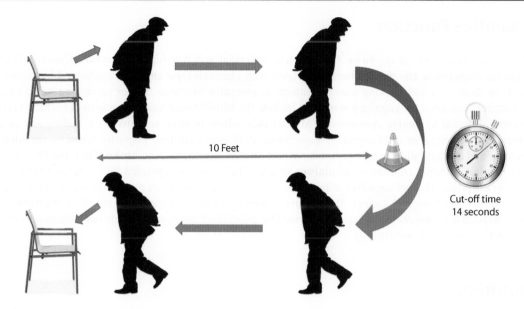

FIGURE 11.1 Timed Up and Go test.

Fall Risk Assessment

Falls are a major health concern in the older population, they are related to the ability of living independently and are associated with worse outcomes, including increased risk of chemotherapy toxicity (36). Falls are typically multifactorial and need to be thoroughly evaluated using a multidisciplinary approach with the goal of minimizing risks (37). They may also be manifestations of an underlying disease, such as infections, and require immediate evaluation.

Comorbidity

An assessment of comorbidity should be included in every CGA. Comorbidity impacts non-cancer specific life expectancy, tolerance to cancer treatment, disease-free and overall survival, and functional decline (27). Comorbidity burden is often measured using standardized indices, including the Charlson Comorbidity Index (CCI) (38) and the Cumulative Illness Rating Scale – Geriatrics (CIRS-G) (39) (Table 11.2).

TABLE 11.2 Tools to measure comorbidity

TOOL	MAIN CHARACTERISTICS
Charlson Comorbidity Index	• Created originally in 1987 to predict 10-year mortality • Points added for age and for several chronic conditions, including cancer • Validated as a prognostic marker for several index diseases • Can be used to predict 10-year survival
Cumulative Illness Rating Scale-Geriatrics (CIRS-G)	• Quantifies burden of disease, no cut-off point (higher scores indicate higher severity) • Validated in primary care, residential settings, nonagenarians, and hospitalized older adults • Predictive capacity for mortality and hospitalization

Cognitive Function

The impact of cancer on cognitive function has important survivorship implications. Cancer-related cognitive impairment has mainly been associated with chemotherapy and is characterized by impairments in short-term and working memory, attention, executive functions, and/or processing speed (40). Instruments validated for cognitive screening include the Mini-Mental State Examination (MMSE) (41) and the Montreal Cognitive Assessment (MoCA) (42), which is more sensitive as it is designed as a screening instrument for mild cognitive impairment. Both assess multiple cognitive domains, including attention and concentration, language, memory, and executive function. Another brief test, the Mini-Cog (43), requires minimal training to administer so it can be easily incorporated into general practice. It remains uncertain whether cognitive impairments in older cancer survivors result from treatment, cancer itself, and/or psychological factors. If cognitive screening raises suspicions for cognitive impairment, more detailed neuropsychological tests performed by a specialist are needed to rule out Alzheimer's disease and/or vascular dementia (40).

Nutrition

An increase in obesity among older cancer survivors has been reported and, as with all cancer survivors, maintaining or obtaining a healthy weight should be a priority since obesity leads to functional decline, comorbidity, and reduced QoL (44). In addition, the incidence of malnutrition among older adults is higher than in their younger counterparts, and is associated with worse outcomes and with increased mortality (27, 44). Screening tools for nutritional status in older survivors include body mass index (BMI), unintentional weight loss, or validated tools such as the Mini Nutritional Assessment (MNA). The MNA has high correlation with clinical assessment and objective indicators of nutritional status and has the highest validity and reliability to detect malnutrition (45). An important issue to consider when assessing the nutritional status of an older adult is social support, since a weak social network may lead to decreased access to food.

Psychological Status

Depression is common among older adults, and its presence increases the risk of functional decline, poor QoL, high caregiver burden, and increased healthcare utilization. Brief validated screening tools, such as the Geriatric Depression Scale (GDS), which is specifically designed for the assessment of depression in older individuals (46), and the Patient Health Questionnaire-9 (PHQ-9) which can be used in populations of all ages (47), may help detect patients who are experiencing depression.

Social Support

Patients who are most vulnerable to psychological distress are those with inadequate social support, and social isolation has been linked to an increased risk of mortality (48). Assessment of social support to identify problems can help plan referrals and assess available resources. An essential part of the CGA is identifying direct and indirect caregivers (adult children, friends, and relatives) who provide not only hands-on care but also indirect support (financial, emotional, social), since the presence of a large network of caregivers prevents isolation and leads to improved outcomes (30). Importantly, caregivers should be screened periodically for symptoms of caregiver burden as an essential part of CGA (49).

BOX 1.   POLYPHARMACY CASE STUDY

Mrs. H is a 72-year-old woman with a history of early-stage hormone receptor-positive breast cancer treated with mastectomy 6 years ago who is visiting her primary care physician for a follow-up visit. She was initially treated with adjuvant letrozole but switched to tamoxifen due to arthralgia and is currently receiving extended tamoxifen therapy. Mrs. H's has several comorbidities including type 2 diabetes, hypertension, chronic back pain, and recently diagnosed depression. Physical examination reveals a BMI of 23 kg/m², a blood pressure of 105/65, and mild back pain. Upon reviewing Mrs. H's medication list, they identify she is taking the following drugs, which have been prescribed by various physicians: aspirin, metformin, pioglitazone, acetaminophen, lisinopril, amlodipine, gabapentin, omeprazole, diclofenac, and paroxetine. Mrs. H's primary care physician decides to reduce pain control medications by discontinuing gabapentin, since she does not seem to have neuropathic pain, and diclofenac. Furthermore, Mrs. H's current blood pressure measurements do not seem to warrant two hypertensives, leading to the discontinuation of amlodipine. After checking drug-drug interactions, the primary care physician reaches out to Mrs. H's oncologist, and they decide to discontinue paroxetine due to potential interactions with tamoxifen, and to substitute for escitalopram.

Polypharmacy

Older cancer survivors have a higher burden of comorbidity when compared with age-matched cancer-free older adults (50). This burden increases with age, going from 27% in survivors aged between 66 and 69 years to 47% in those aged ≥85 years. In turn, these comorbidities are associated with an increased need for the use of medications, leaving cancer survivors at risk of polypharmacy (concurrent use of ≥5 medications) and of receiving potentially inappropriate medications (51). Other definitions of polypharmacy include using a drug without indication, using inadequate dosing, and using a drug that caused adverse effects (AEs) in the past (52).

Prescription medication use is significantly higher in cancer survivors compared with patients without a history of cancer (50). Data from the US show a prevalence of polypharmacy among cancer survivors of 30–60% (53, 54). In these studies, polypharmacy was found to be strongly associated with age, with almost 80% of cancer survivors aged ≥80 years taking ≥5 prescription medications (53). In addition, 40% of cancer survivors are at risk of potential drug interactions (55).

The National Comprehensive Cancer Network (NCCN) Older Adult Oncology Guidelines recommend a comprehensive evaluation of medication-associated issues followed by the discontinuation of non-essential or potentially inappropriate medications (56). Tools such as Beers criteria (57) and Screening Tool of Older People's Prescriptions (STOPP) and the Screening Tool to Alert to Right Treatment (START) (58) can help identify potentially inappropriate medications. Strategies for successful deprescribing among older adults include the involvement of other healthcare professionals, such as geriatricians and/or pharmacists. The inclusion of pharmacists in the multidisciplinary team taking care of older survivors has been recommended by the Cancer and Aging Research Group (CARG), since they can conduct a comprehensive evaluation of all medications, recommend the discontinuation of potentially inappropriate drugs, and help reduce treatment complexity (59).

FRAILTY IN OLDER CANCER SURVIVORS

Frailty describes a state of reduced physiologic reserve that might be conceptualized as a way of aging; however, frailty is also a dynamic construct (60). Older persons may move in and out of frailty, and subsequently in and out of vulnerability. For research purposes, it can be operationalized as a biological

TABLE 11.3   Frequently used models for the definition of frailty

BIOLOGICAL PHENOTYPE MODEL	*DEFICIT ACCUMULATION MODEL*
1. **Shrinking** Unintentional weight loss (>10 lbs. in the prior year)	1. Ratio of existing deficits to total number of deficits assessed.
2. **Weakness** Grip strength in the lowest 20%, (by gender and body mass index)	2. Deficits may include symptoms, signs, laboratory values, diseases, and other health conditions.
3. **Exhaustion** Self-reported	
4. **Slowness** Walking time/15 feet Slowest 20% (by gender and height)	
5. **Low activity** Lowest 20% <383 kcal/week in females <270 kcal/week in males	
Classification 3 or more → frail 1–2 → prefrail 0 → robust	**Classification** <0.10 → non-frail 0.10–0.21 → prefrail 0.211–0.45 → frail >0.45 → most frail (61)

phenotype characterized by reduced physiologic reserve or as an accumulation of conditions that impact function and longevity (Table 11.3). The usual way to identify frailty is through a CGA.

In older cancer survivors, frailty is extremely frequent (59%) (62). Its presence is related to age, gender, cancer type, treatment exposure (particularly radiation to the brain, abdomen and pelvis, extremity amputation, platinum exposure (63, 64), lung surgery, hematopoietic stem cell transplantation (65–67), androgen deprivation therapy) (68, 69), and lifestyle factors (such as smoking and sedentarism) (70), among others.

Frail cancer survivors are at higher risk for early morbidity or mortality. Associations between frailty at the time of diagnosis and adverse health-related outcomes across the disease trajectory have been reported in survivors of breast, colorectal, and other types of cancer. Pre-frailty and frailty are associated with a significantly increased risk of hospital and long-term care admissions (71). In addition, in women with non-metastatic BC, frailty has been negatively associated with cognition at the time of diagnosis and with self-reported cognitive decline (72, 73). An association between frailty and life expectancy among older cancer survivors has also been reported (13.9 years among non-frail survivors vs. 2.5 years among frail survivors) (Figure 11.2) (74).

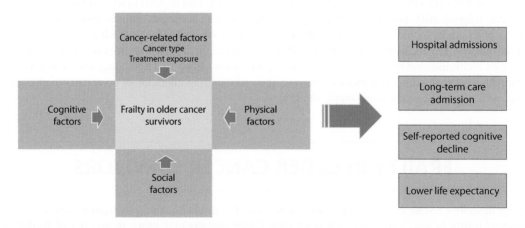

FIGURE 11.2   Determinants and outcomes of frailty in older cancer survivors.

Since frailty is a multicomponent construct, interventions to prevent/treat it require an interdisciplinary perspective. However, currently there is no evidence on how to prevent or treat frailty among older cancer survivors, and oncologists or primary care physicians who identify frailty in a patient should refer him/her to a geriatrician or to a center where geriatric expertise is available (60). In addition, the implementation of nutritional and lifestyle interventions could also prove useful at mitigating frailty. A recent review of studies targeting prevention and treatment of frailty in adult populations with and without chronic disease demonstrated that physical activity and nutritional supplementation were the two interventions most likely to reduce frailty (75). Several promising pharmaceutical approaches are also under investigation, including compounds mimicking caloric restriction, increasing nicotinamide adenine dinucleotide (NAD+) levels, eliminating senescent cells, and inhibiting the receptor for advanced glycation end-products (75).

SYMPTOM MANAGEMENT IN OLDER CANCER SURVIVORS

The clinical and pharmacological management of symptoms among older cancer survivors is complex, since it may be influenced by physiological changes associated with aging. Aging modifies the different systems and organs of the body, usually leading to a reduction in function. These changes mostly impact pharmacokinetics (Table 11.4), while pharmacodynamics are usually only slightly changed, with many alterations caused by drug-drug interactions and polypharmacy. When prescribing to an older person it is a good idea to "*start low, go slow, but go*": start at lower doses, conduct careful titration, and avoid underprescription.

Fatigue

To prevent or reduce fatigue, older adults should do at least 30 minutes of moderate-intensity aerobic activity ≥5 days per week. If they cannot tolerate this intensity, they should do the amount that is possible according to their abilities. Older adults should also engage in progressive muscle-strengthening activity on at least two nonconsecutive days per week and include balance training regularly (76, 77). In older adults, physical activity not only helps with fatigue but also reduces the risk of falls, sarcopenia, and hip fracture. Evidence showing physical activity reduces the risk of cognitive impairment is also substantial (78). A challenging issue for the primary care physician is how to motivate an older cancer survivor to

TABLE 11.4   Changes in pharmacokinetics

PROCESS	CHANGES
Absorption	• Rate and extent are usually unaffected. • Drug-drug and drug-food interactions are common. • Some older adults may have diminished acid secretion in the stomach which may interfere with drug absorption.
Distribution	• Body composition changes, there is an increase in the fat/water ratio, which combined with a decrease in albumin levels causes fat-soluble drugs to have larger distribution volume. • Highly protein-bound drugs have a greater "free" concentration.
Metabolism	• Liver mass and blood flow decrease, with a slight reduction in cytochrome activity, which may cause lower dosages to be therapeutic. • Drugs metabolized through phase II pathways are not affected by aging.
Elimination	• Liver changes and decreased glomerular filtration may cause longer drug half-life. • Cockroft-Gault formula recommended for dose adjustments.

engage in physical activity. It is important to provide guidance regarding activities that are both safe and inspiring, and to encourage truly personalized goal setting taking into account each patient's preferences, habits, social context, and hobbies. Self-management should be promoted, and physical activity should not be presented as a goal in itself, but rather as a tool to stay healthy and to remain socially active.

Pharmacological interventions for fatigue are scarce and include modafinil and methylphenidate. In older adults, these drugs have been studied mainly in the palliative context, with mixed results. Response rate is decreased compared to younger adults (79), and AEs can be severe (agitation or restlessness, sinus tachycardia or palpitations, delirium or confusion, and insomnia). If the decision is made to use psychostimulants, we recommend starting with lower doses than those recommended for adults with a slow upward titration, for the introduction of the drug and a slow taper at the time of discontinuation of the drug (80).

Since fatigue is a geriatric syndrome we recommend that it should lead to a careful evaluation to identify probable underlying causes or triggers. The most common causes of fatigue are thyroid disease, anemia, malnutrition, depression, heart failure, diabetes, and electrolyte imbalance (81).

Pain

In older cancer survivors the appearance of new pain should prompt a diagnostic work-up. On the other hand, chronic pain in older adults (cancer related or not) often develops via a multifactorial pathway, resulting in various sequelae including poor self-reported health and QoL, disability, impaired ambulation, depression, and decreased socialization, as well as falls, low energy, and impaired sleep (82).

The approach to pain management in older persons differs from that for younger people. Clinical manifestations of persistent pain are often complex, and older people may underreport pain. Concurrent illnesses and multiple problems make pain evaluation and treatment more difficult (83, 84). Older persons are more likely to experience medication-related side effects and have a higher potential for complications related to diagnostic and invasive procedures.

Topical agents are ideal for localized pain. Some topical non-steroidal anti-inflammatory drugs (NSAIDs) have comparable efficacy to oral formulations. Even if less effective, these agents may be a reasonable option because their safety profile is superior (85). Topical agents are considered an ideal adjunct for an older adult with localized pain that is uncontrolled with other medications, or when specific medications are contraindicated (86).

Owing to its greater safety than traditional NSAIDs, acetaminophen is recommended as first-line oral therapy for pain (87). In older adults, the maximum dosage is 4 grams per day, and lower doses are preferred (88). NSAID-associated AEs are significant and may be dose-related and time-dependent (89, 90), so they should be used for short periods at the lowest dose possible. In older adults, NSAIDs are preferred for episodic pain, and when it is estimated that the etiology can be corrected leading to the resolution of the symptom. COX-2 inhibitors carry almost the same risk as NSAIDs, so they should be used with the same caution. NSAIDs may adversely affect blood pressure control, renal function, and heart-failure management. Thus, comorbidities should always be considered when prescribing medications for an older adult with pain (91–93).

In cases warranting opioid therapy, optimum management requires a comprehensive treatment program including functional restorative and psychosocial modalities. The potential AEs of opioids represent a barrier to long-term treatment. Although most AEs decrease over time (except for constipation), they can be debilitating lead to therapy discontinuation. Patients should be asked about AEs repeatedly, treatment should be started at low doses and titrated, and a laxative should be prescribed (senna could be an acceptable first option) (83, 94).

Steroids are only recommended in low dose, short-term courses, for patients near the end of life (EOL). Antinociceptive effects have been observed with the use of cannabinoids in animal models and in some clinical trials in patients with persistent pain, but little is known about their effects in older individuals who were not included in clinical trials. Since the therapeutic window for cannabinoids appears to be narrow in older adults due to dysphoria, they are best avoided (95).

Neuropathy

Older adults are at increased risk of neuropathic pain. Age-related diseases/conditions associated with neuropathic pain include diabetes mellitus, postherpetic neuralgia, low back pain (such as lumbar spinal stenosis), limb amputation, and stroke (96). In cancer survivors, these overlap with cancer and treatment-related neuropathy.

Both gabaergics and anti-depressants, typically used for neuropathic pain, should be started at lower doses, and titrated slowly. A good practice is to increase dosage by small amounts every other week. A third consideration is that of AEs: there is general agreement that serotonin and norepinephrine reuptake inhibitors (SNRIs) such as duloxetine and venlafaxine are safe to use among older adults (97). However, the risk of hyponatremia due to SNRI-related syndrome of inappropriate secretion of antidiuretic hormone is greater among older patients. Baseline electrolyte levels should be checked, and sodium levels closely monitored throughout treatment. These drugs can cause sleepiness, dizziness, slowness, and falls, so patients should be advised on fall prevention (98), including wearing appropriate footwear and undertaking household modifications (99, 100).

PREVENTIVE GERONTOLOGY IN OLDER CANCER SURVIVORS

Preventive gerontology is the study of individual and population health strategies across the lifespan aimed at maximizing both the quality and quantity of human longevity. Functional decline, loss of independence, and chronic diseases are not inevitable consequences of aging. Positive habits and behaviors can have an influence on the health and functioning of individuals as they age, making some conditions potentially preventable (101).

Implementing Annual Wellness Visit (AWV) (102) programs for older cancer survivors can help meet needs in prevention. AWVs are yearly appointments with a primary care provider to create or update a personalized prevention plan. AWV can be used to identify potential problems and establish a list of necessary screenings and preventive strategies.

Preventive strategies should be personalized according to a person's age, gender, and risk factor profile. A history of cancer should be considered when establishing preventive interventions, since older cancer survivors have specific psychological, social, and physical health-related issues (5). Older cancer survivors are at increased risk of weight gain, and this can lead to multiple chronic conditions and functional limitations, so special efforts should be geared toward proper nutritional counseling and physical activity. Since substance abuse is associated with multiple diseases, including cancer, individuals of any age can benefit from quitting tobacco and moderating alcohol consumption, and should be advised to do so. Social connections and continuing cognitive activity should be encouraged, as they are both associated with positive health outcomes, including decreased cognitive loss.

Immunizations in Older Cancer Survivors

The decline in immune response associated with aging makes older adults more susceptible to infections (103). This is particularly true for respiratory diseases, which can have serious consequences in older adults. Therefore, vaccination programs and guidelines targeting older individuals have been implemented worldwide. One relevant concern regarding the efficacy of vaccines among older individuals is immunosenescence, or the decline of immune response associated with aging, which may lead to a reduced antibody and cell-mediated immunity after vaccination (104). This is also a concern among cancer survivors, particularly those who received chemotherapy or bone marrow transplantation, since immunizations may not trigger the desired protective response (105).

TABLE 11.5 Recommended vaccinations for older adults aged ≥65 years in the United States, 2020 (adapted from CDC recommendations)

DISEASE	VACCINE	DOSING
Influenza	• Influenza inactivated (IIV) • Influenza recombinant (RIV)	One dose annually
Tetanus, diphtheria, pertussis	• Td • Tdap	Booster every ten years
Pneumococcus	• PPSV23	One dose after age 65
Zoster	• Zoster recombinant (RZV) (preferred) • Zoster live (ZVL) (contraindicated in patients who received treatment in the previous 3 months)	Two doses for RZV One dose for ZVL

Recommended vaccinations (Table 11.5) should be highly encouraged among older cancer survivors (44, 106). However, it is important to mention that live-attenuated viral vaccines, including those for influenza and herpes zoster, should be avoided in patients who received cancer treatment in the previous three months (107). In all cases, recombinant vaccines should be preferred. Primary care physicians should follow usual recommendations for vaccinations in older adults and seek advice from oncologists when making recommendations for patients who have recently completed treatment.

An important consideration is the use of vaccines against COVID-19 among older cancer survivors. As of July, 2021, 22 vaccines had been submitted for approval by the World Health Organization, of which eight had completed the entire assessment and received authorization (108). However, few patients with a history of cancer have been included in studies leading to COVID-19 vaccine approval (only 3.7% in Pfizer's BNT162b2 study) (109), and their efficacy in older cancer survivors is not well understood. Regardless of that, their use in this population at high-risk for severe COVID-19 is warranted.

Cancer Screening

Cancer survivors are at increased risk of subsequent malignancies, including recurrence and development of second neoplasms. The benefit of cancer screening among older survivors needs to be carefully considered in view of competing factors that limit their life expectancy.

Since some older cancer survivors may not live long enough to obtain the potential benefits of screening, it is important to incorporate competing risks and patient preferences into screening decisions. Furthermore, older adults may be at increased risk of harm from the screening test itself, from false positive results, and from the treatment of indolent cancers (112). To better select older cancer survivors who might benefit from screening, a useful strategy is to include an estimation of life expectancy in the shared decision-making process. A practical way to estimate life expectancy is the use of online calculators, which consider age, comorbidities, lifestyle factors and geriatric variables to estimate 5-, 10-, and 14-year life expectancy. Two of those indices are the Lee index (113), which predicts 4- and 10-year all-cause mortality, and the Schonberg index (114), which predicts 5-, 9-, and 14-year all-cause mortality. Both were developed and validated in the US and are available online at eprognosis.org. Importantly, both include a previous cancer diagnosis as a predictive factor for life expectancy.

Although there are no specific recommendations for cancer screening among older cancer survivors, current guidelines are highlighted in Table 11.6. An important component of shared decision-making is determining the best time to stop screening, which generally should occur when harms outweigh benefits. Simulations have shown that the best age for stopping screening for breast, colorectal, and prostate cancer is highly dependent on overall health status and comorbidities, going from 76 years in individuals with no comorbidities to 66 in those with severe comorbid conditions (115). Although deciding whether to stop cancer screening might be a difficult personal choice, older adults are more likely to stop screening in the

TABLE 11.6 Recommendations for cancer screening in older adults in the United States

	BREAST CANCER		COLORECTAL CANCER		LUNG CANCER		PROSTATE CANCER	
	AGE-SPECIFIC RECOMMENDATION	SUGGESTED METHOD	AGE-SPECIFIC RECOMMENDATION	SUGGESTED METHOD	AGE-SPECIFIC RECOMMENDATION	SUGGESTED METHOD	AGE-SPECIFIC RECOMMENDATION	SUGGESTED METHOD
USPSTF (USA)	Screening women aged 50–74 recommended. Current evidence insufficient for women ≥75.	Mammography every 2 years.	Continue regular screening until age 75. Individualize decisions in adults aged 76–85 years depending on health status and comorbidity.	FOBT or endoscopic methods.	Screening until age 80 if 30 pack-year smoking history and current smoker or quit within the past 15 years. Discontinue in case of health problems limiting life expectancy.	Yearly LDCT.	Individual decision between ages 55–69. Do not screen adults aged ≥70.	PSA-based screening, no interval specified.
ACS (USA)	Screen women aged ≥55. Continue as long as a woman is in good health and is expected to live 10 more years or longer.	Mammography every 1–2 years.	Regular screening until age 75. Discuss risks and benefits between age 76 and 85. Stop screening at age 85.	FOBT every 1 to 3 years or endoscopic methods.	Screening until age 74 if fairly good health and currently smoking (at least 30 pack-year) or quit smoking in the past 15 years	Yearly LDCT.	Informed decision beginning at age 50 in men with at least a 10-year life expectancy. No recommendation on when to stop.	PSA every 1–2 years.

Abbreviations: USPSTF: United States Preventive Services Task Force; ACS: American Cancer Society; FOBT: Fecal occult blood test; LDCT: low-dose computed tomography.
Source: Data obtained online from USPSTF Published Recommendations.

context of a trusting patient-physician relationship. Importantly, although patients support using their age and health status (including comorbidities such as cancer) to individualize their screening choices, the utilization of estimated life expectancy as a factor to stop screening might not seem acceptable for many of them (116).

CAREGIVER BURDEN

The tasks of caregivers are diverse: they provide emotional support, personal and medical care, and legal and financial aid. The distress that caregivers experience because of providing care is known as caregiver burden (117). There are several types of caregiver burden (physical, psychosocial, and financial) (118, 119), which are linked to the patient's psychological and health status as well as to their treatment history (such as previous surgery or chemotherapy) (120, 121).

High levels of psychological distress have been reported among the caregivers of cancer survivors. In an Australian study, when compared to population norms, caregivers of older cancer survivors showed higher depression, higher anxiety, increased stress, and lower QoL (122). Caregivers are more likely to suffer from higher burden when survivors have lower education levels, are unemployed or retired, and have lower levels of individual/family resilience (123). In the case of older survivors, caregivers are frequently older adults themselves, placing both elements of the patient-caregiver dyad at high-risk for age-related comorbidities, further increasing burden (124). That being said, it is important to mention that caregiving can also lead to positive experiences, including enhanced relationships, feelings of being rewarded, and personal growth and satisfaction (125). Factors associated with reduced depression among spousal caregivers include increasing patient age and caregiver's perceived spousal support (126).

Although perceived caregiver burden consistently predicts psychological morbidity (127–129), an assessment of the health and well-being of the caregiver is not routinely included in clinical care (130). Ideally, this should involve the physician and social worker, and lead to the identification of factors causing distress. Recommendations include systematically identifying primary and additional caregivers, incorporating the needs and preferences of the caregiver in care planning, improving caregivers' understanding of their role, educating them in the necessary skills for patient care, and recognizing the need for periodical assessment of care outcomes (131, 132). In addition, physicians should explore the caregivers' sense of wellbeing and their need for support.

BOX 2.   OLDER CANCER SURVIVORS AS CAREGIVERS

Mr. P is an 82-year-old man with a history of colon cancer treated with hemicolectomy and adjuvant chemotherapy 5 years ago. His comorbidities include osteoarthritis, hypothyroidism, and atrial fibrillation. He is currently undergoing periodic follow-up with his primary care physician and, up to his last visit 6 months ago he was in excellent health and fully independent. After Mr. P missed two appointments, his primary care physician contacted him to inquire about his health. Mr. P tells him that his wife, who is 78, has recently experienced worsening cognitive decline related to Alzheimer's disease diagnosed 7 years ago. Mr. P has assumed a full-time caregiving role, and this has led to missed appointments and to problems obtaining and taking his medications. He has lost weight, is having trouble sleeping, and has lost interest in his usual activities and hobbies. Mr. P's primary care physician arranges for a visit with a nurse navigator, who provides Mr. P with information aimed at increasing his caregiving skills and puts him in touch with a caregiver support group. Additionally, the nurse navigator sends Mr. P to a financial counselor so he can get information about how to obtain additional help to take care of his wife. His primary care physician also arranges for Mr. P to meet with a mental health professional to assess and treat his recent mood changes.

ADVANCE CARE PLANNING

Advance care planning is the process of making decisions about future medical care to align such care with patient preferences, particularly near the EOL. Engagement in advance care planning leads to improved patient satisfaction and QoL, decreased use of invasive interventions near the EOL, increased hospice use, and reductions in stress, anxiety, and depression among caregivers (133). A key component of the advance care planning process is the completion of advance directives (AD), which allow patients to communicate their choices in a written document. While the completion of AD increases with age, only 50% of older adults in the US have one (134, 135).

There is a lack of information about AD completion rates among older adults with cancer. A study conducted in several US cancer centers found that 42% of older patients did not have an AD, and that those with lower educational levels, Hispanic or African American race/ethnicity, and worse self-reported QoL were less likely to have one. Unfortunately, even less information is available about AD completion or engagement in advance care planning among older cancer survivors. A systematic review of survivorship care plans found that none included a formal recommendation for the discussion of AD (136).

The process of discussing advance care planning and obtaining signed AD is dynamic and complex and should be tailored to the individual needs and characteristics of each older survivor (Figure 11.3). Specific considerations when discussing advance care planning with older adults include assessing cognition and decision-making capacity, identifying surrogates for patients with poor social support, and considering multimorbidity and sensory impairment (which can make it difficult to explain advance care planning) (133). CGA-driven interventions provided by multidisciplinary teams could potentially increase the completion of AD during cancer treatment. A recently published randomized clinical trial conducted in California showed an increase in AD completion of 24% among older adults with cancer treated by a team with geriatric expertise (137).

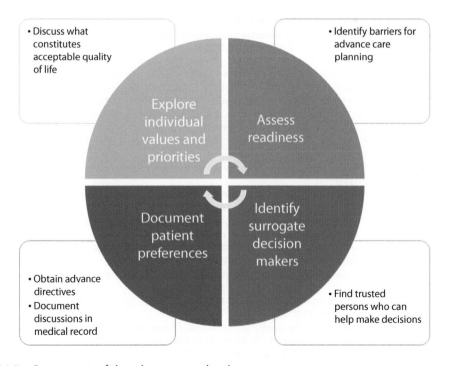

FIGURE 11.3 Components of the advance care planning process.

CONCLUSIONS

Older cancer survivors represent a growing population, and providing them with age-appropriate care should be a priority. Older survivors should be periodically evaluated with a CGA, and interventions aimed at mitigating geriatric syndromes should be implemented by a multidisciplinary team and in shared care models. Likewise, the management of the consequences of treatment should be tailored considering geriatric-specific issues. Finally, survivorship care plans should prioritize the implementation of preventive gerontology interventions to improve overall health and decrease the risk of future disease. Patient-centered geriatric care should be a part of the follow-up of all older cancer survivors and their caregivers.

REFERENCES

1. de Moor JS, Mariotto AB, Parry C, Alfano CM, Padgett L, Kent EE, et al. Cancer survivors in the United States: prevalence across the survivorship trajectory and implications for care. *Cancer Epidemiol Biomarkers Prev.* 2013;22(4):561–70.
2. Sulicka J, Pac A, Puzianowska-Kuźnicka M, Zdrojewski T, Chudek J, Tobiasz-Adamczyk B, et al. Health status of older cancer survivors-results of the PolSenior study. *J Cancer Surviv.* 2018;12(3):326–33.
3. Mohile SG, Xian Y, Dale W, Fisher SG, Rodin M, Morrow GR, et al. Association of a cancer diagnosis with vulnerability and frailty in older Medicare beneficiaries. *J Natl Cancer Inst.* 2009;101(17):1206–15.
4. Deimling GT, Sterns S, Bowman KF, Kahana B. The health of older-adult, long-term cancer survivors. *Cancer Nurs.* 2005;28(6):415–24.
5. Mohile SG, Hurria A, Cohen HJ, Rowland JH, Leach CR, Arora NK, et al. Improving the quality of survivorship for older adults with cancer. *Cancer.* 2016;122(16):2459–568.
6. Tinetti ME, Inouye SK, Gill TM, Doucette JT. Shared risk factors for falls, incontinence, and functional dependence. Unifying the approach to geriatric syndromes. *JAMA.* 1995;273(17):1348–53.
7. Inouye SK, Studenski S, Tinetti ME, Kuchel GA. Geriatric syndromes: clinical, research, and policy implications of a core geriatric concept. *J Am Geriatr Soc.* 2007;55(5):780–91.
8. Given CW, Given B, Azzouz F, Stommel M, Kozachik S. Comparison of changes in physical functioning of elderly patients with new diagnoses of cancer. *Med Care.* 2000;38(5):482–93.
9. Stommel M, Kurtz ME, Kurtz JC, Given CW, Given BA. A longitudinal analysis of the course of depressive symptomatology in geriatric patients with cancer of the breast, colon, lung, or prostate. *Health Psychol.* 2004;23(6):564–73.
10. Ganz PA, Guadagnoli E, Landrum MB, Lash TL, Rakowski W, Silliman RA. Breast cancer in older women: quality of life and psychosocial adjustment in the 15 months after diagnosis. *J Clin Oncol.* 2003;21(21):4027–33.
11. Arndt V, Merx H, Stürmer T, Stegmaier C, Ziegler H, Brenner H. Age-specific detriments to quality of life among breast cancer patients one year after diagnosis. *Eur J Cancer.* 2004;40(5):673–80.
12. King MT, Kenny P, Shiell A, Hall J, Boyages J. Quality of life three months and one year after first treatment for early stage breast cancer: influence of treatment and patient characteristics. *Qual Life Res.* 2000;9(7):789–800.
13. Mor V, Malin M, Allen S. Age differences in the psychosocial problems encountered by breast cancer patients. *J Natl Cancer Inst Monogr.* 1994(16):191–7.
14. Vinokur AD, Threatt BA, Vinokur-Kaplan D, Satariano WA. The process of recovery from breast cancer for younger and older patients. Changes during the first year. *Cancer.* 1990;65(5):1242–54.
15. Wenzel LB, Fairclough DL, Brady MJ, Cella D, Garrett KM, Kluhsman BC, et al. Age-related differences in the quality of life of breast carcinoma patients after treatment. *Cancer.* 1999;86(9):1768–74.
16. Yancik R, Wesley MN, Ries LA, Havlik RJ, Edwards BK, Yates JW. Effect of age and comorbidity in postmenopausal breast cancer patients aged 55 years and older. *JAMA.* 2001;285(7):885–92.
17. Cimprich B, Ronis DL, Martinez-Ramos G. Age at diagnosis and quality of life in breast cancer survivors. *Cancer Pract.* 2002;10(2):85–93.
18. Avis NE, Smith KW, McGraw S, Smith RG, Petronis VM, Carver CS. Assessing quality of life in adult cancer survivors (QLACS). *Qual Life Res.* 2005;14(4):1007–23.
19. Avis NE, Ip E, Foley KL. Evaluation of the Quality of Life in Adult Cancer Survivors (QLACS) scale for long-term cancer survivors in a sample of breast cancer survivors. *Health Qual Life Outcomes.* 2006;4:92.
20. Keating NL, Nørredam M, Landrum MB, Huskamp HA, Meara E. Physical and mental health status of older long-term cancer survivors. *J Am Geriatr Soc.* 2005;53(12):2145–52.

21. Hewitt M, Rowland JH, Yancik R. Cancer survivors in the United States: age, health, and disability. *J Gerontol A Biol Sci Med Sci*. 2003;58(1):82–91.

22. Sweeney C, Schmitz KH, Lazovich D, Virnig BA, Wallace RB, Folsom AR. Functional limitations in elderly female cancer survivors. *J Natl Cancer Inst*. 2006;98(8):521–9.

23. Blair CK, Jacobs DR, Jr., Demark-Wahnefried W, Cohen HJ, Morey MC, Robien K, et al. Effects of cancer history on functional age and mortality. *Cancer*. 2019;125(23):4303–9.

24. Ommundsen N, Wyller TB, Nesbakken A, Jordhøy MS, Bakka A, Skovlund E, et al. Frailty is an independent predictor of survival in older patients with colorectal cancer. *Oncologist*. 2014;19(12):1268–75.

25. Clough-Gorr KM, Stuck AE, Thwin SS, Silliman RA. Older breast cancer survivors: geriatric assessment domains are associated with poor tolerance of treatment adverse effects and predict mortality over 7 years of follow-up. *J Clin Oncol*. 2010;28(3):380–6.

26. Pilotto A, Cella A, Daragjati J, Veronese N, Musacchio C, Mello AM, et al. Three decades of comprehensive geriatric assessment: evidence coming from different healthcare settings and specific clinical conditions. *J Am Med Dir Assoc*. 2017;18(2):192.e1–.e11.

27. Korc-Grodzicki B, Holmes HM, Shahrokni A. Geriatric assessment for oncologists. *Cancer Biol Med*. 2015;12(4):261–74.

28. Stuck AE, Iliffe S. Comprehensive geriatric assessment for older adults. *BMJ*. 2011;343:d6799.

29. Alexander K, Korc-Grodzicki B. Comprehensive Geriatric Assessment (CGA) for cancer patients. In: Extermann M, editor. *Geriatric Oncology*. Cham: Springer International Publishing; 2020. pp. 419–32.

30. Extermann M, Hurria A. Comprehensive geriatric assessment for older patients with cancer. *J Clin Oncol*. 2007;25(14):1824–31.

31. Katz S. Assessing self-maintenance: activities of daily living, mobility, and instrumental activities of daily living. *J Am Geriatr Soc*. 1983;31(12):721–7.

32. Lawton MP, Brody EM. Assessment of older people: self-maintaining and instrumental activities of daily living. *Gerontologist*. 1969;9(3):179–86.

33. Cesari M, Kritchevsky SB, Newman AB, Simonsick EM, Harris TB, Penninx BW, et al. Added value of physical performance measures in predicting adverse health-related events: results from the Health, Aging and Body Composition Study. *J Am Geriatr Soc*. 2009;57(2):251–9.

34. Studenski S, Perera S, Patel K, Rosano C, Faulkner K, Inzitari M, et al. Gait speed and survival in older adults. *JAMA*. 2011;305(1):50–8.

35. Shumway-Cook A, Brauer S, Woollacott M. Predicting the probability for falls in community-dwelling older adults using the Timed Up & Go Test. *Phys Ther*. 2000;80(9):896–903.

36. Magnuson A, Sattar S, Nightingale G, Saracino R, Skonecki E, Trevino KM. A practical guide to geriatric syndromes in older adults with cancer: a focus on falls, cognition, polypharmacy, and depression. *Am Soc Clin Oncol Educ Book*. 2019;39:e96–e109.

37. Gillespie LD, Robertson MC, Gillespie WJ, Sherrington C, Gates S, Clemson LM, et al. Interventions for preventing falls in older people living in the community. *Cochrane Database Syst Rev*. 2012(9):Cd007146.

38. Charlson ME, Pompei P, Ales KL, MacKenzie CR. A new method of classifying prognostic comorbidity in longitudinal studies: development and validation. *J Chronic Dis*. 1987;40(5):373–83.

39. Salvi F, Miller MD, Grilli A, Giorgi R, Towers AL, Morichi V, et al. A manual of guidelines to score the modified cumulative illness rating scale and its validation in acute hospitalized elderly patients. *J Am Geriatr Soc*. 2008;56(10):1926–31.

40. Lange M, Joly F, Vardy J, Ahles T, Dubois M, Tron L, et al. Cancer-related cognitive impairment: an update on state of the art, detection, and management strategies in cancer survivors. *Ann Oncol*. 2019;30(12):1925–40.

41. Folstein MF, Folstein SE, McHugh PR. "Mini-mental state". A practical method for grading the cognitive state of patients for the clinician. *J Psychiatr Res*. 1975;12(3):189–98.

42. Nasreddine ZS, Phillips NA, Bédirian V, Charbonneau S, Whitehead V, Collin I, et al. The Montreal Cognitive Assessment, MoCA: a brief screening tool for mild cognitive impairment. *J Am Geriatr Soc*. 2005;53(4):695–9.

43. Ketelaars L, Pottel L, Lycke M, Goethals L, Ghekiere V, Santy L, et al. Use of the Freund clock drawing test within the Mini-Cog as a screening tool for cognitive impairment in elderly patients with or without cancer. *J Geriatr Oncol*. 2013;4(2):174–82.

44. National Comprehensive Cancer Network. Survivorship (Version 2.2020). https://www.nccn.org/professionals/physician_gls/pdf/survivorship.pdf. Accessed January 16, 2020.

45. Oster P, Rost BM, Velte U, Schlierf G. Comparative nutrition evaluation with the Mini Nutritional Assessment and the Nutritional Risk Assessment Scale. *Nestle Nutr Workshop Ser Clin Perform Programme*. 1999;1:35–9; discussion 9–40.

46. Yesavage JA, Brink TL, Rose TL, Lum O, Huang V, Adey M, et al. Development and validation of a geriatric depression screening scale: a preliminary report. *J Psychiatr Res*. 1982;17(1):37–49.

47. Kroenke K, Spitzer RL, Williams JB. The PHQ-9: validity of a brief depression severity measure. *J Gen Intern Med*. 2001;16(9):606–13.

48. Ikeda A, Kawachi I, Iso H, Iwasaki M, Inoue M, Tsugane S. Social support and cancer incidence and mortality: the JPHC study cohort II. *Cancer Causes Control*. 2013;24(5):847–60.

49. Bellizzi KM, Mustian KM, Palesh OG, Diefenbach M. Cancer survivorship and aging: moving the science forward. *Cancer*. 2008;113(12 Suppl):3530–9.

50. Keats MR, Cui Y, DeClercq V, Grandy SA, Sweeney E, Dummer TJB. Burden of multimorbidity and polypharmacy among cancer survivors: a population-based nested case-control study. *Support Care Cancer*. 2021;29(2):713–723.

51. Sharma M, Loh KP, Nightingale G, Mohile SG, Holmes HM. Polypharmacy and potentially inappropriate medication use in geriatric oncology. *J Geriatr Oncol.* 2016;7(5):346–53.
52. Masnoon N, Shakib S, Kalisch-Ellett L, Caughey GE. What is polypharmacy? A systematic review of definitions. *BMC Geriatr.* 2017;17(1):230.
53. Murphy CC, Fullington HM, Alvarez CA, Betts AC, Lee SJC, Haggstrom DA, et al. Polypharmacy and patterns of prescription medication use among cancer survivors. *Cancer.* 2018;124(13):2850–7.
54. Hsu CD, Lund JL, Nichols H. Polypharmacy risk among five-year cancer survivors. *J Clin Oncol.* 2019;37(15_suppl):11565.
55. Chen L, Cheung WY. Potential drug interactions in patients with a history of cancer. *Curr Oncol.* 2014;21(2):e212–20.
56. National Comprehensive Cancer Network. Older Adult Oncology (Version 1.2020). https://www.nccn.org/professionals/physician_gls/pdf/senior.pdf. Accessed January 16, 2020.
57. American Geriatrics Society 2019 Updated AGS Beers Criteria® for potentially inappropriate medication use in older adults. *J Am Geriatr Soc.* 2019;67(4):674–94.
58. O'Mahony D, O'Sullivan D, Byrne S, O'Connor MN, Ryan C, Gallagher P. STOPP/START criteria for potentially inappropriate prescribing in older people: version 2. *Age Ageing.* 2015;44(2):213–8.
59. Guerard EJ, Nightingale G, Bellizzi K, Burhenn P, Rosko A, Artz AS, et al. Survivorship care for older adults with cancer: U13 conference report. *J Geriatr Oncol.* 2016;7(4):305–12.
60. Morley JE, Vellas B, van Kan GA, Anker SD, Bauer JM, Bernabei R, et al. Frailty consensus: a call to action. *J Am Med Dir Assoc.* 2013;14(6):392–7.
61. Blodgett J, Theou O, Kirkland S, Andreou P, Rockwood K. Frailty in NHANES: comparing the frailty index and phenotype. *Arch Gerontol Geriatr.* 2015;60(3):464–70.
62. Owusu C, Koroukian SM, Schluchter M, Bakaki P, Berger NA. Screening older cancer patients for a Comprehensive Geriatric Assessment: a comparison of three instruments. *J Geriatr Oncol.* 2011;2(2):121–9.
63. Ness KK, Krull KR, Jones KE, Mulrooney DA, Armstrong GT, Green DM, et al. Physiologic frailty as a sign of accelerated aging among adult survivors of childhood cancer: a report from the St Jude Lifetime cohort study. *J Clin Oncol.* 2013;31(36):4496–503.
64. Hayek S, Gibson TM, Leisenring WM, Guida JL, Gramatges MM, Lupo PJ, et al. Prevalence and predictors of frailty in childhood cancer survivors and siblings: a report from the childhood cancer survivor study. *J Clin Oncol.* 2020;38(3):232–47.
65. Eissa HM, Lu L, Baassiri M, Bhakta N, Ehrhardt MJ, Triplett BM, et al. Chronic disease burden and frailty in survivors of childhood HSCT: a report from the St. Jude Lifetime Cohort Study. *Blood Adv.* 2017;1(24):2243–6.
66. Vatanen A, Hou M, Huang T, Söder O, Jahnukainen T, Kurimo M, et al. Clinical and biological markers of premature aging after autologous SCT in childhood cancer. *Bone Marrow Transplant.* 2017;52(4):600–5.
67. Arora M, Sun CL, Ness KK, Teh JB, Wu J, Francisco L, et al. Physiologic frailty in nonelderly hematopoietic cell transplantation patients: results from the bone marrow transplant survivor study. *JAMA Oncol.* 2016;2(10):1277–86.
68. Bylow K, Hemmerich J, Mohile SG, Stadler WM, Sajid S, Dale W. Obese frailty, physical performance deficits, and falls in older men with biochemical recurrence of prostate cancer on androgen deprivation therapy: a case-control study. *Urology.* 2011;77(4):934–40.
69. Winters-Stone KM, Moe E, Graff JN, Dieckmann NF, Stoyles S, Borsch C, et al. Falls and frailty in prostate cancer survivors: current, past, and never users of androgen deprivation therapy. *J Am Geriatr Soc.* 2017;65(7):1414–9.
70. Wilson CL, Chemaitilly W, Jones KE, Kaste SC, Srivastava DK, Ojha RP, et al. Modifiable factors associated with aging phenotypes among adult survivors of childhood acute lymphoblastic leukemia. *J Clin Oncol.* 2016;34(21):2509–15.
71. Williams GR, Dunham L, Chang Y, Deal AM, Pergolotti M, Lund JL, et al. Geriatric assessment predicts hospitalization frequency and long-term care use in older adult cancer survivors. *J Oncol Pract.* 2019;15(5):e399–e409.
72. Mandelblatt JS, Small BJ, Luta G, Hurria A, Jim H, McDonald BC, et al. Cancer-related cognitive outcomes among older breast cancer survivors in the thinking and living with cancer study. *J Clin Oncol.* 2018;36(32):Jco1800140.
73. Mandelblatt JS, Clapp JD, Luta G, Faul LA, Tallarico MD, McClendon TD, et al. Long-term trajectories of self-reported cognitive function in a cohort of older survivors of breast cancer: CALGB 369901 (Alliance). *Cancer.* 2016;122(22):3555–63.
74. Brown JC, Harhay MO, Harhay MN. The prognostic importance of frailty in cancer survivors. *J Am Geriatr Soc.* 2015;63(12):2538–43.
75. Negm AM, Kennedy CC, Thabane L, Veroniki AA, Adachi JD, Richardson J, et al. Management of frailty: a systematic review and network meta-analysis of randomized controlled trials. *J Am Med Dir Assoc.* 2019;20(10):1190–8.
76. Jansen FM, Prins RG, Etman A, van der Ploeg HP, de Vries SI, van Lenthe FJ, et al. Physical activity in non-frail and frail older adults. *PLoS One.* 2015;10(4):e0123168.
77. Weber M, Belala N, Clemson L, Boulton E, Hawley-Hague H, Becker C, et al. Feasibility and effectiveness of intervention programmes integrating functional exercise into daily life of older adults: a systematic review. *Gerontology.* 2018;64(2):172–87.
78. Pahor M, Guralnik JM, Ambrosius WT, Blair S, Bonds DE, Church TS, et al. Effect of structured physical activity on prevention of major mobility disability in older adults: the LIFE study randomized clinical trial. *JAMA.* 2014;311(23):2387–96.
79. Sassi KLM, Rocha NP, Colpo GD, John V, Teixeira AL. Amphetamine use in the elderly: a systematic review of the literature. *Curr Neuropharmacol.* 2020;18(2):126–35.
80. Rao AV, Cohen HJ. Fatigue in older cancer patients: etiology, assessment, and treatment. *Semin Oncol.* 2008;35(6):633–42.
81. Morelli V. Fatigue and chronic fatigue in the elderly: definitions, diagnoses, and treatments. *Clin Geriatr Med.* 2011;27(4):673–86.

82. Patel KV, Guralnik JM, Dansie EJ, Turk DC. Prevalence and impact of pain among older adults in the United States: findings from the 2011 National Health and Aging Trends Study. *Pain.* 2013;154(12):2649–57.

83. Pharmacological management of persistent pain in older persons. *J Am Geriatr Soc.* 2009;57(8):1331–46.

84. Schneiderhan J, Clauw D, Schwenk TL. Primary care of patients with chronic pain. *JAMA.* 2017;317(23):2367–8.

85. Makris UE, Kohler MJ, Fraenkel L. Adverse effects of topical nonsteroidal antiinflammatory drugs in older adults with osteoarthritis: a systematic literature review. *J Rheumatol.* 2010;37(6):1236–43.

86. Marcum ZA, Duncan NA, Makris UE. Pharmacotherapies in geriatric chronic pain management. *Clin Geriatr Med.* 2016;32(4):705–24.

87. Wegman A, van der Windt D, van Tulder M, Stalman W, de Vries T. Nonsteroidal antiinflammatory drugs or acetaminophen for osteoarthritis of the hip or knee? A systematic review of evidence and guidelines. *J Rheumatol.* 2004;31(2):344–54.

88. Makris UE, Abrams RC, Gurland B, Reid MC. Management of persistent pain in the older patient: a clinical review. *JAMA.* 2014;312(8):825–36.

89. Ofman JJ, Maclean CH, Straus WL, Morton SC, Berger ML, Roth EA, et al. Meta-analysis of dyspepsia and nonsteroidal antiinflammatory drugs. *Arthritis Rheum.* 2003;49(4):508–18.

90. Richy F, Bruyere O, Ethgen O, Rabenda V, Bouvenot G, Audran M, et al. Time dependent risk of gastrointestinal complications induced by non-steroidal anti-inflammatory drug use: a consensus statement using a meta-analytic approach. *Ann Rheum Dis.* 2004;63(7):759–66.

91. Juhlin T, Björkman S, Höglund P. Cyclooxygenase inhibition causes marked impairment of renal function in elderly subjects treated with diuretics and ACE-inhibitors. *Eur J Heart Fail.* 2005;7(6):1049–56.

92. Niccoli L, Bellino S, Cantini F. Renal tolerability of three commonly employed non-steroidal anti-inflammatory drugs in elderly patients with osteoarthritis. *Clin Exp Rheumatol.* 2002;20(2):201–7.

93. Juhlin T, Björkman S, Gunnarsson B, Fyge A, Roth B, Höglund P. Acute administration of diclofenac, but possibly not long term low dose aspirin, causes detrimental renal effects in heart failure patients treated with ACE-inhibitors. *Eur J Heart Fail.* 2004;6(7):909–16.

94. Luthra P, Burr NE, Brenner DM, Ford AC. Efficacy of pharmacological therapies for the treatment of opioid-induced constipation: systematic review and network meta-analysis. *Gut.* 2019;68(3):434–44.

95. Abuhasira R, Ron A, Sikorin I, Novack V. Medical cannabis for older patients-treatment protocol and initial results. *J Clin Med.* 2019;8(11).

96. Schmader KE, Baron R, Haanpää ML, Mayer J, O'Connor AB, Rice AS, et al. Treatment considerations for elderly and frail patients with neuropathic pain. *Mayo Clin Proc.* 2010;85(3 Suppl):S26–32.

97. Gilron I, Baron R, Jensen T. Neuropathic pain: principles of diagnosis and treatment. *Mayo Clin Proc.* 2015;90(4):532–45.

98. Voermans NC, Snijders AH, Schoon Y, Bloem BR. Why old people fall (and how to stop them). *Pract Neurol.* 2007;7(3):158–71.

99. Hatton AL, Rome K. Falls, footwear, and podiatric interventions in older adults. *Clin Geriatr Med.* 2019;35(2):161–71.

100. Cuevas-Trisan R. Balance problems and fall risks in the elderly. *Clin Geriatr Med.* 2019;35(2):173–83.

101. Tazkarji B, Lam R, Lee S, Meiyappan S. Approach to preventive care in the elderly. *Can Fam Physician.* 2016;62(9):717–21.

102. Colburn JL, Nothelle S. The medicare annual wellness visit. *Clin Geriatr Med.* 2018;34(1):1–10.

103. Coll PP, Costello VW, Kuchel GA, Bartley J, McElhaney JE. The prevention of infections in older adults: vaccination. *J Am Geriatr Soc.* 2020;68(1):207–14.

104. Sasaki S, Sullivan M, Narvaez CF, Holmes TH, Furman D, Zheng NY, et al. Limited efficacy of inactivated influenza vaccine in elderly individuals is associated with decreased production of vaccine-specific antibodies. *J Clin Invest.* 2011;121(8):3109–19.

105. Small TN, Zelenetz AD, Noy A, Rice RD, Trippett TM, Abrey L, et al. Pertussis immunity and response to tetanus-reduced diphtheria-reduced pertussis vaccine (Tdap) after autologous peripheral blood stem cell transplantation. *Biol Blood Marrow Transplant.* 2009;15(12):1538–42.

106. Centers for Disease Control. Recommended Adult Immunization Schedule for ages 19 years or older. 2020. https://www.cdc.gov/vaccines/schedules/downloads/adult/adult-combined-schedule.pdf. Accessed January 5, 2021.

107. Denlinger CS, Ligibel JA, Are M, Baker KS, Demark-Wahnefried W, Dizon D, et al. Survivorship: immunizations and prevention of infections, version 2.2014. *J Natl Compr Canc Netw.* 2014;12(8):1098–111.

108. World Health Organization. *Status of Covid-19 Vaaccines within WHO EUL/PQ evaluation process. 02 July 2021.* 2021. https://extranet.who.int/pqweb/sites/default/files/documents/Status_COVID_VAX_02July2021.pdf. Accessed July 5, 2021.

109. Polack FP, Thomas SJ, Kitchin N, Absalon J, Gurtman A, Lockhart S, et al. Safety and efficacy of the BNT162b2 mRNA Covid-19 vaccine. *N Engl J Med.* 2020.

110. Chao C, Bhatia S, Xu L, Cannavale KL, Wong FL, Huang PS, et al. Incidence, risk factors, and mortality associated with second malignant neoplasms among survivors of adolescent and young adult cancer. *JAMA Netw Open.* 2019;2(6):e195536.

111. Turcotte LM, Liu Q, Yasui Y, Henderson TO, Gibson TM, Leisenring W, et al. Chemotherapy and risk of subsequent malignant neoplasms in the childhood cancer survivor study cohort. *J Clin Oncol.* 2019;37(34):3310–9.

112. Eckstrom E, Feeny DH, Walter LC, Perdue LA, Whitlock EP. Individualizing cancer screening in older adults: a narrative review and framework for future research. *J Gen Intern Med.* 2013;28(2):292–8.

113. Lee SJ, Lindquist K, Segal MR, Covinsky KE. Development and validation of a prognostic index for 4-year mortality in older adults. *JAMA.* 2006;295(7):801–8.

114. Schonberg MA, Li V, Marcantonio ER, Davis RB, McCarthy EP. Predicting mortality up to 14 years among community-dwelling adults aged 65 and older. *J Am Geriatr Soc*. 2017;65(6):1310–5.

115. Lansdorp-Vogelaar I, Gulati R, Mariotto AB, Schechter CB, de Carvalho TM, Knudsen AB, et al. Personalizing age of cancer screening cessation based on comorbid conditions: model estimates of harms and benefits. *Ann Intern Med*. 2014;161(2):104–12.

116. Schoenborn NL, Lee K, Pollack CE, Armacost K, Dy SM, Bridges JFP, et al. Older adults' views and communication preferences about cancer screening cessation. *JAMA Intern Med*. 2017;177(8):1121–8.

117. Rha SY, Park Y, Song SK, Lee CE, Lee J. Caregiving burden and the quality of life of family caregivers of cancer patients: the relationship and correlates. *Eur J Oncol Nurs*. 2015;19(4):376–82.

118. Deshields TL, Rihanek A, Potter P, Zhang Q, Kuhrik M, Kuhrik N, et al. Psychosocial aspects of caregiving: perceptions of cancer patients and family caregivers. *Support Care Cancer*. 2012;20(2):349–56.

119. Stenberg U, Ruland CM, Miaskowski C. Review of the literature on the effects of caring for a patient with cancer. *Psychooncology*. 2010;19(10):1013–25.

120. Govina O, Kotronoulas G, Mystakidou K, Katsaragakis S, Vlachou E, Patiraki E. Effects of patient and personal demographic, clinical and psychosocial characteristics on the burden of family members caring for patients with advanced cancer in Greece. *Eur J Oncol Nurs*. 2015;19(1):81–8.

121. Johansen S, Cvancarova M, Ruland C. The effect of cancer patients' and their family caregivers' physical and emotional symptoms on caregiver burden. *Cancer Nurs*. 2018;41(2):91–9.

122. Jones SB, Whitford HS, Bond MJ. Burden on informal caregivers of elderly cancer survivors: risk versus resilience. *J Psychosoc Oncol*. 2015;33(2):178–98.

123. Li Y, Wang K, Yin Y, Li S. Relationships between family resilience, breast cancer survivors' individual resilience, and caregiver burden: a cross-sectional study. *Int J Nurs Stud*. 2018;88:79–84.

124. Given B, Sherwood PR. Family care for the older person with cancer. *Semin Oncol Nurs*. 2006;22(1):43–50.

125. Li Q, Loke AY. The positive aspects of caregiving for cancer patients: a critical review of the literature and directions for future research. *Psychooncology*. 2013;22(11):2399–407.

126. Goldzweig G, Schapira L, Baider L, Jacobs JM, Andritsch E, Rottenberg Y. Who will care for the caregiver? Distress and depression among spousal caregivers of older patients undergoing treatment for cancer. *Support Care Cancer*. 2019;27(11):4221–4227.

127. Carey PJ, Oberst MT, McCubbin MA, Hughes SH. Appraisal and caregiving burden in family members caring for patients receiving chemotherapy. *Oncol Nurs Forum*. 1991;18(8):1341–8.

128. Compas BE, Worsham NL, Epping-Jordan JE, Grant KE, Mireault G, Howell DC, et al. When mom or dad has cancer: markers of psychological distress in cancer patients, spouses, and children. *Health Psychol*. 1994;13(6):507–15.

129. Given CW, Stommel M, Given B, Osuch J, Kurtz ME, Kurtz JC. The influence of cancer patients' symptoms and functional states on patients' depression and family caregivers' reaction and depression. *Health Psychol*. 1993;12(4):277–85.

130. Collins LG, Swartz K. Caregiver care. *Am Fam Physician*. 2011;83(11):1309–17.

131. Family Caregiver Alliance. *Caregiver scount too! A toolkit to help practitioners assess the needs of family caregivers*. 2020. https://www.caregiver.org/caregivers-count-too-toolkit. Accessed January 5, 2021.

132. Family Caregiver Alliance. *Caregiver assessment: principles, guidelines and strategies for change, Volume 1*. 2020 https://www.caregiver.org/sites/caregiver.org/files/pdfs/v1_consensus.pdf. Accessed January 5, 2021.

133. Lum HD, Sudore RL, Bekelman DB. Advance care planning in the elderly. *Med Clin North Am*. 2015;99(2):391–403.

134. Rao JK, Anderson LA, Lin FC, Laux JP. Completion of advance directives among U.S. consumers. *Am J Prev Med*. 2014;46(1):65–70.

135. Alshanberi A. Advance directives in patients over 60 years old: assessment of perceived value and need for education in the outpatient setting. *Arch Med*. 2018;10.

136. O'Caoimh R, Cornally N, O'Sullivan R, Hally R, Weathers E, Lavan AH, et al. Advance care planning within survivorship care plans for older cancer survivors: a systematic review. *Maturitas*. 2017;105:52–7.

137. Li D, Sun CL. Geriatric assessment-driven intervention (GAIN) on chemotherapy toxicity in older adults with cancer: a randomized controlled trial. *J Clin Oncol* 2020 38;(15_suppl):12010.

Cardiovascular Complications of Cancer Therapy in Cancer Survivors

12

Susan Dent, Ioannis Milioglou, Harsh Patolia, Brandy Patterson, and Avirup Guha

---

EPIDEMIOLOGY

Cancer survivorship in the United States has increased with advances in detection, surveillance, and treatment.[1] According to the National Cancer Institute's Surveillance, Epidemiology, and End Results (SEER) database, there are over 16.9 million Americans with a history of cancer, with greater than two-thirds diagnosed more than 5 years ago.[2] It is estimated that cancer survivorship will increase to over 22.1 million by the beginning of 2030. While these statistics are encouraging, it is important to understand the potential short and long-term consequences of cancer therapy, including cardiovascular (CV) sequelae.

The Childhood Cancer Survivor Study (CCSS) reports that those aged 35 years and older are at increased risk for stroke, myocardial infarction (MI), and congestive heart failure when compared to their siblings.[3] In the same cohort, survivors demonstrated higher rates of metabolic syndrome, especially among those with a sedentary lifestyle or prior radiation exposure.[4] There is limited data on the long-term CV consequences of cancer therapy in adult cancer survivors, although data is beginning to emerge. In a retrospective review of the SEER registry database, cardiovascular disease (CVD) was the leading cause of death among 63,566 women diagnosed with breast cancer between 1992 and 2000. Among those who died of CVD, only 25.5% were known to have CVD at the time of their cancer diagnosis.[5] The presence of a single CVD risk factor was associated with a greater than two-fold increase in experiencing a cardiac event.[6] Furthermore, breast cancer survivors with CVD have lower survival rates than survivors without CVD – even when adjusted for cancer stage, CVD risk factors, and demographic data.[7] Similarly in men receiving prostate cancer treatment (e.g., androgen deprivation therapy), preexisting CVD risk factors (hypertension and diabetes mellitus) augment the risk of all-cause mortality.[8] Further research is needed to ensure that gains in survivorship are not outweighed by cancer treatment related CV toxicities. In this chapter we review the long-term CV consequences of cancer therapy, risk factors associated with CV morbidity, and models of care to mitigate CV toxicities in cancer survivors.

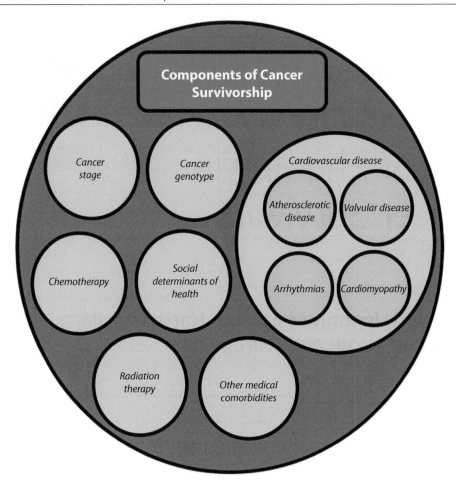

FIGURE 12.1   Components of cancer survivorship.

CARDIOVASCULAR COMPLICATIONS OF CANCER THERAPY IN CANCER SURVIVORS

Patients are at risk of CV complications both during, as well as years after completion of cancer treatment. Cardiovascular events occur later in life in cancer survivors at a much higher rate than the general population, due to shared risk factors such as hypertension and diabetes (known to increase with age) and previous cancer therapy exposure (Figure 12.1). Cardiovascular adverse events associated with different cancer therapies and currently approved indications are summarized in Tables 12.1 and 12.2, as well as Figure 12.2.

Cardiomyopathy/Heart Failure

Heart failure is the most common acute CV adverse event associated with cancer therapy. Cancer survivors remain at risk of developing cardiomyopathy or heart failure years after completion of cancer treatment. An epidemiological study from the United Kingdom showed an increased likelihood of heart failure at 1-year follow-up in cancer survivors (hematologic and solid tumors).[9] This study, encompassing over 120,000 patients, demonstrated that this risk rose over a period of 10 years. For childhood cancer

TABLE 12.1   Cancer drug and arrhythmias

CANCER DRUG CLASS	TYPE OF ARRHYTHMIA
mTOR Inhibitors (except for Everolimus)	SVT, catecholamine polymorphic ventricular tachycardia, QT prolongation, Torsades de Pointes, and bradycardia
Histone deacetylase inhibitors	QT prolongation (romidepsin), ventricular tachycardia, Torsades de pointes, AF
Antimicrotubule gents	Asymptomatic bradycardia SVT, ventricular tachycardia, QT (eribulin)
Tyrosine kinase inhibitors	AF bradycardia (ceritinib, crizotinib), QTc prolongation (nilotinib, alectinib), AF/SVT (ibrutinib/dasatinib)
Alkylating agents	PACs, PVCs, SVT, AF (cyclophosphamide), Sinus bradycardia (cisplatin)
Proteasome inhibitors	Bradycardia, AV block
VEGF inhibitors	QTc prolongation

Abbreviations: mTOR, mammalian target of rapamycin; VEGF, vascular endothelial growth factor: SVT, supraventricular tachycardia; AF, atrial fibrillation; PAC, premature atrial contraction; PVC, premature ventricular contraction.

survivors, the DCOG-LATER study,[10] the St Jude Lifetime Cohort,[11] and the CCSS[12,13] demonstrated a prevalence of heart failure between 4% and 7%.

Targeted HER2-neu therapies

Trastuzumab-related cardiotoxicity varies between 5% and 10%, with up to 28% being reported with concomitant administration of anthracyclines.[14,15] Trastuzumab-related cardiotoxicity ranges from mild to moderate left ventricular (LV) dysfunction to cardiomyopathy, which is usually reversible.[16] Patients often present with mild symptoms; cardiac function improvement is usually observed within 4–6 weeks after discontinuation of the drug.[17] In a recent retrospective study of 49 patients with trastuzumab-related cardiomyopathy, significant recovery was noticed in 79% of patients after trastuzumab discontinuation and initiation of goal-directed medical therapy (GDMT).[18] Age, obesity, and prior heart failure are risk factors for new or worsening heart failure in patients started on trastuzumab.[16]

New generation HER2 inhibitors demonstrate a more favorable cardiovascular profile, with lapatinib causing milder forms of cardiomyopathy. Pertuzumab does not appear to increase the risk of cardiomyopathy when given in combination with trastuzumab.[19,20] Long-term cardiac dysfunction is rare; however, research on the long-term CV consequences of exposure to newer *HER2* targeted therapies is lacking.

VEGF inhibitors (bevacizumab, sunitinib, and sorafenib)

Bevacizumab-induced cardiomyopathy has been sporadically reported, especially when administered in conjunction with anthracyclines or paclitaxel in women with metastatic breast cancer – an indication that no longer exists for these patients.[21]

Interestingly, 28% of patients on sunitinib monotherapy have been reported to have a clinically significant decrease in cardiac function with 8% developing severe heart failure.[22] In a meta-analysis of 6,935 patients treated with sunitinib, the incidence of heart failure was 4.1%, with a relative risk of 1.81 compared to placebo.[23]

Sorafenib has been associated with a 4% risk of mild LV dysfunction and a 1% risk of symptomatic heart failure. Overall, VEGF inhibitor-related cardiomyopathy was reversible with treatment cessation.[14]

Anthracyclines

Anthracyclines are associated with the highest risk of heart failure among chemotherapeutic agents. The cumulative 10-year incidence of heart failure in cancer survivors who received anthracyclines is 38% compared to 32.5% for non-anthracycline chemotherapy.[24] In a large meta-analysis with a pool of

TABLE 12.2   Cancer drug and indication

CANCER DRUG CLASS	INDICATION OF USE
HER2 inhibitors	
Trastuzumab	HER2+ breast, gastric, and endometrial cancer
Lapatinib	HER2+ breast cancer
Pertuzumab	HER2+ breast cancer
VEGF inhibitors	
Bevacizumab	Metastatic colorectal cancer
Sunitinib	Gastrointestinal stromal tumor (GIST)
Sorafenib	Hepatocellular carcinoma
Anthracyclines	
Doxorubicin	Breast cancer, bladder cancer, sarcoma, ALL, NHL
Mitoxantrone	Relapsed ALL, AML
Alkylating agents	
Cyclophosphamide	ALL, breast cancer, HL, NHL, HSCT
Ifosfamide	Testicular cancer, bladder cancer, HL, and NHL
Antimetabolites	
Fluorouracil	Colorectal, esophageal, and gastric cancer
Capecitabine	Metastatic breast and colorectal cancer
Gemcitabine	Metastatic breast and pancreatic cancer, NSCLC
BTK inhibitors	
Ibrutinib	CLL, refractory mantle cell lymphoma
TKI	
Imatinib	Ph+ ALL, Ph+ CML, GIST
Proteasome inhibitors	
Carfilzomib	Refractory/relapsed multiple myeloma
mTOR inhibitors	
Temsirolimus	Endometrial cancer, RCC advanced
Histone deacetylase inhibitors	
Romidepsin	Peripheral and cutaneous T cell lymphoma
Antimicrotubules	
Paclitaxel	Breast cancer, NSCLC
Docetaxel	Breast cancer, head and neck cancer, NSCLC, Castration resistant prostate cancer

Abbreviations: HER2, human epidermal growth factor receptor; VEGF, vascular endothelial growth factor; TKI, tyrosine kinase inhibitor; BTK, Bruton's tyrosine kinase; mTOR, mammalian target of rapamycin; ALL, acute lymphoblastic leukemia; AML, acute myelogenous leukemia, HL, Hodgkin lymphoma; NHL, non-Hodgkin lymphoma; CLL, chronic lymphocytic lymphoma; CML, chronic myelogenous leukemia; RCC, renal cell carcinoma; NSCLC, non-small cell lung cancer; HSCT, hematopoietic stem cell transplant.

patients of more than 50,000 under treatment with modern chemotherapeutic agents, the reported incidence of anthracycline clinical and subclinical cardiotoxicity was 6% (95% CI 3%–9%) and 18% (95% CI 12%–24%), respectively.[25] Anthracycline cardiotoxicity is cumulative and dose-dependent; data from the pooled analysis of three clinical trials demonstrate an increased incidence of heart failure with increasing cumulative doses (3%–5% with 400 mg/m^2, 7%–26% at 550 mg/m^2, and 18%–48% at 700 mg/m^2).[26] Risk factors for anthracycline-induced cardiomyopathy include age >65 years or very young age (<4 years old), female gender, preexisting CV disorders, radiation, and exposure to trastuzumab. It usually manifests within the first year after exposure; however, later manifestations due to compensatory mechanisms have also been reported.[27]

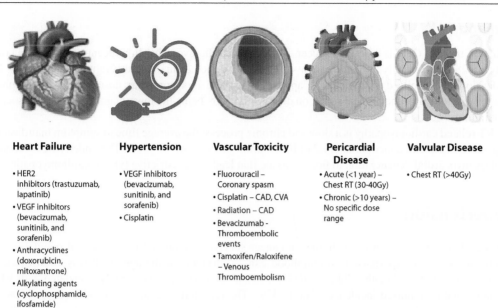

Heart Failure	Hypertension	Vascular Toxicity	Pericardial Disease	Valvular Disease
• HER2 inhibitors (trastuzumab, lapatinib) • VEGF inhibitors (bevacizumab, sunitinib, and sorafenib) • Anthracyclines (doxorubicin, mitoxantrone) • Alkylating agents (cyclophosphamide, ifosfamide) • Fluoropyrimidines (Fluorouracil, Capecitabine) • TKI (imatinib) • Proteasome inhibitors (carfilzomib) • Radiation	• VEGF inhibitors (bevacizumab, sunitinib, and sorafenib) • Cisplatin	• Fluorouracil – Coronary spasm • Cisplatin – CAD, CVA • Radiation – CAD • Bevacizumab - Thromboembolic events • Tamoxifen/Raloxifene – Venous Thromboembolism	• Acute (<1 year) – Chest RT (30-40Gy) • Chronic (>10 years) – No specific dose range	• Chest RT (>40Gy)

FIGURE 12.2   Cancer therapy associated with cardiovascular toxicity. *Abbreviations*: HER2: human epidermal growth factor receptor 2; VEGF: vascular endothelial growth factor; TKI: tyrosine kinase inhibitor; RT: radiation therapy; CAD: coronary artery disease; CVA; cerebral vascular accident.

Nonetheless, not all anthracyclines are equally cardiotoxic. Relative cardiotoxic doses of daunorubicin, idarubicin, epirubicin, and mitoxantrone compared to doxorubicin have been quantitated, and cutoffs of each of the agents are used in monitoring guidelines.[28,29]

Alkylating agents

Cyclophosphamide is an alkylating agent associated with an increased risk of heart failure. Cardiotoxicity can occur acutely (within 1–2 weeks from administration) and with high dose protocols. The reported incidence with high dose protocols has been reported to up to 28%.[14] In a prospective cohort study, 9 of the 32 patients treated with high dose cyclophosphamide over four days (>180 mg/kg) developed heart failure within three weeks, with 6 of them eventually dying.[30] Aggravating factors included prior exposure to anthracyclines and chest irradiation.[14]

Other agents

Bruton tyrosine kinase inhibitors have a more favorable risk profile than other medications; 363 out of 13,572 patients in an observational study developed heart failure.[31] Imatinib was one of the first TKIs reported to cause cardiomyopathy. Currently, there is no epidemiologic data on the incidence of imatinib-induced cardiomyopathy. Murine models of imatinib-resistant c-abl protein are protected from heart failure when exposed to imatinib.[32] Carfilzomib is a proteasome inhibitor recently shown to be associated with adverse cardiac events. In a trial of 266 patients, heart failure (3.8%), cardiac arrest (1.5%), and MI (0.8%) were associated with carfilzomib. Heart failure was reversible after discontinuation of carfilzomib and initiation of GDMT.[22]

Radiation

Radiation therapy (RT) is a potent inducer of diastolic cardiomyopathy. In a recent retrospective cohort study of 282 Hodgkin lymphoma patients treated with mediastinal radiotherapy (minimum 35 Gy), 40 developed diastolic dysfunction.[33] It appears that there is a nonlinear dose–response relationship between diastolic dysfunction and radiation dose, with 25 Gy being the lowest cumulative dose associated with findings.[34]

RT-related cardiomyopathy is a slow and chronic process; the average time to symptom manifestation is up to 18 years, with a median interval of heart failure to death of 3.6 years. The underlying mechanism involves myocardial degeneration to fibrotic tissue that leads to a restrictive type of cardiomyopathy.[34]

Hypertension

The prevalence of hypertension is higher in cancer survivors compared to the general population. The overall incidence of hypertension in childhood cancer survivors at the age of 50 was almost twice as high compared to their healthy siblings (40% vs. 26%).[35] Hypertension is strongly associated with VEGF inhibitors, with a reported incidence of up to 47%. The reported mechanism includes reduced levels of nitric oxide, as well as increased levels of endothelin-1.[24] Hypertension, which is also one of the late adverse effects of cisplatin, was observed in about 20%–50% of patients.[36] In a study where bevacizumab was used for treatment of patients with breast cancer, bevacizumab carried a fivefold risk for hypertension compared to the control arm.[37]

Vascular Toxicity

The reported cumulative incidence of CAD in cancer survivors ranges between 3.8% and 5.3%, according to CCSS and St. Jude cohort studies.[13]

Antimetabolites

High doses of 5-flourouracil (5-FU) (>800 mg/m^2) have been recognized as a significant risk factor for CAD. The reported incidence of 5-FU vascular cardiotoxicity is up to 18%. This adverse effect is acute, with most events manifesting as early as 6 hours post-infusion up to 5 days. Patients may present with chest pain with EKG changes and cardiac markers may or may not be elevated. The overall mortality ranges between 2.2% and 13%. Coronary spasm at the level of preexisting plaques is one of the supported mechanisms of cardiotoxicity and infusional regimens of 5-FU carry greater risk than bolus administration.[14]

Capecitabine, the oral formulation of 5-FU, has been linked with cardiotoxicity, with an incidence ranging between 3% and 9%.[14] In a prospective study of 644 patients without prior CAD history, capecitabine has been reported to induce symptomatic ischemic changes on the ECG in 5.4% of patients.[38] There are no known long-term CV effects of these agents.

VEGF inhibitors

An increased risk for arterial thromboembolic events (stroke, MI, other) in patients receiving chemotherapy plus bevacizumab compared to chemotherapy alone was observed in a meta-analysis with a patient pool of 1,745 patients (HR = 2.0, 95% confidence interval [CI] = 1.05–3.75; $P = 0.031$). Nonetheless, there was no difference between the two groups in venous thromboembolism rates.[39] The pathophysiology of bevacizumab-induced vascular toxicity includes decreased regenerative potential of endothelial cells in response to stress, increased blood viscosity via overproduction of erythropoietin, and decreased endothelial nitric oxide production.[40]

Other agents

Paclitaxel is an antimicrotubular agent that has been found to have minimal risk of MI with incidence rates between 0.2% and 0.5%. The majority of events occur within two weeks from administration in patients with preexisting risk factors (HTN, CAD).[14] Docetaxel has been associated with MI in one study with an incidence of 1.6% compared to the control arm 0.6%.[41]

Sorafenib is associated with MI in multiple studies, with an average reported incidence of MI of 3%.[42]

Carfilzomib was shown in two large trials to be associated with CV events. In both the ENDEAVOR and ASPIRE trials, MI incidence was 3% and 5.9%, respectively.[43,44]

Radiation

Chest RT is a strong risk factor for the later onset of symptomatic CAD in cancer survivors. The cumulative incidence of CAD in patients with a prior history of chest RT for Hodgkin's lymphoma (cumulative dose >35 Gy) was 20% higher than their healthy siblings.[45] In another study of 2,524 survivors of Hodgkin's Lymphoma treated with RT, a 40-year cumulative incidence for CAD of 23% (95% CI 21%–25%) was reported.[46]

Coronary disease is linearly dependent on RT dose.[45] Radiation-induced coronary lesions are usually located proximally, raising the risk for severe MI. Sudden cardiac death (SCD) in the setting of severe asymptomatic CAD is one of the manifestations of RT induced CAD.[47]

Most of the data on RT-related later outcomes come from studies based on obsolete RT protocols. More contemporary radiation techniques (deep inspiration breath-hold, gating, accelerated partial breast irradiation, 3D planning) have improved RT's overall adverse event profile. Nonetheless, the incidence of late-onset CV adverse events with these more recent techniques is yet to be reported.[36]

The exact mechanism is not well described; however, it seems that it differs from atherosclerotic disease. Postmortem analysis of plaques of irradiated patients revealed more fibrous and smooth plaques compares to those of classic CAD patients.[47]

Arrhythmias

Cancer survivors have a higher prevalence of cardiac arrhythmias compared to that of the general population. In 10,724 CCSS patients, the cumulative incidence of grade 3–5 arrhythmias was 1.3%. Hypertension, dyslipidemia, prior anthracycline exposure, and chest RT dose 35 Gy were significant predisposing factors for arrhythmias in these patients.[35]

Anthracyclines

Anthracyclines are strongly associated with QTc interval prolongation, especially with subsequent chemotherapy cycles and prolonged exposure. Approximately 11.5% of patients present with QTc > 450 ms after the first chemotherapy cycle.[48] Anthracycline induced arrhythmias can be secondary to cardiomyopathy, with malignant ventricular arrhythmias occurring even before the onset of ventricular systolic dysfunction.[49]

The mechanism of arrhythmogenesis includes abnormalities in various myocardial cell components, such as the L-type calcium channels, sarcoplasmic calcium, and potassium channels.[50]

Antimetabolites

Fluorouracil causes a broad spectrum of ventricular arrhythmias ranging from premature ventricular contractions (PVCs) to life-threatening arrhythmias and SCD. The incidence of ventricular tachycardia (VT) can be up to 7.4%. Supraventricular tachycardia is rarely linked to 5-FU, and gemcitabine and clofarabine can cause atrial fibrillation.[49]

Coronary spasm and microvasculature dysfunction is the primary proposed mechanism of arrhythmogenesis in these patients.

Other

Valvular abnormalities

Radiation-associated valvulopathy is often seen in cancer survivors, with a reported prevalence of up to 31% in certain survivorship studies.[35] In a recent study, enrolling Hodgkin's lymphoma patients, valvular disease was reported in 20% of the patients who underwent mediastinal RT.[47]

A dose-dependent model is currently supported. Prior exposure to anthracyclines, preexisting hypertension, congenital heart disease, and RT dose >30 Gy are all risk factors that potentiate RT cardiotoxicity. Direct chest irradiation with subsequent irradiation of the valve cusps and leaflets leads to valvular damage followed by thickening, fibrosis, and increased calcium deposition.[13,51] Mild to moderate tricuspid and mitral valve regurgitation were the most prominent lesions in survivorship studies, monitoring patients 5 and 10 years post-treatment.[13] Nonetheless, a recent childhood lymphoma cohort study reported a higher prevalence of mitral and aortic valve abnormalities than right heart valvular lesions.[52] The first signs of radiation-induced valvulopathy on ECHO, evidenced by valvular retraction and shortening, can be noticed within the first year of RT. The progressive fibrotic valvular changes lead to regurgitation and infrequently stenosis 10–20 years post-RT. The characteristic pattern includes calcifications in both aortic and mitral valves sparing the valves' tips and commissures.[47]

Pericardial disease

Acute and chronic pericardial disease is often seen in cancer survivors. According to CCSS, there is a 10-fold higher risk of pericardial disease in patients who underwent chest RT.[53]

It can manifest as acute pericarditis, pericardial effusion, or constrictive pericarditis, with the latter having the worst prognostic outcome. The majority of the patients are diagnosed with asymptomatic pericardial effusion, which may resolve spontaneously, with rare tamponade cases still being reported.[54] Acute pericarditis occurs within days to weeks after RT and is usually expected with doses greater than 36–40 Gy. It is usually a self-limiting process. Chronic pericarditis, which is the most common complication of RT, varies with a range of three months to over a decade.[55] The overall incidence of chronic pericarditis has decreased since the 1970s with the development of more precise RT protocols.[54]

CARDIOVASCULAR RISK AND MONITORING IN CANCER SURVIVORS

Given the potential increased risk of CV morbidity and mortality in cancer survivors, multiple organizations have developed position statements and guidelines assessing CV risk during and following completion of cancer therapy (see Table 12.3). While these statements offer healthcare providers some guidance on evaluating CV risk in this patient population, their applicability is hampered by the variability in definitions of CV toxicity.[56] Furthermore, these guidelines have focused primarily on the CV toxicity of anthracycline and/or trastuzumab-based therapy, although other systemic therapies may cause cancer therapy related cardiac dysfunction (i.e., VEGF therapies). There is also limited guidance on management of patients with known CVD or those with preexisting CV risk factors after completion of cancer therapy.

TABLE 12.3 Comparison of guidelines on cardiovascular monitoring

RECOMMENDATION	SIOG[60]	ESMO[58]	NCCN[59]	ASE/EACVI[56]	ASCO[57]
Management of CV RF prior to, during and after tx	YES	YES	YES	YES	YES
Monitor for CTRCD with ECHO	YES	YES	YES	YES	YES
Monitor for CTRCD with cardiac biomarkers	NO	YES	NO	YES	YES
Timing of cardiac imaging in asymptomatic patients with normal ejection fraction	q 2–3 cycles of anthracycline exposure	*Baseline AC:* q 3–6 weeks before each cycle and reassess after 250 mg/m² dox, after each additional 100 mg/m², and end of tx *Adjuvant Trastuzumab:* q 3 months	Consider in high-risk patients[a] within 1 year after the last anthracycline dose given	*Trastuzumab:* every 3 months *Anthracycline:* at completion of therapy, then 6 months after for doses <240 mg/m²	Echocardiogram 6–12 months after completion of cancer therapy; additional cardiac imaging as clinically indicated

Abbreviations: AC, adriamycin/cyclophosphamide; CV, cardiovascular; RF, risk factor; tx, treatment; CTRD, cancer treatment related cardiac dysfunction; ECHO, echocardiogram; SIOG, International Society of Geriatric Oncology; ESMO, European Society of Medical Oncology; NCCN, National Comprehensive Cancer Network; ASE/EACVI, the American Society of Echocardiography and European Association of Cardiovascular Imaging; ASCO, American Society of Clinical Oncology.

[a] High dose AC (doxorubicin >250 mg/m² or high dose radiation (>30 Gy); combination AC and radiation; tx lower dose AC (doxorubicin <250 mg/m²) and trastuzumab (sequential therapy); treatment with lower dose AC or trastuzumab alone and any one of the following: two CV risk factors or more (smoking, hypertension, diabetes, dyslipidemia, obesity), or age > 60, or baseline compromised cardiac function (EF < 50%–55%), h/o MI, and/or > moderate valvular heart disease, sequential therapy.

American Society of Clinical Oncology

In 2017, the American Society of Clinical Oncology (ASCO) published recommendations on preventing and monitoring cardiac dysfunction in survivors of adult cancers. This guideline focused mainly on CV risk assessment for cancer patients before, during, and following exposure to anthracyclines and/or trastuzumab and/or RT. They recommend an echocardiogram 6–12 months after completion of cancer therapy for asymptomatic adult cancer survivors considered to be at increased risk of CV dysfunction. They were unable to make any recommendations on frequency and duration of surveillance in patients with no cardiac dysfunction. These guidelines stressed the importance of evaluation and management of CV risk factors, as well as a heart-healthy lifestyle, including the role of diet and exercise, as part of long-term follow-up care. This guideline did not provide recommendations on monitoring for LV systolic dysfunction in patients exposed to kinase inhibitors, immune checkpoint inhibitors, lower dose anthracyclines, or trastuzumab alone without CV risk factors, or for lower dose RT (<30 Gy) where the heart is in the treatment field and there are no additional cardiotoxic therapeutic exposures or risk factors.[57]

European Society for Medical Oncology

This position statement, updated in 2020, provides guidance regarding prevention, screening, monitoring, and CV toxicity treatment while emphasizing the need for individualized care.

The guidelines consider EKG and biomarkers' use in following patients undergoing active anthracycline and trastuzumab-based therapy apart from echocardiographic follow-up (see Table 12.3). Unlike other guidelines, European Society for medical Oncology (ESMO) addresses the role of global longitudinal strain (GLS) measurements, anti-VEGF inhibitors, and other cancer therapies that are associated with hypertension. They recommend establishing a baseline blood pressure (BP) measurement and performing serial BP monitoring along with a cardiac physical exam, cardiac biomarkers, and/or cardiac imaging during therapy. ESMO guidelines also address immune checkpoint inhibitor-associated cardiotoxicity and provide management recommendations, although they are formulated from mostly expert opinion given that it is an ongoing area of research.

Asymptomatic post-treatment survivors who have received cardiotoxic therapy and have normal function should be periodically screened for the development of new asymptomatic LV dysfunction with cardiac biomarkers and potentially cardiac imaging 6–12 months and 2 years post-treatment. However, for those who developed LV dysfunction due to any HER2 targeted therapy, anthracyclines, or other anticancer therapy, CV care, including treatment with cardioprotective agents, and annual cardiology evaluation if asymptomatic (more frequently if symptomatic), should be continued indefinitely regardless of improvement in LVEF or symptoms.

For patients with a history of mediastinal chest RT, evaluation for CAD, vascular, and valve disease is recommended, even if asymptomatic, starting at 5 years post-treatment then at least every 3–5 years after that.

Finally, ESMO recommends that cancer patients should be encouraged to exercise regularly, maintain average weight, and consume a healthy diet.[58]

Joint Expert Consensus Statement from the American Society of Echocardiography (ASE) and European Association of Cardiovascular Imaging (EACVI)

This committee focused on guidelines to direct care during and after potentially cardiotoxic therapy. The committee specifically defined cardiotoxicity or cancer therapy-related cardiac dysfunction (CTRCD) as a decrease in LVEF > 10% to a value <53%, which is the standard reference value for a two-dimensional echocardiogram. They also have precise guidelines regarding the use and interpretation of strain imaging. A reduction in GLS of >15% from baseline immediately after or during anthracycline therapy may be predictive of cardiotoxicity. A drop of <8% may not be clinically significant. There is information regarding the pros and cons of utilizing echocardiogram vs. multigated acquisition (MUGA) scan vs. cardiac magnetic resonance (CMR) imaging for studying cardiotoxicity with a heavy emphasis on using echocardiogram as the first modality. During therapy, the overall risk assessment is similar to the ESMO guidelines, but a differential plan is laid out based on ejection fraction above and below 53%. There was little guidance on cardiac surveillance for survivors of cancer.[56]

National Comprehensive Cancer Network (NCCN) Clinical Practice Guidelines on Survivorship

These recommendations were updated in 2020 and are based on an integrated approach between cardiology and oncology based on the American College of Cardiology and American Heart Association's progressive heart failure (HF) stages (A to D). Although the risk factors identified are similar, the difference lies in the approach whereby having a history of either anthracycline exposure or any potentially cardiotoxic chemotherapy and/or chest radiation places survivors in stage B HF. A history of anthracycline use plus CV risk factors increases the risk of developing cardiomyopathy and HF and is thus classified as stage A. The guidelines emphasize management of underlying comorbidities and health behaviors to optimize risk reduction with recommendations for cardiology referral for those with or suspected to have more advanced stages (stage B, C, D) of disease.

NCCN recommends considering a two-dimensional echocardiogram with Doppler flow study within 1 year after completion of anthracycline therapy for survivors with high cumulative anthracycline dose (doxorubicin > 250 mg/m^2 or equivalent) or low cumulative anthracycline dose and one or more heart failure risk factors (e.g., hypertension). If there is no evidence of structural heart disease on the echocardiogram and the patient is asymptomatic (stage A), continue regular surveillance for underlying risk factors. However, if the patient is symptomatic or has any structural disease, the patient is referred to a cardio-oncologist for further evaluation. These recommendations are level 2A and are based upon lower-level evidence; however, there is uniform NCCN consensus that the intervention is appropriate.[59]

The International Society of Geriatric Oncology

The International Society of Geriatric Oncology (SIOG) focuses on elderly patients with particular attention to those above the age of 70 who are considered for anthracycline-based therapy. Overall, the guidelines advocate for rigorous screening for CV risk factors, CVD, prior anthracycline exposure, and/or cardiotoxic chemotherapy. Although the guidelines have robust recommendations for those undergoing anthracycline treatment, there are no specific guidelines for cancer survivors exposed to anthracycline-based therapy.[60]

CARDIORESPIRATORY FITNESS

There is growing recognition of increased CV mortality in cancer survivors related to underlying CVD risk factors and poor cardiac reserve coupled with the direct effects of anticancer therapy.[61,62] Reduced cardiac reserve stems from cancer-specific treatment, leading to cardiomyocyte damage, hypertension, arrhythmias, myocardial and vascular ischemia, and indirect effects of unhealthy lifestyle such as decreased physical activity, poor diet, and body mass.[63]

Cardiorespiratory fitness (CRF) refers to the circulatory and respiratory systems' ability to supply oxygen to skeletal muscles during sustained physical activity.[64] The primary measure of CRF is vital oxygen capacity (VO_2) max. Low levels of CRF are associated with a high risk of CVD, all-cause mortality, and mortality rates attributable to various cancers, especially breast and colon/digestive tract.[65] Importantly, improvements in CRF are associated with reduced mortality risk.[64] CRF has been shown to be up to 36% lower in cancer survivors than age and sex-matched sedentary individuals, without a history of cancer, following the typical 10% decline every decade in normal aging.[66,67] This accelerated CV aging may predispose cancer survivors to excess cancer and non-cancer competing morbidity and mortality.[67]

Exercise therapy has been found to improve CRF in cancer patients, improve the anti-tumor effects of cancer therapy, and attenuate the cardiotoxic effects.[68] There is evidence suggesting that breast tumors reside in hypoxic microenvironments associated with poor survival. By improving VO_{2max}, greater blood flow will reduce hypoxia, leading to improved antitumor efficacy of chemotherapy. Furthermore, increasing tissue oxygenation may slow tumor progression through direct action on tumor intrinsic factors, improve immunosurveillance and immunotherapy.[69]

Scott et al. performed a meta-analysis of 48 randomized control trials (the most prevalent being breast cancer), looking at the effects of a structured exercise intervention on VO_{2max}.[70] There was a general consensus that exercise is safe and tolerable for cancer patients and that exercise improves VO_{2max} and therefore CRF and survival.[69,70] However, many variables will impact whether VO_{2max} improves and to what extent: results may vary based on differences in adjuvant therapy regimens (taxane, non-taxane based, androgen deprivation therapy), baseline profile of patients (pre-existing CVD risk factors), exercise approach (standard vs. non-linear) or intensity (moderate, high-intensity interval training), and underlying patient genetics (variability of sedentary VO_{2max} and trainability of VO_{2max}).[65,67–71] There is also a suggestion that the magnitude of the decline in peak VO_2 may be related to the type of cancer and/or cancer treatment.[66] Jones et al. found that breast and lung cancer survivors were likely to have a VO_{2max} below 18 ml/kg/min, signifying low physical function.[72,73] A consequence of the reduced VO_{2max} is that it is a predictor of survival in breast and lung cancer survivors.[66] By contrast, Cramer et al. and Scott et al. reported that colorectal and prostate cancer survivors typically maintain a VO_{2max} above the 18 ml/kg/min threshold.[74,75]

The current data supports that exercise programs improve CRF and, most importantly, improve survival in cancer patients during and after oncologic therapy.[65] Currently, there is a wide variety of cardiac and pulmonary conditions that insurers will cover for exercise rehabilitation. Neither cancer nor treatment with known cardiotoxic regimens are qualifying conditions for exercise rehabilitation in North America. Therefore, exercise is not currently considered a standard aspect of cancer management or part of survivorship care. Various care models have been developed that incorporate exercise at low cost or reimbursed by insurance. There is a need to spread awareness about these programs, their benefits, and their necessity among patients, oncologists, and policymakers.[76]

SURVIVORSHIP ACROSS THE UNITED STATES: A PROPOSED MODEL OF CARE

As the number of cancer survivors in North America and globally continues to increase, survivorship programs have emerged, emphasizing overall health by managing late treatment-related effects and promoting healthy lifestyle behaviors.[77] However, there is a paucity of information on monitoring strategies for CV health. The risk of cancer therapy-related CV morbidity and mortality extends well beyond the completion of cancer therapy (see Figure 12.3), and yet there is currently little guidance on the best strategies to proactively monitor adult cancer survivors for late CV manifestations of cancer therapy. Long-term follow-up guidelines are available from the Children's Oncology Group for survivors of childhood, adolescent, and young adult cancers that include specific recommendations for CV monitoring after chemotherapy and radiation based on the CCSS that can be incorporated into survivorship plans. In contrast, in survivors of adult cancers, there is minimal evidence to guide clinicians on CV surveillance and monitoring strategies

Given the paucity of data, we propose a pragmatic approach to the CV care of adult cancer survivors that can be easily incorporated into survivorship care plans (see Figure 12.4).

Recommendations are based on cardiovascular risk as follows:

Low risk (group A): no cardiovascular risk factors and no exposure to cardiotoxic cancer therapy
Intermediate risk (group B): ≥2 cardiovascular risk factors but no exposure to cardiotoxic cancer therapy
High risk (group C): ≥2 cardiovascular risk factors and exposure to chronic cardiotoxic cancer therapy (e.g., Ibrutinib for chronic lymphocytic leukemia)

Patients in the *low-risk group* can be followed by their primary care provider (PCP) annually to screen for CV risk factors including Body Mass Index (BMI), metabolic syndrome, lipids, fasting glucose and/or HbA1C, TSH, CBC, and ambulatory blood pressure monitoring (see https://reporter.nih.gov/search/OD_wE-8gDUK2qRwkOMBU5Q/project-details/10159878).

In addition to previous recommendations, for those in the *intermediate risk group*, we recommend a visit with a cardio-oncologist at 2 years and then at 5 years for optimal management of CV risk factors with support from their cancer care team and yearly EKG unless symptoms dictate earlier testing.

For the *highest risk group*, we recommend co-management between the PCP, the cancer multidisciplinary team, and a cardio-oncologist. These patients need annual EKG's unless symptoms dictate earlier

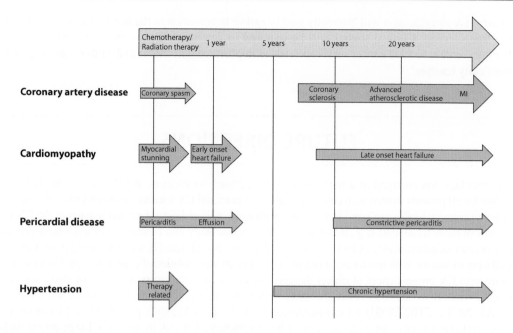

FIGURE 12.3   Timeline for cardiovascular disease in cancer survivors.

testing, optimization of myocardial infarction risk factors, and cardiac imaging to screen for cardiomyopathy annually unless symptoms dictate otherwise.

All cancer survivors should have ambulatory blood pressure measurements annually or bi-annually, and a calcium score performed at 3 to 5 years after the last cancer treatment. Given the likelihood of reduced CRF, consider providing a prescription for an exercise program and possibly a referral to an exercise physiologist. If exercise capacity is severely reduced, consider referral to cardio-oncology rehabilitation. Nutritionists, mental health counselors, smoking cessation programs, and medication reconciliation pharmacists should also be considered at each of these visits.

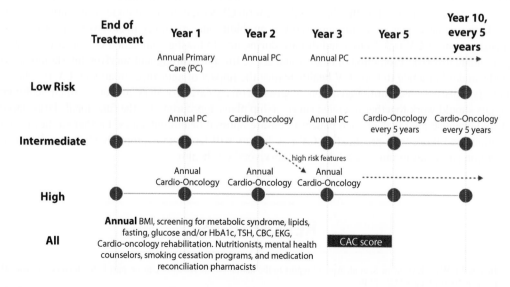

FIGURE 12.4   Cardio-oncology survivorship model of care. *Abbreviations*: PC, primary care; BMI, body mass index; EKG, electrocardiogram; CAC score, coronary artery calcium score.

Early risk identification will hopefully lead to earlier intervention in the hopes of extending CV and cancer-free survival. Clinical studies will be required to determine if increased CV surveillance and earlier intervention in adult cancer survivors leads to improvement in cancer and cardiac outcomes and is economically feasible.

FUTURE DIRECTIONS

Cardio-oncology has emerged as a multidisciplinary approach to attenuate the risk of CV morbidity and mortality for all patients treated with cancer therapy with potential CV toxicity. As novel cancer therapeutics continue to emerge, healthcare providers will be challenged with understanding and managing the CV consequences of these treatments (e.g., metabolic syndrome). Oncology and cardiology societies have provided guidelines on mitigation strategies for CV risk. Still, they have been limited in scope, focusing mainly on strategies during treatment, with less focus on risk management after completion of cancer therapy. Understanding the long-term CV consequences of cancer therapies in adult cancer survivors is an area of study that needs urgent attention. If we are to maintain the gains we are making in cancer-specific survival, studies such as UPBEAT (NCT NCT02791581), a longitudinal cohort study of CV health in patients treated for breast cancer, are needed to increase our understanding of how to attenuate CV risk in survivors. Large cohort studies in patients with hematological and solid cancers assessing CV risk and analyses of cost effectiveness and outcomes of early medical intervention in asymptomatic survivors will define future goals for this patient population. Access to care (Do they have a primary care physician?), insurance coverage, and neighborhood deprivation index (income, education, employment, and housing quality) will be important considerations.

CONCLUSION

Improved screening strategies and novel cancer therapeutics have led to an increasing population of adult cancer survivors. Understanding the short- and long-term CV toxicities of cytotoxic drugs, targeted agents, and radiation is necessary to avoid increased CV morbidity and mortality in survivorship. Attention to the management of CV risk factors and disease during and following completion of cancer therapy will help attenuate this risk. Promotion of healthy and active lifestyles throughout survivorship should be considered standard practice to buoy CV health against the impact of anticancer treatment, CV risk factors, and lifestyle disruptions. Cardiologists, oncologists, primary care providers, and other allied health professionals should work together to create survivorship plans appropriate for the functional status, fatigue level, and exercise tolerance of each patient to ensure optimal health outcomes. Further studies in older populations and those with pre-existing CV risk factors will facilitate appropriate CV surveillance and intervention strategies to improve adult cancer survivors' CV health.

REFERENCES

1. Henley SJ, Ward EM, Scott S, et al. Annual report to the nation on the status of cancer, part I: National cancer statistics. *Cancer.* 2020;126(10):2225–2249.
2. Miller KD, Nogueira L, Mariotto AB, et al. Cancer treatment and survivorship statistics, 2019. *CA Cancer J Clin.* 2019;69(5):363–385.

3. Armstrong GT, Kawashima T, Leisenring W, et al. Aging and risk of severe, disabling, life-threatening, and fatal events in the childhood cancer survivor study. *J Clin Oncol*. 2014;32(12):1218–1227.

4. Meacham LR, Chow EJ, Ness KK, et al. Cardiovascular risk factors in adult survivors of pediatric cancer—A report from the Childhood Cancer Survivor Study. *Cancer Epidemiol Biomarkers Prev*. 2010;19(1):170–181.

5. Patnaik JL, Byers T, DiGuiseppi C, Dabelea D, Denberg TD. Cardiovascular disease competes with breast cancer as the leading cause of death for older females diagnosed with breast cancer: A retrospective cohort study. *Breast Cancer Res*. 2011;13(3):R64.

6. Hershman DL, Till C, Shen S, et al. Association of cardiovascular risk factors with cardiac events and survival outcomes among patients with breast cancer enrolled in SWOG clinical trials. *J Clin Oncol*. 2018;36(26):2710–2717.

7. Armenian SH, Xu L, Ky B, et al. Cardiovascular disease among survivors of adult-onset cancer: A community-based retrospective cohort study. *J Clin Oncol*. 2016;34(10):1122–1130.

8. Nanda A, Chen MH, Moran BJ, Braccioforte MH, D'Amico AV. Cardiovascular comorbidity and mortality in men with prostate cancer treated with brachytherapy-based radiation with or without hormonal therapy. *Int J Radiat Oncol Biol Phys*. 2013;85(5):e209–e215.

9. Strongman H, Gadd S, Matthews A, et al. Medium and long-term risks of specific cardiovascular diseases in survivors of 20 adult cancers: A population-based cohort study using multiple linked UK electronic health records databases. *Lancet*. 2019;394(10203):1041–1054.

10. Feijen E, Font-Gonzalez A, Van der Pal HJH, et al. Risk and temporal changes of heart failure among 5-year childhood cancer survivors: A DCOG-LATER study. *J Am Heart Assoc*. 2019;8(1):e009122.

11. Chow EJ, Chen Y, Kremer LC, et al. Individual prediction of heart failure among childhood cancer survivors. *J Clin Oncol*. 2015;33(5):394–402.

12. Yan AP, Chen Y, Henderson TO, et al. Adherence to surveillance for second malignant neoplasms and cardiac dysfunction in childhood cancer survivors: a Childhood Cancer Survivor Study. *J Clin Oncol*. 2020;38(15):1711–1722.

13. Mulrooney DA, Armstrong GT, Huang S, et al. Cardiac outcomes in adult survivors of childhood cancer exposed to cardiotoxic therapy: A cross-sectional study. *Ann Intern Med*. 2016;164(2):93–101.

14. Chang HM, Moudgil R, Scarabelli T, Okwuosa TM, Yeh ETH. Cardiovascular complications of cancer therapy: Best practices in diagnosis, prevention, and management: Part 1. *J Am Coll Cardiol*. 2017;70(20):2536–2551.

15. Bowles EJ, Wellman R, Feigelson HS, et al. Risk of heart failure in breast cancer patients after anthracycline and trastuzumab treatment: A retrospective cohort study. *J Natl Cancer Inst*. 2012;104(17):1293–1305.

16. Keefe DL. Trastuzumab-associated cardiotoxicity. *Cancer*. 2002;95(7):1592–1600.

17. Ewer MS, Vooletich MT, Durand JB, et al. Reversibility of trastuzumab-related cardiotoxicity: New insights based on clinical course and response to medical treatment. *J Clin Oncol*. 2005;23(31):7820–7826.

18. Guarneri V, Lenihan DJ, Valero V, et al. Long-term cardiac tolerability of trastuzumab in metastatic breast cancer: The M.D. Anderson Cancer Center experience. *J Clin Oncol*. 2006;24(25):4107–4115.

19. Perez EA, Koehler M, Byrne J, Preston AJ, Rappold E, Ewer MS. Cardiac safety of lapatinib: Pooled analysis of 3689 patients enrolled in clinical trials. *Mayo Clin Proc*. 2008;83(6):679–686.

20. Baselga J, Gelmon KA, Verma S, et al. Phase II trial of pertuzumab and trastuzumab in patients with human epidermal growth factor receptor 2-positive metastatic breast cancer that progressed during prior trastuzumab therapy. *J Clin Oncol*. 2010;28(7):1138–1144.

21. Choueiri TK, Mayer EL, Je Y, et al. Congestive heart failure risk in patients with breast cancer treated with bevacizumab. *J Clin Oncol*. 2011;29(6):632–638.

22. Moslehi JJ. Cardiovascular toxic effects of targeted cancer therapies. *N Engl J Med*. 2016;375(15):1457–1467.

23. Richards CJ, Je Y, Schutz FA, et al. Incidence and risk of congestive heart failure in patients with renal and nonrenal cell carcinoma treated with sunitinib. *J Clin Oncol*. 2011;29(25):3450–3456.

24. Curigliano G, Cardinale D, Dent S, et al. Cardiotoxicity of anticancer treatments: Epidemiology, detection, and management. *CA Cancer J Clin*. 2016;66(4):309–325.

25. Lotrionte M, Biondi-Zoccai G, Abbate A, et al. Review and meta-analysis of incidence and clinical predictors of anthracycline cardiotoxicity. *Am J Cardiol*. 2013;112(12):1980–1984.

26. Swain SM, Whaley FS, Ewer MS. Congestive heart failure in patients treated with doxorubicin: A retrospective analysis of three trials. *Cancer*. 2003;97(11):2869–2879.

27. Cardinale D, Colombo A, Bacchiani G, et al. Early detection of anthracycline cardiotoxicity and improvement with heart failure therapy. *Circulation*. 2015;131(22):1981–1988.

28. Feijen EA, Leisenring WM, Stratton KL, et al. Equivalence ratio for daunorubicin to doxorubicin in relation to late heart failure in survivors of childhood cancer. *J Clin Oncol*. 2015;33(32):3774–3780.

29. Feijen EAM, Leisenring WM, Stratton KL, et al. Derivation of anthracycline and anthraquinone equivalence ratios to doxorubicin for late-onset cardiotoxicity. *JAMA Oncol*. 2019;5(6):864–871.

30. Gottdiener JS, Appelbaum FR, Ferrans VJ, Deisseroth A, Ziegler J. Cardiotoxicity associated with high-dose cyclophosphamide therapy. *Arch Intern Med*. 1981;141(6):758–763.

31. Salem JE, Manouchehri A, Bretagne M, et al. Cardiovascular toxicities associated with ibrutinib. *J Am Coll Cardiol*. 2019;74(13):1667–1678.

32. Kerkela R, Grazette L, Yacobi R, et al. Cardiotoxicity of the cancer therapeutic agent imatinib mesylate. *Nat Med*. 2006;12(8):908–916.

33. Heidenreich PA, Hancock SL, Vagelos RH, Lee BK, Schnittger I. Diastolic dysfunction after mediastinal irradiation. *Am Heart J.* 2005;150(5):977–982.

34. van Nimwegen FA, Ntentas G, Darby SC, et al. Risk of heart failure in survivors of Hodgkin lymphoma: Effects of cardiac exposure to radiation and anthracyclines. *Blood.* 2017;129(16):2257–2265.

35. Leerink JM, Baat ECd, Feijen EAM, et al. Cardiac disease in childhood cancer survivors. *JACC: CardioOncology.* 2020;2(3):363–378.

36. Okwuosa TM, Anzevino S, Rao R. Cardiovascular disease in cancer survivors. *Postgrad Med J.* 2017;93(1096):82–90.

37. Rossari JR, Metzger-Filho O, Paesmans M, et al. Bevacizumab and breast cancer: A meta-analysis of first-line phase III studies and a critical reappraisal of available evidence. *J Oncol.* 2012;2012:417673.

38. Kosmas C, Kallistratos MS, Kopterides P, et al. Cardiotoxicity of fluoropyrimidines in different schedules of administration: A prospective study. *J Cancer Res Clin Oncol.* 2008;134(1):75–82.

39. Scappaticci FA, Skillings JR, Holden SN, et al. Arterial thromboembolic events in patients with metastatic carcinoma treated with chemotherapy and bevacizumab. *J Natl Cancer Inst.* 2007;99(16):1232–1239.

40. Kamba T, McDonald DM. Mechanisms of adverse effects of anti-VEGF therapy for cancer. *Br J Cancer.* 2007;96(12):1788–1795.

41. Vermorken JB, Remenar E, van Herpen C, et al. Cisplatin, fluorouracil, and docetaxel in unresectable head and neck cancer. *N Engl J Med.* 2007;357(17):1695–1704.

42. Schmidinger M, Zielinski CC, Vogl UM, et al. Cardiac toxicity of sunitinib and sorafenib in patients with metastatic renal cell carcinoma. *J Clin Oncol.* 2007;26(32):5204–5212.

43. Dimopoulos MA, Goldschmidt H, Niesvizky R, et al. Carfilzomib or bortezomib in relapsed or refractory multiple myeloma (ENDEAVOR): An interim overall survival analysis of an open-label, randomised, phase 3 trial. *Lancet Oncol.* 2017;18(10):1327–1337.

44. Stewart AK, Rajkumar SV, Dimopoulos MA, et al. Carfilzomib, lenalidomide, and dexamethasone for relapsed multiple myeloma. *N Engl J Med.* 2015;372(2):142–152.

45. van Nimwegen FA, Schaapveld M, Janus CP, et al. Cardiovascular disease after Hodgkin lymphoma treatment: 40-year disease risk. *JAMA Intern Med.* 2015;175(6):1007–1017.

46. Mulrooney DA, Nunnery SE, Armstrong GT, et al. Coronary artery disease detected by coronary computed tomography angiography in adult survivors of childhood Hodgkin lymphoma. *Cancer.* 2014;120(22):3536–3544.

47. Naaktgeboren WR, Linschoten M, de Graeff A, et al. Long-term cardiovascular health in adult cancer survivors. *Maturitas.* 2017;105:37–45.

48. Horacek JM, Jakl M, Horackova J, Pudil R, Jebavy L, Maly J. Assessment of anthracycline-induced cardiotoxicity with electrocardiography. *Exp Oncol.* 2009;31(2):115–117.

49. Buza V, Rajagopalan B, Curtis AB. Cancer treatment-induced arrhythmias: Focus on chemotherapy and targeted therapies. *Circ Arrhythm Electrophysiol.* 2017;10(8).

50. Geisberg C, Pentassuglia L, Sawyer DB. Cardiac side effects of anticancer treatments: New mechanistic insights. *Curr Heart Fail Rep.* 2012;9(3):211–218.

51. Desai MY, Windecker S, Lancellotti P, et al. Prevention, diagnosis, and management of radiation-associated cardiac disease: JACC scientific expert panel. *J Am Coll Cardiol.* 2019;74(7):905–927.

52. Christiansen JR, Hamre H, Massey R, et al. Left ventricular function in long-term survivors of childhood lymphoma. *Am J Cardiol.* 2014;114(3):483–490.

53. Mulrooney DA, Hyun G, Ness KK, et al. Major cardiac events for adult survivors of childhood cancer diagnosed between 1970 and 1999: Report from the Childhood Cancer Survivor Study cohort. *BMJ.* 2020;368:l6794.

54. Cuomo JR, Sharma GK, Conger PD, Weintraub NL. Novel concepts in radiation-induced cardiovascular disease. *World J Cardiol.* 2016;8(9):504–519.

55. Andratschke N, Maurer J, Molls M, Trott KR. Late radiation-induced heart disease after radiotherapy. Clinical importance, radiobiological mechanisms and strategies of prevention. *Radiother Oncol.* 2011;100(2):160–166.

56. Plana JC, Galderisi M, Barac A, et al. Expert consensus for the multimodality imaging evaluation of adult patients during and after cancer therapy: A report from the American Society of Echocardiography and the European Association of Cardiovascular Imaging. *J Am Soc Echocardiogr.* 2014;27:911–939.

57. Armenian SH, Lacchetti C, Barac A, et al. Prevention and monitoring of cardiac dysfunction in survivors of adult cancers: American Society of Clinical Oncology clinical practice guideline. *J Clin Oncol.* 2017;35:893–911.

58. Curigliano G, Lenihan D, Fradley M, Ganatra S, et al. Management of cardiac disease in cancer patients throughout oncological treatment: ESMO consensus recommendations. *Ann Oncol.* 2020;31(2):171–189.

59. National Comprehensive Cancer Network. Survivorship: Cardiovascular Disease Risk Assessment. Version 2. 2020.

60. Aapro M, Bernard-Marty C, Brian EG, et al. Anthracycline cardiotoxicity in the elderly cancer patient: a SIOG expert position paper. *Ann Oncol.* 2011;22:257–267.

61. Venturini E, Iannuzzo G, D'Andrea A, Pacileo M, et al. Oncology and cardiac rehabilitation: An underrated relationship. *J Clin Med.* 2020;9(1810):1–26.

62. Haykowsky MJ, Pituskin E, Paterson I. Physical health and exercise in cancer. *Am Coll Cardiol.* 2016;(Aug):1–7.

63. Denlinger CS, Sanft T, Moslehi JJ, Overholser L, et al. Survivorship, version 2.2020. featured updates to the NCCN guidelines. *J Natl Compr Canc Netw.* 2020;18(8):1016–1023.

64. Raghuveer G, Hartz J, David LR, Timothy T, et al. Cardiorespiratory Fitness in youth: An important marker of health: A scientific statement from the American Heart Association. *Circulation.* 2020;142(7):e101–e118.
65. Ross R, Blair SN, Arena R, Church TS, et al. Importance of assessing cardiorespiratory fitness in clinical practice: A case for fitness as a clinical vital sign. American Heart Association scientific statement. *Circulation.* 2016;134:e653–e699.
66. Jones LW, Haykowsky MJ, Swartz JJ, et al. Early breast cancer therapy and cardiovascular injury. *J Am Coll Cardiol.* 2007;50:1435–1441.
67. Scott JM, Nilsen T, Gupta D, Jones LW. Therapy and cardiovascular toxicity in cancer. *Circulation.* 2018;137(11):1176–1191.
68. Tong C, Lau B, Davis MK. Exercise training for cancer survivors. *Curr Treat Options Oncol.* 2020;21(7):53.
69. Lamkin DR, Garland T Jr. Translating preclinical research for exercise oncology: Take it to the VO_{2max}. *Front Oncol.* 2020;10:1–7.
70. Scott J, Zabor EC, Schwitzer E, Koelwyn GJ, et al. Efficacy of exercise therapy on cardiorespiratory fitness in patients with cancer: A systemic review and meta-analysis. *J Clin Oncol.* 2018;36:2297–2305.
71. Hoppeler H. Deciphering VO_{2max}: Limits of the genetic approach. *J Exp Biol.* 2018;221:1–7.
72. Jones LW, Watson D, Herndon JE 2nd, et al. Peak oxygen consumption and long term all-cause mortality in nonsmall cell lung cancer. *Cancer.* 2010;116:4825–4832.
73. Jones LW, Courtney KS, Mackey JR, et al. Cardiopulmonary function and age related decline across the breast cancer survivorship continuum. *J Clin Oncol.* 2012;30:2530–2537.
74. Cramer L, Hildebrandt B, Kung T et al. Cardiovascular function and predictors of exercise capacity in patients with colorectal cancer. *J Am Coll Cardiol.* 2014;64:1310–1309.
75. Scott JM, Hornsby WE. Lane A. Kenjale AA et al. Reliability of maximal cardiopulmonary exercise testing in men with prostate cancers. *Med Sci Sports Exerc.* 2015;47:27–32.
76. Ellahham, SH. Exercise before, during and after cancer therapy. *Am Coll Cardiol.* 2019:1–14.
77. Shapiro CL, Jacobsen PB, Henderson T, et al. ReCap: ASCO core curriculum for cancer survivorship education. *J Oncol Pract.* 2016;12(2):145, e108–e117.

Cancer Rehabilitation
Optimizing Function for Cancer Survivors

13

Cristina Kline-Quiroz, Raman Sharma, and Michael D. Stubblefield

INTRODUCTION

Cancer rehabilitation is the process of restoring cancer survivors to the highest possible level of function and quality of life.[1,2] As many of the late effects of cancer and its treatment, particularly radiation, are not only chronic but progressive, optimal rehabilitation efforts should also focus on maintaining function. Comprehensive cancer rehabilitation is a multidisciplinary endeavor that includes physiatrists (physical medicine and rehabilitation physicians), physical therapists, occupational therapists, speech language pathologists, the oncology team as well as generalists and specialists who share in the care of cancer survivors. While the primary goal of cancer rehabilitation is to facilitate restoration and maintenance of function and quality of life, there are many other valuable aspects to consider, particularly in the era of value-based care.[3] Though data are just now emerging, comprehensive cancer rehabilitation has the potential to not only help keep patients out of the emergency room and hospital, support their ability to tolerate oncologic therapy, improve their pain control and minimize opioid use, but ultimately to save money and lessen the workload of cancer clinicians. This chapter will discuss the principles and practice of cancer rehabilitation including the common impairments likely to benefit from rehabilitation interventions. Certain cancers, such as head and neck and breast cancers, will be discussed in detail to illustrate the complexity of rehabilitation needs in these survivors.[4,5]

CANCER-RELATED FATIGUE

Cancer-related fatigue (CRF) is the most common symptom reported by cancer survivors. It can be associated with cancer itself and/or its treatments.[6] It is characterized by a persistent and functionally limiting subjective sense of physical, emotional, and cognitive exhaustion. Unlike general somatic

DOI: 10.1201/9781003055426-13

fatigue which may improve with rest, CRF is not related to recent exertional activity. In a recent study, up to 98% of cancer survivors reported experiencing fatigue and 58% reported fatigue impacted their daily life more than pain during chemotherapy.[7] Symptoms of CRF may persist for years after treatment in about 30% of survivors.[8] There is a role for screening for fatigue throughout the continuum of cancer care since studies have shown CRF is both underdiagnosed and undertreated by health care providers.[9–11]

CRF is a recognized diagnosis in the tenth edition of the International Classification of Diseases (ICD-10) listed as "neoplastic (malignant) related fatigue."[12] Given the multifactorial nature, the assessment of CRF begins with a comprehensive history and physical examination of various organ systems potentially affected by the underlying cancer processes and treatments. The American Society of Clinical Oncology (ASCO) and the National Comprehensive Cancer Network (NCCN) recommend screening for CRF in patients with malignant disease at the initial visit, end of primary therapy, at the diagnosis of advanced disease, at every chemotherapy visit, and at least annually during follow-up survivorship care.[6,13] Because CRF has both subjective and objective components, it may require measures that are multidimensional including self-reports and performance on testing tools such as the Functional Assessment of Chronic Illness Therapy-Fatigue (FACIT-F) (16) and the Short Form-36 (SF-36) Vitality Sub-Scale.

Potentially reversible causes of CRF such as medical comorbidities (anemia, electrolyte abnormalities, endocrine dysfunction, substance abuse, cardiac, pulmonary, or renal dysfunction), medication adverse effects, pain, psychological distress, sleep dysfunction, nutritional/caloric deficiencies, and deconditioning should be investigated and treated appropriately.[6] The most common reversible cause of CRF is anemia, and its resolution was shown to improve both quality of life and diminish fatigue.[14]

A systematic review recommended exercise after finding favorable data to support improvement of CRF symptoms that persisted despite addressing reversible causes.[1,15] Patients with cancer, especially those undergoing active treatment, are often fatigued and sometimes encouraged to rest rather than start or continue exercising. Since inactivity may lead to deconditioning, reduced muscle mass, loss of physical strength, endurance and function, exercise should be encouraged.[16] Among interventions for CRF during and after treatment, the NCCN guidelines found category 1 evidence for physical activity, yoga, cognitive behavioral therapy, and mindfulness-based stress reduction.[17,18]

CANCER-RELATED COGNITIVE IMPAIRMENT/ MILD COGNITIVE IMPAIRMENT

Cancer-related cognitive impairment (CRCI) differs from CRF in that it has a significant cognitive component.[19] CRCI is also known as mild cognitive impairment. Commonly referred to as "chemobrain" and "chemofog," these terms are not appropriate or accurate, since symptoms can occur without chemotherapy.[20] CRCI may present with impairments in concentration, attention, visual/verbal memories, processing ability, executive function, and language which may persist for years after treatment.[21] Incidence of CRCI is estimated as high as 75% for non-CNS cancers and about 90% for CNS cancers.[19] CRCI rates may vary over the continuum of disease; in the pretreatment phase approximately 20%–40% of patients report symptoms, 65%–75% noted symptoms during treatment, and 30%–60% of survivors reported long-term symptoms after treatments were completed in a study of patients with breast cancer.[21]

Risk factors for CRCI include fatigue, psychological functioning, health behaviors, and certain medical comorbidities. In general, non-modifiable risk factors are related to genetics, demographics, disease, and treatment characteristics.[21] Multiple studies have documented a negative impact on quality of life and activities of daily living in patients with CRCI.[22–24] Studies have also shown a negative impact on school and work performance. Approximately 25% of survivors may continue to experience CRCI 20 years following completion of treatment resulting in impaired work performance and the need to change jobs.[19,25,26] Another study showed impaired social functioning related to decreased productivity, community involvement, and reluctance to seek social support.[27] A study of 360 patients showed that those with CRCI had a worse survival, even when stratified by indolent cancer ($p < 0.01$) and aggressive cancer ($p < 0.001$).[28]

The potential mechanisms contributing to CRCI include compromised integrity of the blood-brain barrier,[29] cell death in the hippocampus and corpus collosum,[30] genetic variability/polymorphisms,[31] DNA damage, cytokine production,[32] telomere shortening,[33] neural repair defects, hormone dysregulation, and neurotransmitter defects.[29] The neurotoxicity of whole brain radiation has been well documented, especially in acute lymphoblastic leukemia (ALL) in children[34] and primary CNS lymphoma.[35] CRCI is also associated with radiotherapy to other parts of the body, although the effects do not seem to be as severe as with chemotherapy.[36] There is a growing body of research evaluating how emotional factors, fatigue, stress, depression, and sleep quality relate to CRCI and extends our knowledge of how loneliness influences perceived cognitive function in survivors.[37,38] Loneliness was found to impact perceived cognitive function via a psychosocial mechanism through feelings of anxiety and fatigue in a study of breast cancer survivors.[37] CRF is a common comorbidity with CRCI and should also be addressed since data suggests cancer-related psychological or biological processes negatively influence cognitive functioning and associated aspects of brain structure and function.[20] Cognitive rehabilitation can help mitigate CRCI and can be implemented in a variety of settings including outpatient, inpatient, home-based, and virtually via telehealth.[39]

PAIN

Cancer and its treatments are responsible for a variety of complex pain disorders resulting in significant functional impairment and reduced quality of life.[40] Cancer pain has been reported by up to 90% of patients with advanced disease.[41] Pain may be due to direct local tumor invasion, metastases, side effects of treatment, or issues unrelated to cancer or its treatment such as arthritis.[41]

It should not be assumed that pain in patients with active cancer, even those with metastatic disease, or a history of cancer is "cancer pain." Identification of the exact etiology of pain is often key to safe and effective pain reduction, function optimization, quality of life improvement, caregiver burden reduction and reduced healthcare costs.[42] Analgesics, such as opioids, should generally not be the primary modality used to treat pain in cancer survivors. Clinicians should consider the risks and benefits of other interventions such as non-opioid medications, physical modalities, exercise, and interventional procedures.[40] If other modalities have failed to provide adequate pain relief, then opioids should be considered. For patients with bone pain from metastatic disease, NSAIDS, bone modifying agents (bisphosphonates and RANKL inhibitors such as denosumab), or radiation therapy may be considered as adjunctive therapy.[43] It is critical to incorporate open patient/physician communication so that specific types of pain can be assessed regularly throughout the continuum of cancer care, as adjustments may be necessary to the treatment plan as dictated by disease progression, treatment toxicity, and medical comorbidity.[44]

Rehabilitation treatment plans focus on modulating nociception, stabilizing and unloading painful structures, influencing pain perception, and alleviating soft tissue musculotendinous pain.[40] Physiatrist-directed physical therapy has been found to effectively help stabilize painful areas and improve myofascial pain.[45] These exercise programs have been found to be effective before, during, and after treatments for improving function and quality of life.[46,47] A number of interventional procedures such as intrathecal anesthesia, radiofrequency nerve ablation, electrical nerve stimulation and vertebroplasty may be considered for pain that remained refractory to medications or in which analgesic medications would be contraindicated due to adverse effects. There are an increasing number of studies in the palliative care population for patients with terminal disease, focused on significantly improving a patient's mobility, safety, and quality of life by encouraging early evaluation by a physiatrist.[48]

NEUROPATHY

There are many etiologies of nerve dysfunction in the general population and cancer survivors. Chemotherapy-induced peripheral neuropathy (CIPN) is the most common neurologic complication of cancer treatment and can have a profound impact on quality of life and survivorship.[49] An accurate assessment of the incidence and prevalence of neuromuscular disorders in cancer patients is not currently available due to variability in etiology, underlying comorbidities, assessment measures, and varying clinical presentation.[1,50] Although considered a conservative estimate, it is thought that approximately one-third of adult chronic cancer pain patients, across all tumor types and stages, have cancer-related neuropathic pain (pain due to direct damage to the nervous system from primary tumor or metastases, or from treatments such as chemotherapy).[51,52]

Patients with CIPN may experience numbness, tingling, paresthesias, burning pain, weakness, impaired proprioception or gait abnormalities in addition to dysesthesias and allodynia.[1] Symptoms are typically dose-dependent and often associated with cumulative exposure to one or more anticancer medications over the course of a chemotherapy regimen.[50,53] Studies have shown that CIPN symptoms can occur with many agents, but certain classes of chemotherapeutics are especially prone to causing neuropathy including the vinca alkaloids, the taxanes, and the platinum-based compounds.[52]

When CIPN develops outside the pattern expected for a given neurotoxic agent, then referral to physiatry or neurology for evaluation should be considered.[52] Regular monitoring during chemotherapy is recommended as new symptoms may appear or existing symptoms progress. Evaluation can help clarify the source of neuropathic symptoms and identify potentially reversible or treatable causes of neural dysfunction.[1]

The 2020 ASCO Guideline Update reconfirmed that no agents have been shown to be effective to prevent CIPN. However, the authors concluded there was sufficient evidence to recommend duloxetine to treat pain in patients with established painful CIPN.[54] The magnitude of the benefit of duloxetine appears to be limited and may still not provide full control of symptoms in some patients.[54] In addition to duloxetine, there is some evidence to support the use of pregabalin, gabapentin, venlafaxine, amitriptyline, valproate, opioids, and capsaicin.[43] Interventions such as electrical stimulation and acupuncture have also been shown to provide additional relief for some patients who did not benefit from other measures.[55–57]

LYMPHEDEMA

Lymphedema is the regional accumulation of protein-rich fluid with resultant inflammation, adipose deposition, and fibrosis as a result of damage or dysfunction of the lymphatic system.[58] Cancer and its treatment can lead to impairments of the lymphatic system resulting in secondary lymphedema. Depending on the location of lymphatic injury, swelling can present in the limbs, face, neck, trunk, or genitalia. This local swelling can further impact physical symptoms, functional impairments, and quality of life.[59,60]

The prevalence of lymphedema in cancer survivors varies by cancer diagnosis and the modalities used in treatment. In breast cancer survivors, a meta-analysis found that 21% develop arm lymphedema[61] and in head and neck cancer survivors, lymphedema incidence has been reported to be as high as 75%–90%.[62] Although lymphedema is common in cancer survivors, it is essential to consider a broad differential and perform appropriate clinical evaluation as indicated for other potential causes of swelling such as hypo-proteinemia, heart failure, venous insufficiency, deep vein thrombosis, or tumor recurrence.[63]

Lymphedema can be evaluated with imaging and volume measurements. Lymphoscintigraphy, per-formed by injecting a radiolabeled tracer, is the standard imaging technique utilized in diagnosing lym-phatic dysfunction.[64] Near infrared fluorescence imaging with indocyanine green is an emerging imaging modality also in use to identify lymphatic dysfunction.[65] There are several methods routinely used to obtain volume measurements for surveillance and monitoring of progression. These include circumferen-tial tape measurements, water displacement, perometry, and bioimpedance spectroscopy.[66] Additionally, soft tissue composition can be assessed with tissue dielectric constant[67] and ultrasound.[66]

Clinically, lymphedema is commonly graded on a 3-stage scale. In stage I, the fluid is high in protein and swelling is improved with elevation of the affected limb. By stage II, elevation is no longer effective in reducing tissue swelling, along with progression of fibrosis and subcutaneous fat. Stage III is character-ized by trophic skin changes, fibrosis, and warty overgrowth. There is increasing attentiveness to stage 0 or 1a which is a subclinical presentation of damaged lymphatics with subtle changes in tissue without apparent swelling.[68]

Early identification and treatment are crucial to help prevent lymphedema progression and further complications. Specifically, in breast cancer survivors there is a growing body of evidence from retrospec-tive, prospective, and randomized trials to support that prospective surveillance and early intervention decreases progression to clinical lymphedema and chronic breast cancer related lymphedema (BCRL)[69–72] and decreases the direct treatment costs.[73] Although risk reduction practices for BCRL have been contro-versial, studies support that venipunctures, blood pressure measurements, and air travel were not associ-ated with BCRL.[74,75] The National Comprehensive Cancer Network Survivorship guidelines states these precautionary measures are likely unnecessary and that when necessary venipuncture and blood pressure measurements may be done on the at-risk arm but if possible to utilize the non-at-risk limb.[76]

Complete decongestive therapy (CDT) and compression garments are the cornerstones of treatment. CDT is effective in reducing lymphedema volume and consists of manual lymphatic drainage, short stretch compression bandage, exercises, skin hygiene, and maintenance compression garments.[77] Skin hygiene is imperative to prevent infections and there is evidence that exercise, including resistance train-ing which was previously discouraged, can be implemented.[68,78] Additionally, there are surgical treatment options which vary from microsurgical procedures, suction-assisted lipectomies, and surgical resection.[68]

IMPAIRMENTS IN ACTIVITIES OF DAILY LIVING AND MOBILITY

Activities of daily living (ADLs) refer to tasks people perform on a daily basis such as bathing, toileting, dressing, feeding, and functional transfers.[79] Functional transfers are the transitions that enable a person to navigate their environment such as getting out of bed or getting into the shower. Additionally, instru-mental activities of daily living (IADLs) can include community mobility, shopping, meal preparation, managing their finances, medication, and health management.[79] Community mobility encompasses the ability to negotiate the community such as going to a store, a physician visit or recreational activity, which requires additional skills including walking longer distances, traversing uneven terrain, and maneuvering around the traffic from other persons.[80] Functional impairments and symptoms such as fatigue, pain, neu-ropathy, and cognitive impairment can hinder the ability to perform ADLs. Despite appropriate treatment, impairments in ADLs can persist and are an opportunity to intervene to optimize function.

The prevalence of impairments in ADLs and IADLs vary from 8% to 57% and 38% to 65%, respec-tively.[81] This may be underrecognized clinically. In a study of patients undergoing outpatient cancer treatment, 30% endorsed insufficient strength to perform ADLs and 27% required assistance; however, providers only noted these in 1.6% and 0%.[82] This unmet need is an opportunity to provide valuable contributions to patient care. Functional impairments were associated with shorter survival time[83] and the ability to perform IADLs is associated with improved quality of life in cancer patients.[84] To address these needs physical and occupational therapy can provide education, therapeutic exercise, compensatory strategies, and adaptive equipment to optimize functional independence and enhance quality of life.[85,86]

As fatigue is common in cancer survivors, utilizing energy conservation principles for ADLs can maximize tolerance.[86] These can be taught by an occupational therapist and may include using assistive devices, placing frequently used items at easy to reach heights, minimizing overexertion and prioritizing the activities that contribute most to their quality of life.[86]

When functional impairments are present, assistive devices can enhance functional independence in household and self-care tasks.[87] There is an expansive array of assistive devices and adaptive equipment available. For example, long-handled reachers, button hooks, and sock aids can facilitate dressing and grasping items to decrease the exertion and coordination required.[86] Adaptive utensils can enable feeding and grab bars in the bathroom can assist with toilet and shower transfers.

The prevalence of impaired mobility and falls in cancer survivors varies from 20% to 55%.[81] The risk of falls is affected by deconditioning, impaired physical function, and neurologic deficits.[88] Assistive devices for mobility include single point canes, four pronged canes, and walkers which can enhance balance and mobility.[89] Furthermore, balance and endurance training was found to improve function and quality of life.[90]

FUNCTIONAL IMPAIRMENTS IN HEAD AND NECK CANCER SURVIVORS

Head and neck cancer is the seventh most common cancer worldwide,[91] and comprises a heterogenous collection of malignancies that can involve the oral cavity, pharynx, larynx, salivary glands, and paranasal sinuses. Sixty to 70% are diagnosed at an advanced stage frequently requiring multimodal treatment.[92] Head and neck cancer survivors may experience shoulder dysfunction, spinal accessory nerve palsy, cervical dystonia, dysphagia, dysarthria, trismus, lymphedema, and many other disorders (Figure 13.1).[93]

The prevalence of shoulder dysfunction varies broadly, but has been reported as high as 100% for loss of range of motion in abduction and pain.[94] A radical neck dissection involves sacrificing the spinal accessory nerve which provides innervation to the trapezius. However, even when spared, an electrodiagnostic study found that the spinal accessory nerve was always impaired in all cases of neck dissection.[95] Furthermore, critical structures for shoulder function, such as cervical nerve roots and brachial plexus, may be within the radiation field and damage can result in weakness of the rotator cuff muscles.[96] These altered biomechanics with abnormal scapular and glenohumeral motion deleteriously impact shoulder function and pain.[97] This can present as rotator cuff tendinopathies and adhesive capsulitis[96] for which physical or occupational therapy is the cornerstone of treatment.[98,99]

Neck dysfunction is experienced by a majority of head and neck cancer survivors and can present with pain and deficits in range of motion in any plane.[100] A unique presentation in this population is cervical dystonia due to injury of either the spinal accessory nerve or cervical nerve roots, and radiation fibrosis.[96] Patients may experience pain and spasms in the neck muscles, particularly the sternocleidomastoid, scalenes, and trapezius.[96] Treatment can include physical therapy to restore and maintain range of motion with a life-long home exercise program,[96] medications for neuropathic pain,[93] and botulinum toxin injections.[101]

When mouth opening is restricted to less than 35 mm, it is referred to as trismus.[102] Almost one-half of head and neck cancer survivors experience this and, for one-third, trismus can persist

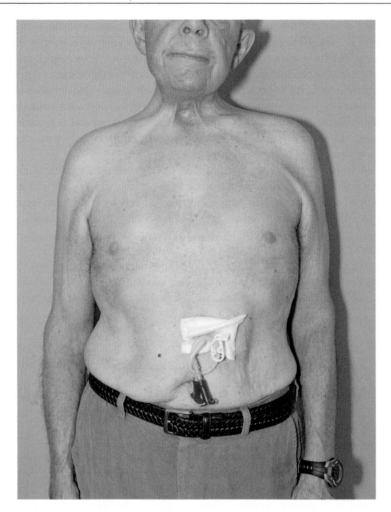

FIGURE 13.1 A 76-year-old man with a history of squamous cell carcinoma of the base of the left tongue diagnosed in 2005. He was treated with cisplatin and parotid – sparing IMRT 5400 cGy in 30 fractions to the tongue base and upper cervical lymphatics and 5000 cGy in 25 fractions to the low anterior neck. He now has severe radiation fibrosis syndrome with cervical dystonia, trismus, face and neck lymphedema, dysphagia, and dysphonia. Though complex, his impairments are typical for head and neck cancer survivors. A multidisciplinary approach that includes not only the physician but physical therapy, occupational therapy, and speech language pathology is critical to optimal rehabilitation. Initial therapy will likely require 6–8 weeks for the patient's functional level to maximize and plateau. A life-long exercise program is critical to maintaining the benefits of therapy. Because radiation late effects will continue to progress indefinitely, the patient will also require life-long surveillance by a physician and periodic (e.g., yearly) courses of therapy to optimize function.

for years.[103] It is important to address this complaint because it can negatively impact eating and oral hygiene, and may contribute to anxiety, depression, and reduced quality of life.[104] It is also important to address anxiety and depression when present as they can deleteriously impact somatic symptoms.[105] Treatment to improve range of motion may involve physical therapy and jaw stretching devices,[106,107] such as TheraBite® Jaw Motion Rehabilitation System™ or Dynasplint® Trismus System. Botulinum toxin injections, although not found to increase jaw opening, ameliorate pain, and muscle spasms for several months.[108] Medication options include nerve stabilizing agents[93] to address neuropathic pain and pentoxifylline[109] if trismus is related to radiation fibrosis. The effect of pentoxifylline is minimal at best.

Lymphedema[110,111] in head and neck cancer survivors can also be internal, with swelling localized to the soft tissue and mucosa of the upper airway and digestive tracts. In addition to swelling, this has broad implications on function by impacting swallowing, voice, cervical range of motion, body image and quality of life.[59] CDT remains the foundation of treatment followed by lifelong self-care maintenance at home.[112]

FUNCTIONAL IMPAIRMENTS IN BREAST CANCER SURVIVORS

Breast cancer is the most commonly diagnosed cancer in women.[91] Survivors frequently experience musculoskeletal and neuromuscular symptoms as well as functional impairments. Common presentations include shoulder dysfunction, post mastectomy pain syndrome, aromatase inhibitor induced musculoskeletal symptoms and lymphedema (Figure 13.2), fatigue, cognitive impairment, and CIPN, which are also prevalent in this population and were discussed above.

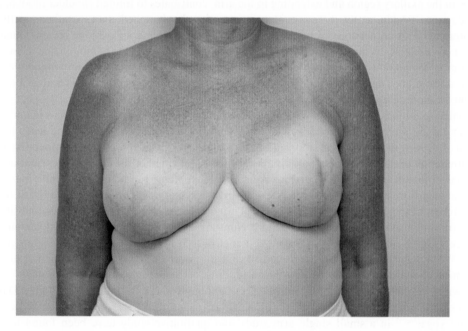

FIGURE 13.2 A 60-year-old woman diagnosed with stage IIA left-sided and stage I right-sided breast cancer in 2015. She underwent bilateral skin sparing mastectomy with tissue expander reconstruction. This was followed by AC-T (doxorubicin, cyclophosphamide, and paclitaxel) chemotherapy. She did not receive radiation. She underwent replacement of her tissue expanders with silicone implants in 2016. She remains in remission from breast cancer, but has multiple functional late effects of her cancer and its treatment including chemotherapy-induced peripheral neuropathy, mild cognitive impairment, and post-mastectomy pain syndrome. Rehabilitation intervention can often mitigate such issues with improvement of function and quality of life. This patient required approximately 8 weeks physical therapy to address her neuropathy and post-mastectomy pain syndrome. Additionally, she required 6 weeks of occupational therapy to provide cognitive rehabilitation services. While the patient's symptoms improved significantly to where she could resume many of her life roles including caring for grandchildren, her symptoms never completely resolved. A home exercise program has been critical in maintaining her function at an optimal level.

Prospective surveillance for lymphedema facilitates early identification and treatment with the benefit of decreased costs and progression to clinically evident and chronic lymphedema.[69,70,73] Unfortunately, lymphedema remains under-diagnosed and disproportionally undiagnosed in African American women with lower income and lower levels of social support.[113]

Postmastectomy pain syndrome, or post breast surgery pain syndrome, refers to chronic pain following any breast surgery. The prevalence has varied widely from 20% to 68%.[114,115] It refers to a cluster of diagnostic subgroups that can result from various etiologies.[116] Diagnostic subgroups include shoulder dysfunction, chest wall pain, axillary web syndrome, intercostobrachial neuralgia, and phantom breast pain.[116] Identification of the etiologic pain generator is essential to guide treatment recommendations. Treatment may include physical therapy,[117] pharmacotherapy,[118] injection procedures, and autologous fat grafting.[118] Depending on the etiology of pain, procedures may include intercostobrachial nerve block,[119] serratus plane block,[120] or botulinum toxin injections.[121]

Shoulder dysfunction in breast cancer survivors can present with pain, limited range of motion, stiffness, weakness, and impaired function commonly due to rotator cuff pathology and adhesive capsulitis.[122] Shoulder morbidity not only occurs in the shoulder ipsilateral to the breast cancer. The contralateral shoulder is also detrimentally impacted with findings of altered kinematics and muscle activity following treatment when compared to healthy controls.[123] In addition to the biomechanical impact of surgery and radiation fibrosis on shoulder function, comorbidities experienced in breast cancer survivors can also have deleterious impacts. For example, axillary web syndrome, which refers to a rope like structure that develops in the axillary region and extending to the arm, contributes to limited shoulder motion, particularly abduction.[124] Additionally, there is evidence suggesting that lymphedema can pathologically impact the rotator cuff.[125] A cornerstone of treatment is physical therapy, and a Cochrane review found that in breast cancer, exercise resulted in significant improvement in shoulder range of motion and recommended consideration for prompt implementation post operatively.[126] Nonsteroidal anti-inflammatories can be considered for mild to moderate pain, while corticosteroid injections may be considered as a temporary treatment for more severe pain.[127]

Aromatase inhibitor induced musculoskeletal symptoms (AIMSS) may occur in as many as 82%[128] of women taking aromatase inhibitors (AIs) for hormone sensitive breast cancer and leads to discontinuation of therapy in 24%.[129] Therefore, addressing musculoskeletal complaints is imperative to facilitate continuation of AIs. Treatment paradigms vary based on whether the clinical presentation is focal arthralgias or tendinopathies versus diffuse pain. Focal symptoms can be managed individually based on their standard treatment outside AIMSS. For diffuse symptoms, care is geared toward the entire body. In breast cancer survivors with AIMSS, 150 minutes of aerobic exercise per week and supervised strength training was found to decrease pain.[130] Nonsteroidal anti-inflammatories and acetaminophen have been utilized empirically.[128] A randomized control trial found that duloxetine decreased pain in AIMSS.[131] Supplements have also been studied and improvements in pain and function noted with glucosamine chondroitin in a single-arm phase II study.[132] Decreased pain with high dose vitamin D was shown in a double-blind placebo controlled trail although additional studies on vitamin D have not shown a significant improvement.[133,134] Additionally, acupuncture[135] in a small randomized controlled study and yoga[136,137] in a small single arm study and qualitative study have been found to improve AIMSS.

CONCLUSION

Restoring function and quality of life to cancer survivors safely and effectively requires a team of clinicians with specialized knowledge, skill, and experience. Ideally, rehabilitation efforts should begin at diagnosis, especially for patients with cancers whose treatment is known to cause predictable morbidity (e.g., breast, head and neck). Patients should be followed prospectively at regular intervals through treatment and into survivorship. Such surveillance may need to be continued indefinitely when late effects (e.g., radiation fibrosis syndrome) are likely to emerge months or years later.

There is no special coding or billing for "cancer rehabilitation." Services are subject to the same ICD-10 codes and reimbursements that any other physician or therapy services are. Despite insurance coverage that is generally equivalent to functional disorders like back pain or shoulder dysfunction, referral to and utilization of rehabilitation in cancer survivors has not become standard care. There are many reasons for this, including lack of awareness and knowledge about cancer rehabilitation services on the part of patients and clinicians, poor access to services, and adoption of and adherence to rehabilitation programs.[138] Overcoming these barriers will require enhancing the knowledge of clinicians caring for cancer survivors. Not only must such clinicians effectively identify and evaluate physical and function limiting disorders, but they also need to appropriately refer survivors to the services they need in a consistent and systematic manner.

Because rehabilitation services specializing in the care of cancer patients are rare, clinicians should take an active part in identifying and developing local rehabilitation services to support their patients. The importance of partnering with and serving as a mentor to rehabilitation clinicians who are developing their knowledge and skill with respect to cancer survivors cannot be overstated. Such partnerships should provide education and feedback to rehabilitation practitioners so they can safely and effectively gain the knowledge, skill, and confidence they need to support the best outcomes for cancer survivors. Regularly scheduled office hours where therapists and others can ask specific questions is one useful approach. Developing cancer rehabilitation team rounds, either in-person or virtually, to formally present and discuss cancer survivors in a manner similar to a tumor board may also be an effective strategy. While there is no panacea to ensure that all cancer survivors get the services they need, identification of rehabilitation needs in cancer survivors and the cultivation of a rehabilitation network to help manage them are critical first steps.

REFERENCES

1. Kline-Quiroz C, Nori P, Stubblefield MD. Cancer rehabilitation: acute and chronic issues, nerve injury, radiation sequelae, surgical and chemo-related, Part 1. *Med Clin North Am.* 2020;104(2):239–250.
2. Nori P, Kline-Quiroz C, Stubblefield MD. Cancer rehabilitation: acute and chronic issues, nerve injury, radiation sequelae, surgical and chemo-related, Part 2. *Med Clin North Am.* 2020;104(2):251–262.
3. Stubblefield MD, Kendig TD, Khanna A. Revitalizing cancer survivors – making cancer rehabilitation the standard of care. *MD Advis.* 12(2):30–33.
4. Cheville AL, Troxel AB, Basford JR, Kornblith AB. Prevalence and treatment patterns of physical impairments in patients with metastatic breast cancer. *J Clin Oncol.* 2008;26(16):2621–2629.
5. Dijkstra PU, van Wilgen PC, Buijs RP, et al. Incidence of shoulder pain after neck dissection: a clinical explorative study for risk factors. *Head Neck.* 2001;23(11):947–953.
6. Berger AM, Mooney K, Alvarez-Perez A, et al. Cancer-related fatigue, version 2.2015. *J Natl Compr Canc Netw.* 2015;13(8):1012–1039.
7. Williams LA, Bohac C, Hunter S, Cella D. Patient and health care provider perceptions of cancer-related fatigue and pain. *Support Care Cancer.* 2016;24(10):4357–4363.
8. Servaes P, Verhagen S, Bleijenberg G. Determinants of chronic fatigue in disease-free breast cancer patients: a cross-sectional study. *Ann Oncol.* 2002;13(4):589–598.
9. Thong MSY, van Noorden CJF, Steindorf K, Arndt V. Cancer-related fatigue: causes and current treatment options. *Curr Treat Options Oncol.* 2020;21(2):17.
10. Jones G, Rutkowski N, Trudel G, et al. Translating guidelines to practice: a training session about cancer-related fatigue. *Curr Oncol.* 2020;27(2):e163–e170.
11. Escalante CP, Manzullo E, Valdres R. A cancer-related fatigue clinic: opportunities and challenges. *J Natl Compr Canc Netw.* 2003;1(3):333–343.
12. World Health Organization. International Statistical Classification of Diseases and Related Health Problems, 10th Revision.

13. Bower JE, Bak K, Berger A, et al. Screening, assessment, and management of fatigue in adult survivors of cancer: an American Society of Clinical Oncology Clinical Practice Guideline Adaptation. *J Clin Oncol.* 2014;32(17):1840–1850.

14. Littlewood TJ, Kallich JD, San Miguel J, Hendricks L, Hedenus M. Efficacy of darbepoetin alfa in alleviating fatigue and the effect of fatigue on quality of life in anemic patients with lymphoproliferative malignancies. *J Pain Symptom Manage.* 2006;31(4):317–325.

15. Cramp F, Byron-Daniel J. Exercise for the management of cancer-related fatigue in adults. *Cochrane Database Syst Rev.* 2012;11:CD006145.

16. Lucía A, Earnest C, Pérez M. Cancer-related fatigue: can exercise physiology assist oncologists? *Lancet Oncol.* 2003;4(10):616–625.

17. National Comprehensive Cancer Network (NCCN). Cancer related fatigue (version 2.2020). 2020.

18. Van der Gucht K, Melis M, Ahmadoun S, et al. A mindfulness-based intervention for breast cancer patients with cognitive impairment after chemotherapy: study protocol of a three-group randomized controlled trial. *Trials.* 2020;21(1):290.

19. Allen DH, Myers JS, Jansen CE, Merriman JD, Von Ah D. Assessment and management of cancer- and cancer treatment-related cognitive impairment. *J Nurse Pract.* 2018;14(4):217–224.e215.

20. Menning S, de Ruiter MB, Veltman DJ, et al. Multimodal MRI and cognitive function in patients with breast cancer prior to adjuvant treatment—the role of fatigue. *Neuroimage Clin.* 2015;7:547–554.

21. Vannorsdall TD. Cognitive changes related to cancer therapy. *Med Clin North Am.* 2017;101(6):1115–1134.

22. Reid-Arndt SA, Hsieh C, Perry MC. Neuropsychological functioning and quality of life during the first year after completing chemotherapy for breast cancer. *Psychooncology.* 2010;19(5):535–544.

23. Von Ah D, Habermann B, Carpenter JS, Schneider BL. Impact of perceived cognitive impairment in breast cancer survivors. *Eur J Oncol Nurs.* 2013;17(2):236–241.

24. Selamat MH, Loh SY, Mackenzie L, Vardy J. Chemobrain experienced by breast cancer survivors: a meta-ethnography study investigating research and care implications. *PLOS ONE.* 2014;9(9):e108002.

25. Wefel JS, Lenzi R, Theriault R, Buzdar AU, Cruickshank S, Meyers CA. 'Chemobrain' in breast carcinoma?: a prologue. *Cancer.* 2004;101(3):466–475.

26. Vardy J, Wefel JS, Ahles T, Tannock IF, Schagen SB. Cancer and cancer-therapy related cognitive dysfunction: an international perspective from the Venice cognitive workshop. *Ann Oncol.* 2008;19(4):623–629.

27. Reid-Arndt SA, Yee A, Perry MC, Hsieh C. Cognitive and psychological factors associated with early posttreatment functional outcomes in breast cancer survivors. *J Psychosoc Oncol.* 2009;27(4):415–434.

28. Hshieh TT, Jung WF, Grande LJ, et al. Prevalence of cognitive impairment and association with survival among older patients with hematologic cancers. *JAMA Oncol.* 2018;4(5):686–693.

29. Ahles TA, Saykin AJ. Candidate mechanisms for chemotherapy-induced cognitive changes. *Nat Rev Cancer.* 2007;7(3):192–201.

30. Dietrich J, Han R, Yang Y, Mayer-Pröschel M, Noble M. CNS progenitor cells and oligodendrocytes are targets of chemotherapeutic agents in vitro and in vivo. *J Biol.* 2006;5(7):22.

31. Jamroziak K, Robak T. Pharmacogenomics of MDR1/ABCB1 gene: the influence on risk and clinical outcome of haematological malignancies. *Hematology.* 2004;9(2):91–105.

32. Fishel ML, Vasko MR, Kelley MR. DNA repair in neurons: so if they don't divide what's to repair? *Mutat Res.* 2007;614(1–2):24–36.

33. Schröder CP, Wisman GB, de Jong S, et al. Telomere length in breast cancer patients before and after chemotherapy with or without stem cell transplantation. *Br J Cancer.* 2001;84(10):1348–1353.

34. Cheung YT, Khan RB, Liu W, et al. Association of cerebrospinal fluid biomarkers of central nervous system injury with neurocognitive and brain imaging outcomes in children receiving chemotherapy for acute lymphoblastic leukemia. *JAMA Oncol.* 2018;4(7):e180089.

35. Doolittle ND, Korfel A, Lubow MA, et al. Long-term cognitive function, neuroimaging, and quality of life in primary CNS lymphoma. *Neurology.* 2013;81(1):84–92.

36. Janelsins MC, Kohli S, Mohile SG, Usuki K, Ahles TA, Morrow GR. An update on cancer- and chemotherapy-related cognitive dysfunction: current status. *Semin Oncol.* 2011;38(3):431–438.

37. Henneghan A, Stuifbergen A, Becker H, Kesler S, King E. Modifiable correlates of perceived cognitive function in breast cancer survivors up to 10 years after chemotherapy completion. *J Cancer Surviv.* 2018;12(2):224–233.

38. Schmidt JE, Beckjord E, Bovbjerg DH, et al. Prevalence of perceived cognitive dysfunction in survivors of a wide range of cancers: results from the 2010 LIVESTRONG survey. *J Cancer Surviv.* 2016;10(2):302–311.

39. Myers JS, Cook-Wiens G, Baynes R, et al. Emerging from the haze: a multicenter, controlled pilot study of a multidimensional, psychoeducation-based cognitive rehabilitation intervention for breast cancer survivors delivered with telehealth conferencing. *Arch Phys Med Rehabil.* 2020;101(6):948–959.

40. Cheville AL, Smith SR, Basford JR. Rehabilitation medicine approaches to pain management. *Hematol Oncol Clin North Am.* 2018;32(3):469–482.

41. Cheville AL. Pain management in cancer rehabilitation. *Arch Phys Med Rehabil.* 2001;82(3 Suppl 1):S84–87.

42. Silver JK, Raj VS, Fu JB, Wisotzky EM, Smith SR, Kirch RA. Cancer rehabilitation and palliative care: critical components in the delivery of high-quality oncology services. *Support Care Cancer.* 2015;23(12):3633–3643.

43. Stubblefield MD. Cancer rehabilitation. *Semin Oncol.* 2011;38(3):386–393.

44. Foust Winton RE, Draucker CB, Von Ah D. Pain management experiences among hospitalized postcraniotomy brain tumor patients. *Cancer Nurs.* 2020.

45. Cheville AL, Basford JR. Role of rehabilitation medicine and physical agents in the treatment of cancer-associated pain. *J Clin Oncol.* 2014;32(16):1691–1702.

46. Silver JK. Cancer rehabilitation and prehabilitation may reduce disability and early retirement. *Cancer.* 2014;120(14):2072–2076.

47. Stout NL, Baima J, Swisher AK, Winters-Stone KM, Welsh J. A systematic review of exercise systematic reviews in the cancer literature (2005–2017). *PM&R.* 2017;9(9S2):S347–S384.

48. Silver JK, Stout NL, Fu JB, Pratt-Chapman M, Haylock PJ, Sharma R. The state of cancer rehabilitation in the United States. *J Cancer Rehabil.* 2018;1:1–8.

49. Kannarkat G, Lasher EE, Schiff D. Neurologic complications of chemotherapy agents. *Curr Opin Neurol.* 2007;20(6):719–725.

50. Stubblefield MD, Burstein HJ, Burton AW, et al. NCCN task force report: management of neuropathy in cancer. *J Natl Compr Canc Netw.* 2009;7(Suppl 5):S1–S26; quiz S27–S28.

51. Garzón-Rodríguez C, Lyras L, Gayoso LO, et al. Cancer-related neuropathic pain in out-patient oncology clinics: a European survey. *BMC Palliat Care.* 2013;12(1):41.

52. Custodio CM. Electrodiagnosis in cancer rehabilitation. *Phys Med Rehabil Clin N Am.* 2017;28(1):193–203.

53. Chen X, Stubblefield MD, Custodio CM, Hudis CA, Seidman AD, DeAngelis LM. Electrophysiological features of taxane-induced polyneuropathy in patients with breast cancer. *J Clin Neurophysiol.* 2013;30(2):199–203.

54. Loprinzi CL, Lacchetti C, Bleeker J, et al. Prevention and management of chemotherapy-induced peripheral neuropathy in survivors of adult cancers: ASCO guideline update. *J Clin Oncol.* 2020:JCO2001399.

55. Bao T, Patil S, Chen C, et al. Effect of acupuncture vs sham procedure on chemotherapy-induced peripheral neuropathy symptoms: a randomized clinical trial. *JAMA Netw Open.* 2020;3(3):e200681.

56. He Y, Guo X, May BH, et al. Clinical evidence for association of acupuncture and acupressure with improved cancer pain: a systematic review and meta-analysis. *JAMA Oncol.* 2020;6(2):271–278.

57. Majithia N, Loprinzi CL, Smith TJ. New practical approaches to chemotherapy-induced neuropathic pain: prevention, assessment, and treatment. *Oncology (Williston Park).* 2016;30(11):1020–1029.

58. Warren AG, Brorson H, Borud LJ, Slavin SA. Lymphedema: a comprehensive review. *Ann Plast Surg.* 2007; 59(4):464–472.

59. Deng J, Murphy BA, Dietrich MS, et al. Impact of secondary lymphedema after head and neck cancer treatment on symptoms, functional status, and quality of life. *Head Neck.* 2013;35(7):1026–1035.

60. Hayes SC, Janda M, Cornish B, Battistutta D, Newman B. Lymphedema after breast cancer: incidence, risk factors, and effect on upper body function. *J Clin Oncol.* 2008;26(21):3536–3542.

61. DiSipio T, Rye S, Newman B, Hayes S. Incidence of unilateral arm lymphoedema after breast cancer: a systematic review and meta-analysis. *Lancet Oncol.* 2013;14(6):500–515.

62. Ridner SH, Dietrich MS, Niermann K, Cmelak A, Mannion K, Murphy B. A prospective study of the lymphedema and fibrosis continuum in patients with head and neck cancer. *Lymphat Res Biol.* 2016;14(4):198–205.

63. Stubblefield MD. *Cancer rehabilitation: principles and practice.* Berlin: Springer Publishing Company; 2018.

64. Yuan Z, Luo Q, Zhu J, Lu H, Zhu R. The role of radionuclide lymphoscintigraphy in extremity lymphedema. *Ann Nucl Med.* 2006;20(5):341–344.

65. O'Donnell TF, Rasmussen JC, Sevick-Muraca EM. New diagnostic modalities in the evaluation of lymphedema. *J Vasc Surg Venous Lymphat Disord.* 2017;5(2):261–273.

66. Paskett ED, Dean JA, Oliveri JM, Harrop JP. Cancer-related lymphedema risk factors, diagnosis, treatment, and impact: a review. *J Clin Oncol.* 2012;30(30):3726–3733.

67. Purcell A, Nixon J, Fleming J, McCann A, Porceddu S. Measuring head and neck lymphedema: the "ALOHA" trial. *Head Neck.* 2016;38(1):79–84.

68. Committee E. The diagnosis and treatment of peripheral lymphedema: 2016 consensus document of the International Society of Lymphology. *Lymphology.* 2016;49(4):170–184.

69. Shah C, Arthur DW, Wazer D, Khan A, Ridner S, Vicini F. The impact of early detection and intervention of breast cancer-related lymphedema: a systematic review. *Cancer Med.* 2016;5(6):1154–1162.

70. Stout Gergich NL, Pfalzer LA, McGarvey C, Springer B, Gerber LH, Soballe P. Preoperative assessment enables the early diagnosis and successful treatment of lymphedema. *Cancer: Interdiscipl Int J Am Cancer Soc.* 2008;112(12):2809–2819.

71. Soran A, Ozmen T, McGuire KP, et al. The importance of detection of subclinical lymphedema for the prevention of breast cancer-related clinical lymphedema after axillary lymph node dissection; a prospective observational study. *Lymphat Res Biol.* 2014;12(4):289–294.

72. Ridner SH, Dietrich MS, Cowher MS, et al. A randomized trial evaluating bioimpedance spectroscopy versus tape measurement for the prevention of lymphedema following treatment for breast cancer: interim analysis. *Ann Surg Oncol.* 2019;26(10):3250–3259.

73. Stout NL, Pfalzer LA, Springer B, et al. Breast cancer-related lymphedema: comparing direct costs of a prospective surveillance model and a traditional model of care. *Phys Therapy.* 2012;92(1):152–163.

74. Ferguson CM, Swaroop MN, Horick N, et al. Impact of ipsilateral blood draws, injections, blood pressure measurements, and air travel on the risk of lymphedema for patients treated for breast cancer. *J Clin Oncol.* 2016;34(7):691–698.

75. Showalter SL, Brown JC, Cheville AL, Fisher CS, Sataloff D, Schmitz KH. Lifestyle risk factors associated with arm swelling among women with breast cancer. *Ann Surg Oncol*. 2012;20(3):842–849.

76. National Comprehensive Cancer Network (NCCN). NCCN Survivorship Guideline 2. 2020. https://www.nccn.org/professionals/physician_gls/pdf/survivorship.pdf. Published 2020.

77. Lasinski BB, McKillip Thrift K, Squire D, et al. A systematic review of the evidence for complete decongestive therapy in the treatment of lymphedema from 2004 to 2011. *PM&R*. 2012;4(8):580–601.

78. Schmitz KH, Ahmed RL, Troxel A, et al. Weight lifting in women with breast-cancer-related lymphedema. *N Engl J Med*. 2009;361(7):664–673.

79. Grov EK, Fosså SD, Dahl AA. Activity of daily living problems in older cancer survivors: a population-based controlled study. *Health Soc Care Community*. 2010;18(4):396–406.

80. Shumway-Cook A, Patla AE, et al. Environmental demands associated with community mobility in older adults with and without mobility disabilities. *Phys Therapy*. 2020;82(7):670–681.

81. Hamaker ME, Schiphorst AH, ten Bokkel Huinink D, Schaar C, van Munster BC. The effect of a geriatric evaluation on treatment decisions for older cancer patients—a systematic review. *Acta Oncol*. 2014;53(3):289–296.

82. Cheville AL, Beck LA, Petersen TL, Marks RS, Gamble GL. The detection and treatment of cancer-related functional problems in an outpatient setting. *Support Care Cancer*. 2009;17(1):61–67.

83. Wedding U, Röhrig B, Klippstein A, Pientka L, Höffken K. Age, severe comorbidity and functional impairment independently contribute to poor survival in cancer patients. *J Cancer Res Clin Oncol*. 2007;133(12):945–950.

84. Wedding U, Röhrig B, Klippstein A, Brix C, Pientka L, Höffken K. Co-morbidity and functional deficits independently contribute to quality of life before chemotherapy in elderly cancer patients. *Support Care Cancer*. 2007;15(9):1097–1104.

85. Silver JK, Baima J, Mayer RS. Impairment-driven cancer rehabilitation: an essential component of quality care and survivorship. *CA Cancer J Clin*. 2013;63(5):295–317.

86. Pergolotti M, Williams GR, Campbell C, Munoz LA, Muss HB. Occupational therapy for adults with cancer: why it matters. *Oncologist*. 2016;21(3):314–319.

87. Cheville A. Rehabilitation of patients with advanced cancer. *Cancer: Interdiscipl Int J Am Cancer Soc*. 2001;92(S4):1039–1048.

88. Holley S. A look at the problem of falls among people with cancer. *Clin J Oncol Nurs*. 2002;6(4):193–197.

89. Bateni H, Maki BE. Assistive devices for balance and mobility: benefits, demands, and adverse consequences. *Arch Phys Med Rehabil*. 2005;86(1):134–145.

90. Kneis S, Wehrle A, Müller J, et al. It's never too late - balance and endurance training improves functional performance, quality of life, and alleviates neuropathic symptoms in cancer survivors suffering from chemotherapy-induced peripheral neuropathy: results of a randomized controlled trial. *BMC Cancer*. 2019;19(1):414.

91. Bray F, Ferlay J, Soerjomataram I, Siegel RL, Torre LA, Jemal A. Global cancer statistics 2018: GLOBOCAN estimates of incidence and mortality worldwide for 36 cancers in 185 countries. *CA Cancer J Clin*. 2018;68(6):394–424.

92. Chow LQM. Head and neck cancer. *N Engl J Med*. 2020;382(1):60–72.

93. Cohen EE, LaMonte SJ, Erb NL, et al. American Cancer Society head and neck cancer survivorship care guideline. *CA: Cancer J Clin*. 2016;66(3):203–239.

94. Gane EM, Michaleff ZA, Cottrell MA, et al. Prevalence, incidence, and risk factors for shoulder and neck dysfunction after neck dissection: a systematic review. *Eur J Surg Oncol*. 2017;43(7):1199–1218.

95. Erisen L, Basel B, Irdesel J, et al. Shoulder function after accessory nerve-sparing neck dissections. *Head Neck*. 2004;26(11):967–971.

96. Stubblefield MD. Radiation fibrosis syndrome: neuromuscular and musculoskeletal complications in cancer survivors. *PM&R*. 2011;3(11):1041–1054.

97. Huang YC, Lee YY, Tso HH, et al. The sonography and physical findings on shoulder after selective neck dissection in patients with head and neck cancer: a pilot study. *Biomed Res Int*. 2019;2019:2528492.

98. Carvalho AP, Vital FM, Soares BG. Exercise interventions for shoulder dysfunction in patients treated for head and neck cancer. *Cochrane Database Syst Rev*. 2012(4):CD008693.

99. Shimada Y, Chida S, Matsunaga T, Sato M, Hatakeyama K, Itoi E. Clinical results of rehabilitation for accessory nerve palsy after radical neck dissection. *Acta oto-laryngologica*. 2007;127(5):491–497.

100. Ghiam MK, Mannion K, Dietrich MS, Stevens KL, Gilbert J, Murphy BA. Assessment of musculoskeletal impairment in head and neck cancer patients. *Support Care Cancer*. 2017;25(7):2085–2092.

101. Bach C-A, Wagner I, Lachiver X, Baujat B, Chabolle F. Botulinum toxin in the treatment of post-radiosurgical neck contracture in head and neck cancer: a novel approach. *Eur Ann Otorhinolaryngol Head Neck Dis*. 2012;129(1):6–10.

102. Dijkstra P, Huisman P, Roodenburg J. Criteria for trismus in head and neck oncology. *Int J Oral Maxillofac Surg*. 2006;35(4):337–342.

103. Watters AL, Cope S, Keller MN, Padilla M, Enciso R. Prevalence of trismus in patients with head and neck cancer: a systematic review with meta-analysis. *Head Neck*. 2019;41(9):3408–3421.

104. Pauli N, Johnson J, Finizia C, Andrell P. The incidence of trismus and long-term impact on health-related quality of life in patients with head and neck cancer. *Acta Oncol*. 2013;52(6):1137–1145.

105. Brown LF, Kroenke K, Theobald DE, Wu J, Tu W. The association of depression and anxiety with health-related quality of life in cancer patients with depression and/or pain. *Psychooncology*. 2010;19(7):734–741.

106. Shulman DH, Shipman B, Willis FB. Treating trismus with dynamic splinting: a cohort, case series. *Adv Therapy*. 2008;25(1):9–16.

107. Cohen EG, Deschler DG, Walsh K, Hayden RE. Early use of a mechanical stretching device to improve mandibular mobility after composite resection: a pilot study. *Arch Phys Med Rehabil*. 2005;86(7):1416–1419.

108. Dana MH, Cohen M, Morbize J, Marandas P, Janot F, Bourhis J. Botulinum toxin for radiation-induced facial pain and trismus. *Otolaryngol Head Neck Surg*. 2008;138(4):459–463.

109. Bensadoun RJ, Riesenbeck D, Lockhart PB, et al. A systematic review of trismus induced by cancer therapies in head and neck cancer patients. *Support Care Cancer*. 2010;18(8):1033–1038.

110. Ridner SH, Dietrich MS, Niermann K, Cmelak A, Mannion K, Murphy B. A prospective study of the lymphedema and fibrosis continuum in patients with head and neck cancer. *Lymphat Res Biol*. 2016;14(4):198–205.

111. Deng J, Ridner SH, Dietrich MS, et al. Prevalence of secondary lymphedema in patients with head and neck cancer. *J Pain Symptom Manag*. 2012;43(2):244–252.

112. Smith BG, Hutcheson KA, Little LG, et al. Lymphedema outcomes in patients with head and neck cancer. *Otolaryngol Head Neck Surg*. 2015;152(2):284–291.

113. Sayko O, Pezzin LE, Yen TW, Nattinger AB. Diagnosis and treatment of lymphedema after breast cancer: a population-based study. *PM&R*. 2013;5(11):915–923.

114. Stevens PE, Dibble SL, Miaskowski C. Prevalence, characteristics, and impact of postmastectomy pain syndrome: an investigation of women's experiences. *Pain*. 1995;61(1):61–68.

115. Peintinger F, Reitsamer R, Stranzl H, Ralph G. Comparison of quality of life and arm complaints after axillary lymph node dissection vs sentinel lymph node biopsy in breast cancer patients. *Br J Cancer*. 2003;89(4):648–652.

116. Wisotzky E, Hanrahan N, Lione TP, Maltser S. Deconstructing postmastectomy syndrome: implications for physiatric management. *Phys Med Rehabil Clin N Am*. 2017;28(1):153–169.

117. De Groef A, Van Kampen M, Dieltjens E, et al. Effectiveness of postoperative physical therapy for upper-limb impairments after breast cancer treatment: a systematic review. *Arch Phys Med Rehabil*. 2015;96(6):1140–1153.

118. Larsson IM, Ahm Sørensen J, Bille C. The post-mastectomy pain syndrome—a systematic review of the treatment modalities. *Breast J*. 2017;23(3):338–343.

119. Wisotzky EM, Saini V, Kao C. Ultrasound-guided intercostobrachial nerve block for intercostobrachial neuralgia in breast cancer patients: a case series. *PM&R*. 2016;8(3):273–277.

120. Zocca JA, Chen GH, Puttanniah VG, Hung JC, Gulati A. Ultrasound-guided serratus plane block for treatment of postmastectomy pain syndromes in breast cancer patients: a case series. *Pain Pract*. 2017;17(1):141–146.

121. O'Donnell CJ. Pectoral muscle spasms after mastectomy successfully treated with botulinum toxin injections. *PM&R*. 2011;3(8):781–782.

122. Stubblefield MD, Keole N. Upper body pain and functional disorders in patients with breast cancer. *PM&R*. 2014;6(2):170–183.

123. Shamley D, Lascurain-Aguirrebeña I, Oskrochi R, Srinaganathan R. Shoulder morbidity after treatment for breast cancer is bilateral and greater after mastectomy. *Acta Oncol*. 2012;51(8):1045–1053.

124. Torres Lacomba M, Mayoral Del Moral O, Coperias Zazo JL, Yuste Sanchez MJ, Ferrandez JC, Zapico Goni A. Axillary web syndrome after axillary dissection in breast cancer: a prospective study. *Breast Cancer Res Treat*. 2009;117(3):625–630.

125. Jang DH, Kim MW, Oh SJ, Kim JM. The influence of arm swelling duration on shoulder pathology in breast cancer patients with lymphedema. *PLOS ONE*. 2015;10(11):e0142950.

126. McNeely ML, Campbell K, Ospina M, et al. Exercise interventions for upper-limb dysfunction due to breast cancer treatment. *Cochrane Database Syst Rev*. 2010(6):Cd005211.

127. Stubblefield MD, Custodio CM. Upper-extremity pain disorders in breast cancer. *Arch Phys Med Rehabil*. 2006;87(3 Suppl 1):S96–99; quiz S100–S101.

128. Lombard JM, Zdenkowski N, Wells K, et al. Aromatase inhibitor induced musculoskeletal syndrome: a significant problem with limited treatment options. *Support Care Cancer*. 2016;24(5):2139–2146.

129. Henry NL, Azzouz F, Desta Z, et al. Predictors of aromatase inhibitor discontinuation as a result of treatment-emergent symptoms in early-stage breast cancer. *J Clin Oncol*. 2012;30(9):936–942.

130. Irwin ML, Cartmel B, Gross CP, et al. Randomized exercise trial of aromatase inhibitor-induced arthralgia in breast cancer survivors. *J Clin Oncol*. 2015;33(10):1104–1111.

131. Henry NL, Unger JM, Schott AF, et al. Randomized, multicenter, placebo-controlled clinical trial of duloxetine versus placebo for aromatase inhibitor-associated arthralgias in early-stage breast cancer: SWOG S1202. *J Clin Oncol*. 2018;36(4):326–332.

132. Greenlee H, Crew KD, Shao T, et al. Phase II study of glucosamine with chondroitin on aromatase inhibitor-associated joint symptoms in women with breast cancer. *Support Care Cancer*. 2013;21(4):1077–1087.

133. Rastelli AL, Taylor ME, Gao F, et al. Vitamin D and aromatase inhibitor-induced musculoskeletal symptoms (AIMSS): a phase II, double-blind, placebo-controlled, randomized trial. *Breast Cancer Res Treat*. 2011;129(1):107–116.

134. Shapiro AC, Adlis SA, Robien K, et al. Randomized, blinded trial of vitamin D3 for treating aromatase inhibitor-associated musculoskeletal symptoms (AIMSS). *Breast Cancer Res Treat.* 2016;155(3):501–512.

135. Crew KD, Capodice JL, Greenlee H, et al. Randomized, blinded, sham-controlled trial of acupuncture for the management of aromatase inhibitor-associated joint symptoms in women with early-stage breast cancer. *J Clin Oncol.* 2010;28(7):1154–1160.

136. Galantino ML, Desai K, Greene L, Demichele A, Stricker CT, Mao JJ. Impact of yoga on functional outcomes in breast cancer survivors with aromatase inhibitor-associated arthralgias. *Integr Cancer Ther.* 2012;11(4):313–320.

137. Galantino ML, Greene L, Archetto B, et al. A qualitative exploration of the impact of yoga on breast cancer survivors with aromatase inhibitor-associated arthralgias. *Explore (NY).* 2012;8(1):40–47.

138. Stubblefield MD. The underutilization of rehabilitation to treat physical impairments in breast cancer survivors. *PM&R.* 2017;9(9S2):S317–S323.

Integrating Cancer Survivorship into Primary Care

14

Karolina Lisy, Jennifer Kim, and Michael Jefford

INTRODUCTION

As described in detail elsewhere, the number of cancer survivors internationally is increasing significantly. The majority of cancer survivors are long-term survivors (diagnosed over 5 years prior), and most are over 70 years of age. With the increasing prevalence of survivors, limited specialist oncology resources and recognition that optimal survivorship care must combine cancer care with whole person, holistic care, there is an increased focus on how to include continuing primary care in the care of cancer survivors. This chapter describes the integral role of primary care in providing optimal care for cancer survivors, covering the key roles of primary care, evidence supporting primary care involvement and specific models, and outlining relevant guidance to support primary care providers (PCPs).

PRIMARY CARE FOR CANCER SURVIVORS

The World Health Organization (WHO) describes primary care as "first-contact, accessible, continued, comprehensive and coordinated care. First-contact care is accessible at the time of need; ongoing care focuses on the long-term health of a person rather than the short duration of the disease; comprehensive care is a range of services appropriate to the common problems in the respective population and coordination is the role by which primary care acts to coordinate other specialists that the patient may need." (1)

Atun (2) notes that the general practitioner (GP) or PCP is "the only clinician who operates at the nine levels of care: prevention, pre-symptomatic detection of disease, early diagnosis, diagnosis of established disease, management of disease, management of disease complications, rehabilitation, palliative care and counselling". PCPs play an important role in the management of cancer (3).

DOI: 10.1201/9781003055426-14

The practice of primary care varies across health care systems worldwide. As such, the current care of cancer survivors is equally varied. In the US, as in most countries, there is no common model of survivorship care nor a routine transition time or hand-off procedure from oncology to primary care-led care. Survivorship visits are most often based in oncology clinics and led by oncology-trained advanced practice providers, such as nurses and physician assistants. Rubin et al. (3) discusses how PCPs functioning as the "gatekeeper" in health care systems can impact preventive care, cancer diagnosis, and survivorship. When a PCP referral is required for access to specialist services, more care is managed solely through primary care.

Importantly, primary care is typically provided by clinicians who are generalists, rather than clinicians with restricted areas of specialty, such as cardiology, or palliative care. Rubin et al. (3) note "the enduring and universal strength of primary care is a core commitment to generalism. This is supported by a continuous longitudinal relationship with patients, and PCP's clinical expertise with the often undifferentiated and ill-defined nature of the problems presented."

PCPs already manage survivors within their clinical practice. The largest groups of long-term survivors are those with a personal history of prostate cancer, breast cancer, colorectal cancer, and melanoma (4). A PCP with 2000 patients has around 70 patients with a personal history of cancer. This number is predicted to double by 2040 (5). Several studies note that survivors have significant contact with PCPs in the years following end of treatment, highlighting that PCPs play a substantial role in the follow up care of survivors (6–9).

Although PCPs may see few new patients with cancer, they play important roles in prevention, detection, and co-management during treatment and also in the post-treatment phase. Many studies indicate that PCPs are willing to be involved in the care of cancer survivors, particularly if they are provided with adequate guidance, support and are able to gain access to specialist oncology care as necessary (10). Likewise, patients are mostly positive about primary care's role in survivorship care (11). Survivors who have experienced PCP-led care, or shared care between oncologists and PCPs are particularly supportive (12–14). It is acknowledged that not every survivor has a PCP. Ideally, all patients/survivors should be linked with a PCP.

GOALS OF SURVIVORSHIP CARE

As noted elsewhere, the pivotal Institute of Medicine report "From cancer patient to cancer survivor, lost in transition" described four key elements of survivorship care (15). The first is a focus on prevention of recurrent and new cancers, as well as late effects. The second is a focus on surveillance: for cancer spread, recurrence, and subsequent cancers, but also surveillance for possible long-term and late effects. The third key element focuses on interventions to deal with the consequences of cancer and treatment including medical problems, such as lymphedema and sexual dysfunction, symptoms such as pain and fatigue, and psychological distress in both survivors themselves as well as caregivers and family members. There should also be attention to practical issues such as employment, insurance and disability. The fourth key element of survivorship care is effective coordination between oncology specialists and PCPs to ensure that survivors' health care needs are met.

Importantly, survivorship care must be seen in the context of the whole person's circumstances. It is important to note that many, indeed the majority of cancer survivors, have comorbid illness. At times, other illnesses may take a greater priority in overall whole-person care. For example, ongoing monitoring for recurrence of a prior melanoma may be deprioritized in someone with end stage renal failure, or severe congestive cardiac failure. A recent Australian study found the majority of cancer patients had at least one other chronic illness, and 21% had three or more chronic diseases (16). Survivors with other chronic conditions experience greater limitations, worse health status, and lost productivity (17).

IMPACT OF CANCER – LONG-TERM AND LATE EFFECTS

While the majority of cancer survivors adjust well to life after cancer, a significant minority may experience a broad range of consequences as a result of cancer and its treatments (18–24). Some of these issues are apparent during treatment or soon after, whereas others may develop months or years later. Common physical issues include fatigue, pain, change in cognition, and sleep disturbance. Emotional and psychological issues are also common, including fear of cancer recurrence or progression, anxiety, and depression. Social and practical consequences include altered relationships, difficulty returning to work or study, and loss of income.

Survivors also report a range of unmet needs. A systematic review examining unmet needs in Australian cancer survivors noted that psychosocial needs predominate, including the need for assistance to deal with the fear of cancer recurrence, feeling uncertain about the future, and worry about partners, family, and friends (25). A study in the UK likewise reported that the most commonly reported unmet needs were regarding fear of cancer recurrence (20). A systematic review examining survivors' health care needs in primary care found the most mentioned needs were psychosocial in nature, including the need for information around the survivorship phase, and support around adjustment (26).

Many of these issues are commonly encountered within primary care practice. Guidelines exist for the management of many of these issues in cancer survivors, including from the American Society of Clinical Oncology (ASCO) and the US National Comprehensive Cancer Network (NCCN). Exercise and psychological therapies can help manage fatigue (27, 28), cognitive behavioral therapy (CBT) can be effective for insomnia (29); CBT, meta-cognitive approaches and mindfulness can help manage anxiety and depression (30, 31). Meta cognitive therapy can assist those with moderately severe fear of cancer recurrence (32). Cognitive training, exercise and mind-body therapies may assist with cognitive impairment (33). Pharmacological and non-pharmacological interventions may assist with pain management (34).

Adult survivors of childhood cancer and adolescent and young adult survivors are at particular risk of long-term consequences. One report from the Childhood Cancer Survivor Study indicates that the relative risk of a chronic condition in a survivor of childhood cancer compared to their sibling was 3.3, and the relative risk of a severe or life-threatening condition compared to a sibling was 8.2 (35). Survivors of childhood cancer are also at risk of developing a second cancer, and may present symptomatically in primary care (36).

PCPs can play a key role in supporting many of the unmet needs of survivors. In a US survey of 127 PCPs from both academic and community practices, the majority were confident in monitoring cancer-related symptoms such as psychosocial issues, pain, fatigue, and bone health, likely as these are also common issues in primary care (37). The majority also agreed that PCPs are important in post-cancer surveillance and treatment-related effect monitoring. Despite this, less than 25% of PCPs felt their training prepared them for survivorship care and many responses highlight the significant ambiguity about the PCP's role in cancer-related follow-up (37). Clear communication between the PCP, oncologist, and survivor may clarify specific roles and risks for late effects in each patient's survivorship care. Specifying these roles may also empower survivors to discuss their unmet needs with their PCP as well as encourage PCPs to take an active role in the management of long-term and late effects.

CAUSES OF DEATH IN CANCER SURVIVORS

A number of studies have reported causes of death in cancer survivors. The index cancer is frequently the cause of death in those with poor prognosis cancers (for example, people with pancreatic or lung cancer). However, in long-term survivors, even of these poor prognosis cancers, other causes are important including deaths from another cancer, cardiovascular disease, pulmonary disease, and suicide (38–44). This highlights the importance of screening for and attention to other cancers, management of comorbid illness, and attention to health risk factors and psychological wellbeing.

A recent study reported by Afifi and colleagues (45), examined causes of death after a breast cancer diagnosis. In total, 754,270 women diagnosed with breast cancer between 2000 and 2015 were included. While the greatest proportion of deaths (46.2%) occurred within 5 years of diagnosis, mostly due to breast or other cancers, the most common non-cancer causes of death within the first 10 years of diagnosis were heart disease and cerebrovascular disease. Mortality for those who survived 10-plus years from their diagnosis was more likely to be from non-cancer causes, largely also cardiac and cerebrovascular disease. This study emphasizes that non-cancer causes of death are not only common, but in terms of long-term survival, more common than breast cancer deaths. Implications of this study illustrate an opportunity for improved survivorship care through PCP-led preventive care and management of comorbid disease and cardiovascular risk factors.

Similarly, a recent study from Australia found that, in people surviving 5 years post diagnosis, causes of death were more commonly from non-cancer causes, including ischemic heart disease and stroke (46).

HEALTH PROMOTION AND BEHAVIOR CHANGE

PCPs have an important role in encouraging behavior change, specifically around tobacco and alcohol use, inactivity, overweight and obesity, and sun exposure. These factors are well known cancer risk factors, and there is growing evidence that attention to these issues may reduce the risk of cancer recurrence and improve survival.

Smoking cessation has been associated with decreased mortality in cancer survivors (47) and greater quality of life (QoL) (48). Despite the known benefits of smoking cessation, a large study in the US found that only 52% of cancer patients who were current smokers reported being counseled to quit smoking within the previous year (49). Brief advice from a PCP can be effective in promoting smoking cessation and is considered affordable, globally (50, 51). Other effective strategies include telephone helplines, automated text messaging, printed materials, cytisine, and nortriptyline; each of which is considered globally affordable (51).

Similarly, brief interventions in primary care have been shown to reduce harmful and hazardous alcohol consumption (52–55). Alcohol is proven to increase risk of recurrence in breast cancer survivors (56), and increase the risk of new primary cancer and mortality in head and neck cancer survivors (57). In those diagnosed with breast or colorectal cancer, moderate alcohol intake is linked with higher cancer-specific mortality (57). One Australian study found that alcohol consumption was not routinely discussed in primary care encounters (58). Increased PCP awareness of the direct impact of alcohol intake in survivors may improve regular re-evaluation of consumption and further patient counseling.

Obesity is a risk factor for some common cancer types, as well as being a risk factor for recurrence and poorer survival after treatment for cancer (59). Health professional advice to lose weight appears to increase motivation to lose weight and result in modest weight loss, however only a minority of overweight or obese adults receive this advice (60–63). Evidence indicates that physical activity can decrease both the risk of developing cancer and the risk of cancer recurrence (64, 65), and a meta-analysis of published studies suggests that physical activity may reduce disease recurrence and cancer deaths in breast cancer survivors (66). Counseling patients on exercise in primary care can be effective in increasing physical activity and may improve QoL (67, 68). Bully et al suggest that lifestyle modification interventions that are underpinned and linked to a strong theoretical framework, in particular the transtheoretical model which seeks to understand how individuals move through different stages of behavior change (specifically pre-contemplation, contemplation, preparation, action, and maintenance), may be most effective (69).

CARING FOR CAREGIVERS

Some studies indicate that caregivers and family members of people diagnosed with cancer can have significant unmet needs, including for information, and may experience similar concerns to survivors, including worry about cancer progression or recurrence, anxiety, and depression (70, 71). Just as survivors often experience test anxiety, associated with getting an imaging or blood test and waiting for results, caregivers also often experience parallel anxiety about the survivor's tests or their own. Caregiver stress can lead to psychological and sleep problems, impaired physical health, impaired immune function, and lower financial wellbeing (70). Interventions may reduce these ill effects, though do not appear to be implemented in practice. As some PCPs may also provide care to caregivers and family members, they are thus well placed to manage how cancer can impact on the broader family unit.

THE ROLE OF PRIMARY CARE IN SURVIVORSHIP

PCPs have an important role in dealing with many of the survivorship issues discussed above, including physical, psychosocial, and practical consequences of cancer and its treatment, comorbidity management, health promotion, and lifestyle behavior change. Indeed, long-term surveillance, screening, and management of these issues are likely to depend on PCP engagement. In countries with a "gatekeeper" system, psychosocial and late effects are more likely to present to PCPs. Figure 14.1 summarizes key survivorship issues that may be managed by PCPs in collaboration with specialists and a patient's support system.

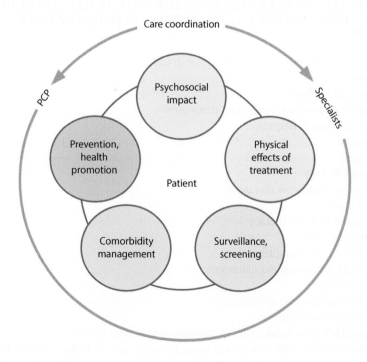

FIGURE 14.1   The survivorship care team and core survivorship care domains.

Survivorship issues that may be managed by PCPs in collaboration with oncology providers and specialist referrals are: surveillance of recurrence and screening for new or secondary malignancy; physical effects of cancer treatment; psychosocial impact including mental health, reproductive and sexual health, financial health; comorbidity management; and health promotion and preventive care. Note that supportive services, family, caregivers, community resources are also part of the care team.

APPROACH TO SURVIVORSHIP CARE BY PCPs

As discussed above, each of the survivorship domains outlined in Figure 14.1 needs to be assessed in order to create an individualized plan and manage the health of patients living with or after cancer. In a time-constrained clinic visit, the breadth and depth of survivorship topics may seem overwhelming to cover. Using a note template can assist by serving both as a guide of questions and talking points, as well as documentation for both the clinician and patient to reference. An example note template in shown in Box 14.1 and incorporates a brief diagnosis and treatment history as well as the core survivorship elements to be addressed. In discussing each element with the patient, the clinician can review and verify the information, enquire about any survivorship issues the patient may be experiencing and provide support for these issues, educate the patient, discuss individualized plans and share decision making. These conversations may also further build rapport between the patient and clinician and ease communication surrounding sensitive topics such as mental, reproductive, and sexual health. As much of cancer care is siloed and specialty-driven, a PCP's uniquely holistic and systematic perspective can be the most comprehensive and actionable approach to survivorship care.

> **BOX 14.1   CANCER SURVIVORSHIP NOTE TEMPLATE: GUIDE**
> **FOR PRIMARY CARE CANCER SURVIVORSHIP VISIT**
>
> 1. Cancer Treatment History and Survivorship Care
>   **Diagnosis [a]:**
>   - Stage (If applies)
>   - Laterality, receptors/important descriptors
>   - Date and age at diagnosis:
>   **Treatment:**
>   - Surgery [b]:
>   - Chemotherapy [c]:
>   - Adjuvant endocrine therapy [d]:
>   - Radiation [e]:
>   - Targeted biologic therapy:
>   - Immunotherapy:
>   - Bone marrow transplant:
>   - Current symptoms and management [f]:
>   - Late effects [g]:
>   - Genetic counseling and testing [h]:
>   - Reproductive health [i]:
>   - Surveillance: includes imaging, laboratory tests, and others [j]:
>   - Follow-up plan with cancer care team, primary care, and other specialists[k]:

2. Health Maintenance
- Vaccines[l]: Tdap, flu, pneumococcal, HPV[m], inactivated zoster[m]
- Pap test[m]: Last, due
- Mammogram[m]: Last, due
- Colonoscopy[m]: Last, due
- DEXA[m]: Last, due
- Lung cancer screening[m]:
- Dental check:
- Screening labs[m]:
- Exercise and nutrition:

3. Supportive Care[n]
- Mood, anxiety, fear of cancer recurrence[o]:
- Coping and support[p]:
- Sexual health[q]:
- Financial health, employment:

4. Resources[r]
- Patient Education & Psychosocial support: Examples include Cancer.Net (ASCO), American Cancer Society, Cancer Support Community, CANCER*care*, National Coalition for Cancer Survivorship
- Meditation, Relaxation: Apps include Mind Shift (designed specifically for teens/young adults), Smiling Mind, UCLA Mindful, Calm, Headspace
- Nutrition guidance: Dietitian referral and/or online resources with consideration to cultural cuisine
- Local support groups:[s]

---

[a] By asking the patient to describe the method of diagnosis (screen detected or symptom based) the PCP engages in a personal conversation and assesses the patient's experience with cancer care
b, Age at diagnosis
[b] Surgery details include only basic information including date
[c] Full names of chemotherapy drugs are listed to remove ambiguity for patient and other healthcare providers around abbreviations and completion date
[d] Applies to patients with hormonally driven diseases (prostate and breast cancer) and should include the drug type, start date of therapy, and intended duration of treatment
[e] Completion date, field, i.e., left breast or pelvic, and dose (if known)
[f] Refers to side effects of cancer treatment that persist after treatment (also known as long term effects)
[g] Risk of subsequent complications due to prior exposures to cancer treatments
[h] Document genetic testing date and result and any additional subsequent cancer screening result. If no genetic testing, take personal and family cancer history, then make appropriate referrals for genetic counseling and testing if needed.
[i] Explore interest in family building
[j] Serves to clarify what tests are needed or not needed (i.e., patient with bilateral mastectomies does not require annual mammograms and this is stated), the frequency, and name of the ordering clinician
[k] States the names of the clinicians involved in the patient's care and follow-up schedule, including name of PCP if different from clinician conducting this visit
[l] Consider additional vaccinations if bone marrow transplant history, surgical or functional asplenia
[m] As indicated
[n] Psychosocial issues
[o] Assessment for psychological distress, anxiety/depression and fear of cancer recurrence; assess satisfaction and/or difficulties with sexual health
[p] Identify primary caretaker or support, how survivorship has impacted relationship
[q] Body image
[r] Not a comprehensive list
[s] Familiarity with local resources is encouraged
Source: Adapted from *Health After Cancer*, Stanford University. https://mededucation.stanford.edu/courses/health-after-cancer/

Surveillance and Screening

Many patients have their surveillance testing ordered and monitored by their cancer care team for several years after diagnosis. PCP visits provide an additional medical touch point for encouraging appropriate survivorship follow-up. PCP awareness of surveillance schedules can help ensure the patient is current on recommended imaging and bloodwork. If a surveillance plan is unclear, PCPs can communicate with the oncology team to confirm follow-up schedules. Such communication may also provide a valuable opportunity to discuss risk for new or secondary malignancy and other late effects from cancer treatment. Important survivorship information can be recorded in a central part of the patient's chart for further reference and patient education.

Clear follow-up schedules are important not only to screen for recurrence, but also because survivors are at greater risk of developing a new cancer compared with the general population. The higher rate of another malignancy in survivors is influenced by factors such as genetic susceptibility, exposure (for example tobacco), and mutagenic effects of previous cancer treatment. For example, certain chemotherapy agents increase risk for therapy-related leukemias, while radiation increases the risk of subsequent cancers in the radiation field such as breast, skin, and colon cancer (72, 73). Therefore, for patients with prior radiation exposure, specific cancer screening may start earlier than routine age-based recommendations. The Children's Oncology Group recommends that survivors of childhood, adolescent, or young adult cancer who received 20 Gy or more of chest irradiation begin high-risk breast screening with mammography and MRI starting at age 25, or 8 years after chest radiotherapy (74). PCPs can assess each individual's treatment-related malignancy risk by understanding the mutagenic effects of cancer treatments. In addition to treatment-related risks, PCPs should assess predisposing factors such as genetic susceptibility. A detailed family history is important in recognizing genetic syndromes (for example, BRCA, Lynch) with referral to cancer genetics clinics as appropriate. PCPs can also seek to foster patient self-advocacy by educating patients about their risks of subsequent cancer and encouraging healthy behaviors such as sun protection and breast exams.

Physical Effects of Treatment

Many PCPs are familiar with the management of a range of long-term and late effects arising from cancer treatment, such as congestive heart failure, osteoporosis, lymphedema, and neuropathy. Chemotherapy-induced peripheral neuropathy (CIPN) is a common acute and long-term effect of many cancer treatments and may have a significant impact on QoL for survivors by disrupting mobility, proprioception, balance, and functional status. When numbness is present with CIPN, patients may describe "clumsiness" such as tripping or dropping objects due to decreased sensation in their hands and feet. Some survivors may not associate these incidents with their cancer treatment, but discussing a possible correlation with CIPN as well as providing guidance may help patients understand unexplained symptoms and prevent potential injury. For those survivors who have chronic, symptomatic neurotoxicity from chemotherapy, PCPs should discuss with patients the overall burden and impact of symptoms on their lives, as well as the risks and benefits of pharmacologic treatment (75). Non-pharmacologic treatment of CIPN should include physical therapy for mobility concerns, targeted exercise, and fall prevention (75). Pharmacologic therapy for painful CIPN may provide modest benefits (76), with evidence supporting the use of duloxetine as a multimodal treatment for patients who also may have anxiety, depression, or chronic musculoskeletal pain (76). CIPN may improve gradually, but neuropathy that is worsening more than a year after the end of active treatment should be evaluated further as other causes of neuropathy may coexist. PCP's are familiar with the multiple etiologies of peripheral neuropathy and should utilize this knowledge in counseling and evaluating patients with neuropathy after cancer treatment.

Late effects can present soon after the end of treatment or, as in the case of radiation, up to decades later. One example is radiation-induced tissue fibrosis that can appear years after treatment and may be detected when patients present with new symptoms to their PCP. PCP awareness of these late effects is important in recognizing symptoms and providing timely diagnosis and targeted management, including referral to specialists.

For example, a patient with a history of laryngeal cancer treated 5 years prior with minimally invasive surgery, chemotherapy, and radiation presents with fatigue and dysphagia. The PCP can easily screen for hypothyroidism and mood disorders, but may also need to refer to a multi-disciplinary team for specialized care. Oropharyngeal radiation late effects such as dry mouth and esophageal strictures can severely impact dental health and the complex coordination required for swallowing. Referrals to speech and swallow therapists and radiation oncologists can guide further evaluation and intervention. Survivors should be counseled on meticulous dental hygiene and referred for frequent dental follow up. Difficulty eating can cause nutritional deficiencies and persistent weight loss, both of which can exacerbate fatigue. Dietician referral is important for the assessment of nutritional needs and how to achieve these if food and fluid consistency needs to be modified. By understanding potential late effects, PCPs can screen for symptoms and impact QoL by initiating early intervention.

Prevalent survivorship issues like fatigue, cognitive dysfunction, and sleep disorders have limited evidence-based treatments, though interventions to address these issues are being developed. The time-course of these symptoms depends on each patient's treatment, and mild to moderate symptoms can last months to 1 year or more after completion of cancer therapy (77). We recommend that patients be screened for reversible factors, including mood and sleep disorders, underlying medical conditions, medication adverse effects, and pain. Management may include increased organizational strategies (for example, physical notes, electronic reminders), timing cognitively demanding tasks to highest energy levels, relaxation, regular exercise, psychotherapy, and occupational therapy. In the case of patients with progressive, persistent fatigue presenting months after completing treatment, further evaluation should be carried out. Insomnia treatment can include sleep hygiene education, CBT, pharmacotherapy, regular exercise, referral to a sleep specialist, and treatment of other underlying causes (29).

A prevalent survivorship issue expressed by many patients is the struggle to feel "normal" again after cancer treatment. PCPs can help keep in perspective the significant physical and psychologic stress of cancer treatment and offer reassurance that finding a "new normal" in some situations is acceptable and even desirable and this process is likely to evolve over time. By introducing the concept of a "new normal", PCPs can reframe post-treatment expectations and reduce feelings of pressure that originate either with the patient or their family and friends to return to their pre-cancer selves. The PCP plays a central role in supporting survivors as they establish their "new normals," not only in evaluating symptoms and navigating health plans, but also in actively listening, guiding, and reassuring as needed.

Finally, PCPs should be sensitive about initiating early discussions regarding reproductive health and family planning (78). Referrals to reproductive specialists can be informative, even if a patient is not yet ready to build their family, particularly as gonadal reserve can decline more rapidly in patients with treatment-related fertility risks. Addressing sexual health is also meaningful to many survivors as sexual dysfunction is common in both female and male survivors, such as those undergoing hormonal deprivation therapy for breast and prostate cancer (79). PCPs are typically comfortable with treatment of menopausal symptoms such as hot flashes and vaginal dryness and should discuss these symptoms with young survivors who may experience menopausal symptoms secondary to prior treatment and those undergoing gonadal suppression.

Psychosocial Impact

The psychosocial impacts of cancer survivorship may affect an individual's physical and mental health. Anxiety, depression, post-traumatic stress disorder (PTSD), and fear of recurrence are critical topics to address for survivors. Fear of recurrence is not only one of the most common problems

BOX 14.2 TIPS FOR MANAGING PSYCHOSOCIAL IMPACTS OF CANCER AND TREATMENT

- Acknowledge and validate the fear of recurrence and anxiety surrounding survivorship. Consider starting the conversation as follows: "Many of my patients tell me that they struggle with fear of recurrence after diagnosis and treatment. You've been through a lot. It is normal to have these thoughts. Have you experienced fear of recurrence?"
- Avoid making assumptions about how worried a patient is, or what they are worried about. Instead of telling patients not to worry or to "be positive," which may discourage open communication, tell them that PCPs are a part of the care team and available to discuss concerns. "Fear of recurrence will come and go and change with time, but please come talk to me when you are worried. We can continue to work through this together."
- Be aware that anxiety is often triggered by testing, clinic visits, and waiting for tests results.
- Inquire about the patient's mood directly during multiple visits.
- Identify patients who need further referral to mental health specialists.

reported by survivors, but it is also one with high unmet need (25, 80). About half of all cancer survivors experience moderate to severe levels of fear of recurrence, with 7% reporting highly disabling symptoms (80). These feelings can be isolating and distressing for many survivors and may trigger further depression and PTSD. Poor mental health has negative impacts on QoL and may contribute to common post-treatment symptoms like fatigue and sleep disturbance. Box 14.2 provides some tips for PCPs in enquiring about psychological or emotional issues that patients may be experiencing.

Many survivors struggle with health anxiety after their cancer diagnosis. For some, health anxiety causes symptom hypervigilance and high health care utilization, but for others, it leads to health care avoidance. Survivors often interpret pain as an indication of a late effect, cancer recurrence, or presentation of a new malignancy. Even minor aches and pains can trigger significant worry and fear of recurrence. PCPs can re-frame some of these concerns with specific guidance for symptoms that may ease health anxiety (for example, see case study in Box 14.3).

Survivors who are parents of non-adult children during treatment may experience marked stress and distress. As Moore et al. discuss, parental cancer diagnosis can change parenting behavior and

BOX 14.3 CASE STUDY: MANAGING HEALTH ANXIETY

CB is 2 years' post-treatment for early stage breast cancer and presents with concerns about 2 days of headache. She is worried that her symptoms may be a sign of brain metastasis. If a thorough history and exam suggest the etiology is most likely a tension headache, it may be reassuring to explain what features of her symptoms make it less likely to be a metastatic recurrence. Discuss that aches and pains are normal after cancer, as is worrying about them. Giving her a specific time frame after which persistent symptoms warrant follow up, as well as specific symptoms that she needs to report urgently will assist and reassure her, in addition to knowing she is being followed carefully. A clear explanation of clinical reasoning and a detailed plan can relieve anxiety and promote appropriate symptom self-management.

parenting efficacy beliefs, namely concern about negative impacts on children and feeling capable to meet their children's needs (81). The physical, functional, and emotional changes of cancer and its treatment including anxiety/depression, fatigue, altered appearance, and decreased mobility can strain the parent's time and capacity for caregiving and alter interactions with their children. Co-parents may also feel significant stress from caregiving and childcare needs. PCPs should consider proactively addressing parenting concerns to help identify parent, co-parent, and child distress. Adult or child psychologists may be able to help parents with counseling and effective communication at a developmentally appropriate level.

The financial consequences of cancer treatment may become a significant source of stress for many survivors and their families. Zafar and Abernethy describe financial toxicity from cancer as both an objective financial burden (direct out-of-pocket costs to the patient) and financial distress (adverse impacts on wellbeing) (82). The financial burden of cancer includes not only the cost of treatment, but also higher medical expenses after treatment. Zafar and Abernethy further report that a large proportion of their studied patients in the US reported "significant" or "catastrophic" financial burden. These costs not only led patients to exhaust savings and accrue excessive debt, but also to alter treatment-related decisions based on cost (83). Some patients may weigh the cost of medication in choosing a treatment, take less medication than prescribed, or forgo basic necessities to afford treatment. Another US study showed that 25% of cancer survivors reported depleting all or most of their savings while being treated for cancer (84). The financial burden of cancer also incorporates reduced income through missed work days, reduced working hours or job loss. Many survivors cannot return to work at the same capacity, if at all, during and after treatment. Household financial support may also be impacted as partners, caregivers, and other family members may miss work due to changes in caregiving roles, transportation to appointments, and childcare.

Prevention and Health Promotion

Within a survivor's health care team, PCPs are the most comfortable with and best equipped to manage preventive care. Vaccination, however, is a common source of confusion for survivors and PCPs. Though hopefully done before immunosuppressive treatments like chemotherapy, most survivors should have their routine vaccinations up-to-date. Typically, non-live vaccines can be given three or more months after chemotherapy while influenza vaccines can be given during chemotherapy. Special considerations should be made for live vaccines (contraindicated in active immunosuppression), timing of vaccines after chemotherapy and B-cell therapy, surgical/functional asplenia, and re-vaccination after stem cell transplant (85). PCPs may communicate with specialists in the care team for specific guidance on vaccination for individual patients.

As discussed earlier, health promotion including regular exercise, healthy nutrition, minimizing alcohol intake, and tobacco cessation is important for survivors. Substance use and poor control of modifiable cardiovascular risk factors such as hypertension, diabetes, and obesity can also amplify the risks of cardiovascular late effects from certain treatments. PCPs are central in helping survivors control these factors through regular follow-up and consistent patient education. These efforts can positively impact a patient's functional status and QoL in addition to minimizing treatment-related effects and, in some cases, recurrence risk (56–58). Increased physical activity may also mitigate ongoing pain, fatigue, emotional distress, and bone loss. Some survivors are deconditioned after treatment, so exercise must be tailored to the ability and limitations of the patient and up-titrated as tolerated. PCPs can suggest supervised exercise programs, aquatic therapy, and social support like a "workout buddy" as appropriate. Setting specific, attainable aerobic and strengthening goals or defining a certain amount of time to exercise per week may help patients stay active every day. The NCCN survivorship guidelines for patients include examples of types of physical activity and goals that patients and PCPs can utilize as a resource (85).

Comorbidity Management

Cancer survivors may be unsure if and how their cancer treatment may affect their other chronic comorbidities. As PCPs are well-versed in managing multiple chronic conditions, primary care is well-placed to provide management of comorbidities. Asking a patient's oncology team (medical, surgical, and/or radiation oncologist) about potential sequelae of prior or ongoing treatments for diseases like diabetes and hypertension may be helpful for both the PCP and the patient. PCPs can be instrumental for central oversight of survivorship care, particularly as some survivors need to see several specialists and may become overwhelmed with appointments, medication changes, and testing. Care coordination and empathic communication, such as distilling complex information from specialists, can be the difference between overwhelming, siloed care and integrated, holistic care.

MODELS OF POST-TREATMENT FOLLOW UP CARE

Traditionally, follow-up care for cancer survivors has been hospital-based and led by specialists, however PCP- or GP-led models, nurse-led models, and shared care models are increasingly being explored and recommended (86–88). A primary care-led survivorship clinic is described in Box 14.4.

BOX 14.4   CASE STUDY: PILOT OF A PRIMARY
CARE CANCER SURVIVORSHIP CLINIC

One of the authors of this chapter (JK) established the Primary Care Cancer Survivorship Clinic at Stanford University in Palo Alto, California. This model was focused on addressing the transition from oncology to primary care-based care after the completion of active cancer treatment.

The pilot started with one internal medicine-trained PCP, who provided both survivorship and ongoing primary care. The scope of practice was initially limited to breast and gynecologic cancers to facilitate development of expertise in specific treatments and survivorship issues in these patient populations. The PCP underwent training through available online survivorship curricula, survivorship-focused national conferences, and observing breast and gynecological oncology visits. The PCP also partnered with a breast oncologist "champion", a colleague who was readily available through email and text message for discussion and questions during the first 3 months of the pilot.

Aims of the initial 1–3 visits were to discuss a treatment summary with the patient as well as a comprehensive plan for any long-term and late effects, surveillance of the primary cancer, screening for secondary malignancy, preventive care, comorbidity management, as well as a number of physical and psychosocial survivorship issues including mood, fear of recurrence, fertility, sexual health, exercise, and nutrition.

In order to maintain sustainability of this clinic, the model evolved into a consultative approach where each patient had between 1 and 6 visits to complete survivorship discussions, then transitioned to another PCP for ongoing care. The final clinic note was provided to the patient and PCP as both a treatment summary and an individualized guide for the survivorship care plan.

A review of this 3-year pilot through 20 patient interviews found that 100% of participants were satisfied with their primary care survivorship experience and felt it was helpful. 70% felt their visits improved their confidence in self-management. 90% felt all cancer survivors should have a visit in a primary care-based cancer survivorship clinic. 70% of participants thought primary care was the right space for this clinic.

EVIDENCE TO SUPPORT PRIMARY CARE

Evidence suggests that follow-up that is led by specialist oncologists, without involving PCPs, results in sub-optimal management of comorbid health conditions, suboptimal health promotion and attention to health risk factors (89–94). A recent audit of hospital-based follow-up for colorectal cancer survivors suggested that essential elements of survivorship care such as primary cancer screening, discussion of psychosocial impacts and social or practical challenges were poorly addressed in hospital appointments with oncology providers (95). This study also indicated evidence of overuse of specialist-led follow-up, with some patients receiving more than the recommended number of hospital visits, suggesting this model represents an inefficient use of limited oncology services.

Compelling evidence, discussed below, suggests that optimal care of cancer survivors must involve PCPs, either via PCP-led care or a shared care model, to ensure that all health care needs are adequately and efficiently met.

Greater Preventive Care

A number of large observational studies using cancer registry and Medicare data in the US have investigated provision of preventive care in primary care, mixed or oncology settings, and have shown that patients receive preventive care at higher rates when PCPs are involved (90, 94, 96, 97).

Two studies of colorectal cancer survivors in the first 5 years post-treatment found that patients exclusively seeing their PCP were more likely to receive influenza vaccination, cholesterol screening, bone densitometry, mammograms, and cervical cancer screening compared with patients exclusively seeing their oncologist for cancer follow-up (90). The group most likely to receive preventive care was patients who visited both their PCP and oncologist for survivorship care. This trend has also been observed in breast cancer survivors between 1 and 5 years post-diagnosis (94). Likewise a further study found that increased rates of preventive care, including influenza vaccination, cholesterol screening, and colorectal cancer screening, were positively associated with PCP visits in prostate cancer survivors in the first 12 months following treatment (96). Longer-term data looking at colorectal cancer survivors 5–10 years post-diagnosis found that, compared with seeing an oncologist only, survivors were more likely to receive influenza and pneumococcal vaccination, cholesterol screening, and bone densitometry when seeing their PCP only, and most likely to receive all of these services when seeing both their PCP and oncologist (97).

Greater Care for Comorbidities

Another critical element of survivorship care is management of comorbidities. Some studies suggest that cancer survivors are less likely than people without a personal cancer history to receive care for comorbid conditions (89, 93). One US study investigated comorbidity care for colorectal cancer survivors 2–3 years post-diagnosis by looking at associations between the type of provider patients visited and a range of comorbidity quality indicators (92). Patients who saw a PCP were more likely to receive recommended care for chronic conditions (including lipid profile, diabetic eye exam, and diabetic monitoring) compared with those who did not see a PCP. Similarly, an additional study of colorectal cancer survivors found that those who received care exclusively from a PCP compared to an oncologist were more likely to receive comorbidity management, and those who saw both were most likely to receive care for comorbid illness (89). A recent Australian audit examined documentation following follow up visits between colorectal survivors and oncology providers, mostly surgeons (95). While there was documentation of aspects such as history and examination, physical effects, and screening for recurrence, there was little focus on management of comorbid disease, health behaviors, and health maintenance (95).

PCP or GP-led vs Oncology-led Follow-up

Landmark studies by Grunfeld and colleagues were the first to show that GP or PCP-led follow-up is a safe, effective and acceptable alternative to hospital (cancer center)-based survivorship care for survivors of stage I–III breast cancer (14, 98–100). Clinical outcomes, such as detection of recurrence and time to diagnosis, and health-related QoL appeared similar (98). Patients assigned to GP-led care reported higher satisfaction (14), and reduced costs at both the patient and health care system level (100).

Subsequently, RCTs have examined GP-led follow-up for survivors of colon cancer (101, 102) and melanoma (103). These trials found no differences between groups in clinical outcomes (number and time to recurrence, death) or patient-reported outcomes including QoL, anxiety, and depression. GP-led care resulted in greater patient satisfaction in one study (103) and reduced costs in another (101).

A recent systematic review has collated the evidence for PCP versus cancer specialist follow up (104). The review found there were no differences in clinical outcomes of survival, or serious clinical events including recurrence (both number and time to diagnosis), disease spread, new cancer or death between primary care compared with hospital-based specialist care, indicating that the two models are equivalent regarding these outcomes. Differences were seen however in two studies that assessed adherence to follow-up guidelines; one UK study found that melanoma survivors receiving follow-up care in primary care more likely to be seen according to guidelines compared to those receiving follow-up care in the hospital (103); and one Australian study of colon cancer survivors found that those in primary care more likely to have fecal occult blood testing and those seeing their surgeon more likely to have ultrasounds and colonoscopies (102).

The review also considered a number of patient-reported outcomes, including QoL, anxiety and depression, physical symptoms, and patient satisfaction. There were no differences in overall QoL between primary and hospital-based care, however one study of colon cancer survivors did find differences in favor of primary care using QoL subscales measuring role functioning, emotional functioning, and pain (101). Four studies looking at anxiety and depression outcomes found no differences, and one study investigating physical symptoms showed that breast cancer patients receiving follow-up in primary care reported less fatigue compared with usual care (105). Results for patient satisfaction were mixed, with two RCTs showing greater satisfaction among patients in primary care, and one study showing outcomes in favor of hospital-based follow-up.

Four studies examining costs unsurprisingly showed lower costs to the health system in primary care vs secondary care, and lower costs to the patient, including time off work, travel, and parking. Overall, evidence indicates equivalent clinical and patient-reported outcomes between hospital-based and primary care models, while primary care incurs lower costs. The generalizability of these results is limited by the fact that most studies focused on breast and colorectal cancer, and were conducted in countries with universal health care (i.e., UK, Canada, and Australia).

Shared Care between Primary Care and Oncology Providers

In addition to transitioning survivorship care entirely to primary care, sharing cancer follow-up care between primary care and oncology providers is a further model of care being investigated (12, 106). One completed randomized controlled trial (RCT) investigated shared care for prostate cancer survivors, where the shared care intervention involved replacing two scheduled hospital follow-up visits with primary care visits, providing GPs with clinical management guidelines, providing both GPs and patients with survivorship care plans and automated appointment reminders, conducting needs assessment and providing patients with information resources. Results indicated that there were no differences between shared and usual care arms regarding adherence to PSA testing or patients' QoL and other patient-reported outcomes, including distress and unmet needs. Importantly, patients who had experienced shared care indicated a preference for shared care compared with usual care. Shared care was also found to cost less per patient compared to usual care (12). A further RCT is currently underway investigating shared care for survivors of colorectal cancer (106). In this trial, shared care similarly involves replacing two scheduled hospital visits with primary care, supporting GPs with information provision such as a survivorship care plan and follow-up guidelines, providing patients with a common concerns checklist and information resources, and an appointment reminder system.

In addition to these studies examining multi-faceted and scheduled shared care interventions, a systematic review of shared survivorship care also included any interventions where GPs were engaged in survivorship care, including by providing GPs with information (107). The review found there were no differences in QoL, psychological distress or physical symptoms for patients receiving shared care compared to usual follow-up, demonstrating that shared care results in equivalent patient-reported outcomes. Participants' attitudes and perceptions of shared care were either equivalent to usual care, with no differences in patient satisfaction, or patients indicated positive attitudes to shared care and their PCPs.

GUIDANCE FOR PRIMARY CARE

Primary care may be more effective at meeting the diverse needs of survivors, however a range of barriers have been identified in engaging and sustaining primary care involvement in cancer and survivorship care.

At a patient level, barriers include not having a known, trusted GP, prior poor experience with a GP, particularly if this involved a delay in cancer diagnosis, reluctance to leave or reduce contact with the hospital team at completion of treatment, patient perceptions that oncologists provide superior care, and patients' expectations and perceptions about the purpose of follow-up care, particularly around detection of recurrent cancer (13, 108–111). PCPs, who may see patients infrequently during active treatment, may feel insufficiently trained in and communicated with about survivorship issues. Furthermore, many countries, including the US, Canada, and Australia, have no billing code associated with survivorship care available for PCPs, so it is not recognized as a reimbursable service. Other barriers to primary care involvement include a lack of communication between hospital-based and PCPs, lack of evidence-based follow-up guidelines for primary care, and inconsistent or absent policy to support primary care involvement (110).

Guidelines

A number of organizations and professional societies have developed guidelines around post-treatment survivorship care. In the US, these include the American Cancer Society (112), ASCO (113), and the NCCN (77). The Children's Oncology Group also have comprehensive guidelines for the long-term follow-up of childhood cancer survivors (74).

Some (though not all) of these guidelines consider survivorship care broadly and holistically, focusing on the four broad goals stated in the IOM report; others focus largely on surveillance testing. The role of PCPs, however, is often unclear within these guidelines. It should be noted that the level of evidence to support recommendations is variable, and often recommendations are based on expert opinion. It will be important to develop guidelines which are shown to result in improved outcomes for cancer survivors, in a sustainable, cost effective manner.

It should be noted that some studies have shown that routine surveillance testing does not lead to improved outcomes. This is true for survivors of diffuse large B cell lymphoma (114), routine CA-125 tumor marker monitoring in ovarian cancer (115) and surveillance for metastases in breast cancer survivors (116). Other studies investigating detection of recurrence suggest that there is no association between intense, hospital-based surveillance and detection of recurrence for breast or colorectal cancer (117, 118).

Guidance for Shared Care

This chapter has discussed various models of follow-up care, including shared care between primary care and oncology providers. In keeping with the growing push for alternative survivorship care models, resources to support shared care have been developed and are becoming increasingly available (87, 110, 119). Evidence-based guidance relevant to primary care to support shared survivorship care is described in Box 14.5.

Improved survivorship care models must be responsive to the needs of individuals, with a shift away from the current one-size-fits-all approach to follow-up; not all patients will be suitable for shared care. For an individual patient, the most suitable model of post-treatment survivorship care will be impacted by a number of factors: type of cancer and type of treatments, time since completing treatment, current and anticipated issues, patient-expressed needs and concerns, comorbid illness, the patient's ability and confidence to self-manage, the patient's relationship with their oncology providers and PCP, and practical considerations such as the distance to and ability to travel to treatment centers and providers.

**BOX 14.5   GUIDANCE TO SUPPORT SHARED
SURVIVORSHIP CARE (ADAPTED FROM (110, 119))**

- Consider which patients might be suitable for shared care based on factors such as risk of recurrence or new cancers; persistent, complex side effects; personal circumstances; and capacity for self-management. Recognizing that patients' circumstances and risk profiles may change over time, it is important to re-assess patients and change the model of care if suitable.
- GPs should be involved as part of the shared care team from the point of diagnosis onwards. This may include GPs attending or dialing in to multidisciplinary meetings if this is practical.
- Provide a direct line of communication between primary care and oncology providers. Avoid placing responsibility on the patient for communication between providers in a shared care team.
- GPs should be provided with information about patients' diagnoses, treatment history, and potential long-term and late effects.
- GPs should be provided with clear and concise guidance regarding their role in cancer follow-up care, including timelines, actions required and communication with specialists or re-referral if recurrence is suspected.
- Additional survivorship training or education courses and resources should be available for GPs but not required.
- Establish rapid referral pathways to oncology providers if recurrence or other serious events are suspected.
- Engage patients in shared care by promoting and communicating the benefits of shared follow-up, such as greater continuity of care with their GP, reduced travel and waiting times.
- Both oncologists and GPs should discuss shared care with patients early so they know to expect shared care and consider this standard. If patients do not have a known or trusted GP, it may be helpful for oncology providers to work with the patient to find a suitable GP for shared care.
- Educate patients on the GP's role in follow-up care and how to navigate which provider to see for specific concerns and symptoms.

Patients treated with complex regimens who have significant symptom burden or multiple physical, emotional and social impacts may require much of their survivorship care to be provided by specialist services. For example, a patient who recently completed combined chemotherapy and radiation for head and neck cancer. In contrast, a patient who has recently had surgical resection only for an early stage melanoma, or someone who completed treatment for an early stage colon cancer 5 years prior may be managed entirely in the primary care setting. Another patient, having ongoing oral hormonal therapy, but who has completed surgery, chemotherapy, biological, and radiotherapy, may be managed in a shared care arrangement between oncology and primary care.

There should be ongoing communication between specialist oncology care and primary care. Rapid and reliable channels of communication (direct phone numbers, email) between cancer center and primary care-based members of a shared care team are recommended. Electronic medical records that can be accessed by different providers across multiple sites may also enhance communication by sharing information in real-time. Finally, survivorship care plans may be useful in communicating expectations around care and follow-up schedules between patients and their providers.

As noted elsewhere in this chapter, PCPs value specific guidance and information from cancer teams. Key recommendations to support primary care involvement in survivorship care include providing PCPs with diagnostic and treatment summaries, information about prognosis and likely outcomes, clear and concise guidance regarding cancer follow-up care, particularly regarding rapid re-access pathways back into the hospital/cancer center if recurrence or another serious event is suspected. The roles and responsibilities of each provider need to be clarified and documented to both providers and patients.

Patient benefits of PCP-led or shared survivorship care include greater continuity of care; more holistic, whole-person care; reduced waiting and travel times; and lower associated costs such as parking and time off work. Some of these benefits may be particularly relevant for patients who live rurally, as the integration of PCPs in cancer treatment is geographically necessary in certain settings. Discussing these benefits with patients may increase acceptance of receiving PCP-led or shared survivorship care.

EDUCATION FOR PCPS

Rubin and colleagues (3) suggest that cancer remains underrepresented in undergraduate and postgraduate medical curricula. US studies have shown limited awareness by PCPs of potential long-term and late effects from cancer treatments (120, 121). Oncology is not commonly offered in GP trainee rotations in the UK, and was rated as the most poorly taught area out ten subspecialty areas in PCP residency programs in Canada (3). Another study from England found that though GPs often provide care to people living beyond cancer, many GPs do not feel confident managing survivors' concerns and express interest in further education to improve knowledge and expertise (9).

It is clear that greater focus should be placed on training of the primary care workforce across the cancer continuum. Joint training between oncology and primary care could build confidence and trust, promote ongoing communication and support shared management. Communication between oncology and primary care is an opportunity for education. Likewise, educational interventions for PCPs can and should be embedded in new models of care.

A number of free online cancer survivorship focused educational courses have been developed, including those focused specifically on PCPs (Box 14.6).

The Australian Cancer Survivorship Centre has also coordinated a placement program for PCPs in Victoria, Australia (122, 123). This involved GPs, primary health care nurses and community based allied health providers spending time with oncology teams with the goals of building trust and collaboration, gaining understanding of each other's roles, building skills around survivorship care, and supporting

BOX 14.6 SURVIVORSHIP EDUCATION COURSES

CANCER SURVIVORSHIP FOR PRIMARY CARE PRACTITIONERS
- Hosted by Future Learn and developed by University of Melbourne and Victorian Comprehensive Cancer Centre, Australia.
- Aimed at primary care providers, this course covers the physical and psychosocial effects of cancer, emerging therapies and approaches to patient care.
- Website: https://www.futurelearn.com/courses/cancer-survivorship

CANCER SURVIVORSHIP COURSE FOR PRIMARY CARE PHYSICIANS
- Developed by Stanford University.
- Presents basic principles of cancer survivorship, the role of primary care, and provides practical tools and tips for patient care targeting to primary care providers.
- Website: https://med.stanford.edu/aftercancer/our-programs/cancer-survivorship-course-primary-care-physicians.html

CANCER SURVIVORSHIP E-LEARNING SERIES FOR PRIMARY CARE PROVIDERS
- Developed by the American Cancer Society and the GW Cancer Centre.
- Covers the role of primary care providers and the purpose of survivorship care, with modules focused on follow-up for prostate, colorectal, breast, and head and neck cancers.
- Website: https://cme.smhs.gwu.edu/gw-cancer-center-/content/cancer-survivorship-e-learning-series-primary-care-providers

CANCER SURVIVORSHIP
- Hosted by eviQ Education at Cancer Institute NSW, Australia and developed by the Australian Cancer Survivorship Centre.
- Introductory course for health professionals that covers the basics of cancer survivorship, as well as models of care and survivorship care plans.
- Website: https://education.eviq.org.au/courses/supportive-care/cancer-survivorship

shared management. The program was feasible at multiple sites in the state and participants felt that it improved their knowledge and skills around survivorship care.

SUMMARY

Primary care has an important role in managing many facets of cancer survivorship care, particularly in the face of the growing cancer survivorship population. Primary care is well-placed to manage late and long-term effects from cancer and its treatment, manage comorbidities, provide holistic support for common survivorship issues, encourage healthy lifestyle behaviors, as well as assist with surveillance for recurrent or subsequent cancers. Evidence supports the importance of primary care in these roles, indicating that survivors who receive some or all of their survivorship care in primary care settings receive greater preventive care and comorbidity management, with equivalent clinical and QoL outcomes. While the role of primary care is not well-documented in current follow-up guidelines, guidance to support increased inclusion of primary care in survivorship is emerging. Opportunities for cancer survivorship education for PCPs may further build capacity.

REFERENCES

1. World Health Organization. Available from: https://www.euro.who.int/en/health-topics/Health-systems/primary-health-care/main-terminology.
2. Atun R. What are the advantages and disadvantages of restructuring a health care system to be more focused on primary care services?: Copenhagen, WHO Regional Office for Europe (Health Evidence Network report; https://www.euro.who.int/__data/assets/pdf_file/0004/74704/E82997.pdf; accessed 21 October 2020); 2004.
3. Rubin G, Berendsen A, Crawford SM, Dommett R, Earle C, Emery J, et al. The expanding role of primary care in cancer control. *Lancet Oncol.* 2015;16(12):1231–72.
4. Miller KD, Nogueira L, Mariotto AB, Rowland JH, Yabroff KR, Alfano CM, et al. Cancer treatment and survivorship statistics, 2019. *CA Cancer J Clin.* 2019;69(5):363–85.
5. Maddams J, Utley M, Moller H. Projections of cancer prevalence in the United Kingdom, 2010–2040. *Br J Cancer.* 2012;107(7):1195–202.
6. Brandenbarg D, Roorda C, Groenhof F, de Bock GH, Berger MY, Berendsen AJ. Primary healthcare use during follow-up after curative treatment for colorectal cancer. *Eur J Cancer Care.* 2017;26(3).
7. Khan NF, Watson E, Rose PW. Primary care consultation behaviours of long-term, adult survivors of cancer in the UK. *Br J Gen Pract.* 2011;61(584):197–9.
8. Roorda C, Berendsen AJ, Groenhof F, van der Meer K, de Bock GH. Increased primary healthcare utilisation among women with a history of breast cancer. *Support Care Cancer.* 2013;21(4):941–9.
9. Walter FM, Usher-Smith JA, Yadlapalli S, Watson E. Caring for people living with, and beyond, cancer: an online survey of GPs in England. *Br J Gen Pract.* 2015;65(640):e761–8.
10. Emery JD, Shaw K, Williams B, Mazza D, Fallon-Ferguson J, Varlow M, et al. The role of primary care in early detection and follow-up of cancer. *Nat Rev Clin Oncol.* 2014;11(1):38–48.
11. O'Brien R, Rose PW, Campbell C, Weller D, Neal RD, Wilkinson C, et al. Experiences of follow-up after treatment in patients with prostate cancer: a qualitative study. *BJU Int.* 2010;106(7):998–1003.
12. Emery JD, Jefford M, King M, Hayne D, Martin A, Doorey J, et al. ProCare Trial: a phase II randomized controlled trial of shared care for follow-up of men with prostate cancer. *BJU Int.* 2017;119(3):381–9.
13. Frew G, Smith A, Zutshi B, Young N, Aggarwal A, Jones P, et al. Results of a quantitative survey to explore both perceptions of the purposes of follow-up and preferences for methods of follow-up delivery among service users, primary care practitioners and specialist clinicians after cancer treatment. *Clin Oncol (R Coll Radiol).* 2010;22(10):874–84.
14. Grunfeld E, Fitzpatrick R, Mant D, Yudkin P, Adewuyi-Dalton R, Stewart J, et al. Comparison of breast cancer patient satisfaction with follow-up in primary care versus specialist care: results from a randomized controlled trial. *Br J Gen Pract.* 1999;49(446):705–10.
15. Hewitt M, Greenfield, S., Stovall, E. *From Cancer Patient to Cancer Survivor: Lost in Transition.* Washington, DC: National Academies Press; 2006.
16. Mahumud RA, Alam K, Dunn J, Gow J. The burden of chronic diseases among Australian cancer patients: evidence from a longitudinal exploration, 2007–2017. *PLOS ONE.* 2020;15(2):e0228744.
17. Dowling EC, Chawla N, Forsythe LP, de Moor J, McNeel T, Rozjabek HM, et al. Lost productivity and burden of illness in cancer survivors with and without other chronic conditions. *Cancer.* 2013;119(18):3393–401.
18. Foster C, Wright D, Hill H, Hopkinson J, Roffe L. Psychosocial implications of living 5 years or more following a cancer diagnosis: a systematic review of the research evidence. *Eur J Cancer Care.* 2009;18(3):223–47.
19. Glaser AW, Fraser LK, Corner J, Feltbower R, Morris EJ, Hartwell G, et al. Patient-reported outcomes of cancer survivors in England 1–5 years after diagnosis: a cross-sectional survey. *BMJ Open.* 2013;3(4).
20. Harrison SE, Watson EK, Ward AM, Khan NF, Turner D, Adams E, et al. Primary health and supportive care needs of long-term cancer survivors: a questionnaire survey. *J Clin Oncol.* 2011;29(15):2091–8.
21. Jefford M, Karahalios E, Pollard A, Baravelli C, Carey M, Franklin J, et al. Survivorship issues following treatment completion—results from focus groups with Australian cancer survivors and health professionals. *J Cancer Surviv.* 2008;2(1):20–32.
22. Jefford M, Ward AC, Lisy K, Lacey K, Emery JD, Glaser AW, et al. Patient-reported outcomes in cancer survivors: a population-wide cross-sectional study. *Support Care Cancer.* 2017;25(10):3171–9.
23. Stein KD, Syrjala KL, Andrykowski MA. Physical and psychological long-term and late effects of cancer. *Cancer.* 2008;112(11 Suppl):2577–92.
24. Watson E, Shinkins B, Frith E, Neal D, Hamdy F, Walter F, et al. Symptoms, unmet needs, psychological well-being and health status in survivors of prostate cancer: implications for redesigning follow-up. *BJU Int.* 2016;117(6B):E10–9.

25. Lisy K, Langdon L, Piper A, Jefford M. Identifying the most prevalent unmet needs of cancer survivors in Australia: a systematic review. *Asia Pac J Clin Oncol.* 2019.
26. Hoekstra RA, Heins MJ, Korevaar JC. Health care needs of cancer survivors in general practice: a systematic review. *BMC Fam Pract.* 2014;15:94.
27. Corbett TK, Groarke A, Devane D, Carr E, Walsh JC, McGuire BE. The effectiveness of psychological interventions for fatigue in cancer survivors: systematic review of randomised controlled trials. *Syst Rev.* 2019;8(1):324.
28. Kessels E, Husson O, van der Feltz-Cornelis CM. The effect of exercise on cancer-related fatigue in cancer survivors: a systematic review and meta-analysis. *Neuropsychiatr Dis Treat.* 2018;14:479–94.
29. Qaseem A, Kansagara D, Forciea MA, Cooke M, Denberg TD, Clinical Guidelines Committee of the American College of Physicians. Management of chronic insomnia disorder in adults: a clinical practice guideline from the American College of Physicians. *Ann Intern Med.* 2016;165(2):125–33.
30. Sun H, Huang H, Ji S, Chen X, Xu Y, Zhu F, et al. The efficacy of cognitive behavioral therapy to treat depression and anxiety and improve quality of life among early-stage breast cancer patients. *Integr Cancer Ther.* 2019;18:1534735419829573.
31. Oberoi S, Yang J, Woodgate RL, Niraula S, Banerji S, Israels SJ, et al. Association of mindfulness-based interventions with anxiety severity in adults with cancer: a systematic review and meta-analysis. *JAMA Netw Open.* 2020;3(8):e2012598.
32. Butow PN, Turner J, Gilchrist J, Sharpe L, Smith AB, Fardell JE, et al. Randomized trial of ConquerFear: a novel, theoretically based psychosocial intervention for fear of cancer recurrence. *J Clin Oncol.* 2017;35(36):4066–77.
33. Mayo SJ, Lustberg M, H MD, Nakamura ZM, Allen DH, Von Ah D, et al. Cancer-related cognitive impairment in patients with non-central nervous system malignancies: an overview for oncology providers from the MASCC Neurological Complications Study Group. *Support Care Cancer.* 2021 Jun;29(6):2821–2840.
34. Paice JA, Portenoy R, Lacchetti C, Campbell T, Cheville A, Citron M, et al. Management of chronic pain in survivors of adult cancers: American Society of Clinical Oncology Clinical Practice Guideline. *J Clin Oncol.* 2016;34(27):3325–45.
35. Oeffinger KC, Mertens AC, Sklar CA, Kawashima T, Hudson MM, Meadows AT, et al. Chronic health conditions in adult survivors of childhood cancer. *N Engl J Med.* 2006;355(15):1572–82.
36. Berendsen AJ, Groot Nibbelink A, Blaauwbroek R, Berger MY, Tissing WJ. Second cancers after childhood cancer—GPs beware! *Scand J Prim Health Care.* 2013;31(3):147–52.
37. Geramita EM, Parker IR, Brufsky JW, Diergaarde B, van Londen GJ. Primary care providers' knowledge, attitudes, beliefs, and practices regarding their preparedness to provide cancer survivorship care. *J Cancer Educ.* 2020;35(6):1219–26.
38. Abdel-Rahman O. Causes of death in long-term lung cancer survivors: a SEER database analysis. *Curr Med Res Opin.* 2017;33(7):1343–8.
39. Anderson C, Lund JL, Weaver MA, Wood WA, Olshan AF, Nichols HB. Noncancer mortality among adolescents and young adults with cancer. *Cancer.* 2019;125(12):2107–14.
40. Fossa SD, Gilbert E, Dores GM, Chen J, McGlynn KA, Schonfeld S, et al. Noncancer causes of death in survivors of testicular cancer. *J Natl Cancer Inst.* 2007;99(7):533–44.
41. Kong J, Diao X, Diao F, Fan X, Zheng J, Yan D, et al. Causes of death in long-term bladder cancer survivors: a population-based study. *Asia Pac J Clin Oncol.* 2019;15(5):e167–e74.
42. Oh CM, Lee D, Kong HJ, Lee S, Won YJ, Jung KW, et al. Causes of death among cancer patients in the era of cancer survivorship in Korea: attention to the suicide and cardiovascular mortality. *Cancer Med.* 2020;9(5):1741–52.
43. Ye Y, Otahal P, Marwick TH, Wills KE, Neil AL, Venn AJ. Cardiovascular and other competing causes of death among patients with cancer from 2006 to 2015: an Australian population-based study. *Cancer.* 2019;125(3):442–52.
44. Zaorsky NG, Churilla TM, Egleston BL, Fisher SG, Ridge JA, Horwitz EM, et al. Causes of death among cancer patients. *Ann Oncol.* 2017;28(2):400–7.
45. Afifi AM, Saad AM, Al-Husseini MJ, Elmehrath AO, Northfelt DW, Sonbol MB. Causes of death after breast cancer diagnosis: a US population-based analysis. *Cancer.* 2020;126(7):1559–67.
46. Koczwara B, Meng R, Miller MD, Clark RA, Kaambwa B, Marin T, et al. Late mortality in people with cancer: a population-based Australian study. *Med J Aust.* 2020.
47. Browman GP, Wong G, Hodson I, Sathya J, Russell R, McAlpine L, et al. Influence of cigarette smoking on the efficacy of radiation therapy in head and neck cancer. *N Engl J Med.* 1993;328(3):159–63.
48. Gritz ER, Carmack CL, de Moor C, Coscarelli A, Schacherer CW, Meyers EG, et al. First year after head and neck cancer: quality of life. *J Clin Oncol.* 1999;17(1):352–60.
49. Ramaswamy AT, Toll BA, Chagpar AB, Judson BL. Smoking, cessation, and cessation counseling in patients with cancer: a population-based analysis. *Cancer.* 2016;122(8):1247–53.
50. Stead LF, Buitrago D, Preciado N, Sanchez G, Hartmann-Boyce J, Lancaster T. Physician advice for smoking cessation. *Cochrane Database Syst Rev.* 2013(5):CD000165.
51. West R, Raw M, McNeill A, Stead L, Aveyard P, Bitton J, et al. Health-care interventions to promote and assist tobacco cessation: a review of efficacy, effectiveness and affordability for use in national guideline development. *Addiction.* 2015;110(9):1388–403.
52. Anderson P, O'Donnell A, Kaner E. Managing alcohol use disorder in primary health care. *Curr Psychiatry Rep.* 2017;19(11):79.
53. Beyer F, Lynch E, Kaner E. Brief interventions in primary care: an evidence overview of practitioner and digital intervention programmes. *Curr Addict Rep.* 2018;5(2):265–73.

54. Beyer FR, Campbell F, Bertholet N, Daeppen JB, Saunders JB, Pienaar ED, et al. The Cochrane 2018 review on brief interventions in primary care for hazardous and harmful alcohol consumption: a distillation for clinicians and policy makers. *Alcohol Alcohol.* 2019;54(4):417–27.

55. O'Donnell A, Anderson P, Newbury-Birch D, Schulte B, Schmidt C, Reimer J, et al. The impact of brief alcohol interventions in primary healthcare: a systematic review of reviews. *Alcohol Alcohol.* 2014;49(1):66–78.

56. Kwan ML, Kushi LH, Weltzien E, Tam EK, Castillo A, Sweeney C, et al. Alcohol consumption and breast cancer recurrence and survival among women with early-stage breast cancer: the life after cancer epidemiology study. *J Clin Oncol.* 2010;28(29):4410–6.

57. LoConte NK, Brewster AM, Kaur JS, Merrill JK, Alberg AJ. Alcohol and cancer: a statement of the American Society of Clinical Oncology. *J Clin Oncol.* 2018;36(1):83–93.

58. Bryant J, Yoong SL, Sanson-Fisher R, Mazza D, Carey M, Walsh J, et al. Is identification of smoking, risky alcohol consumption and overweight and obesity by General Practitioners improving? A comparison over time. *Fam Pract.* 2015;32(6):664–71.

59. Ligibel JA, Alfano CM, Courneya KS, Demark-Wahnefried W, Burger RA, Chlebowski RT, et al. American Society of Clinical Oncology position statement on obesity and cancer. *J Clin Oncol.* 2014;32(31):3568–74.

60. Aveyard P, Lewis A, Tearne S, Hood K, Christian-Brown A, Adab P, et al. Screening and brief intervention for obesity in primary care: a parallel, two-arm, randomised trial. *Lancet.* 2016;388(10059):2492–500.

61. Carvajal R, Wadden TA, Tsai AG, Peck K, Moran CH. Managing obesity in primary care practice: a narrative review. *Ann N Y Acad Sci.* 2013;1281:191–206.

62. de Heer H, Kinslow B, Lane T, Tuckman R, Warren M. Only 1 in 10 patients told to lose weight seek help from a health professional: a nationally representative sample. *Am J Health Promot.* 2019;33(7):1049–52.

63. Jackson SE, Wardle J, Johnson F, Finer N, Beeken RJ. The impact of a health professional recommendation on weight loss attempts in overweight and obese British adults: a cross-sectional analysis. *BMJ Open.* 2013;3(11):e003693.

64. Schmid D, Leitzmann MF. Association between physical activity and mortality among breast cancer and colorectal cancer survivors: a systematic review and meta-analysis. *Ann Oncol.* 2014;25(7):1293–311.

65. World Cancer Research Fund. Physical activity and the risk of cancer. Available from: https://www.wcrf.org/dietandcancer/exposures/physical-activity.

66. Ibrahim EM, Al-Homaidh A. Physical activity and survival after breast cancer diagnosis: meta-analysis of published studies. *Med Oncol.* 2011;28(3):753–65.

67. Elley CR, Kerse N, Arroll B, Robinson E. Effectiveness of counselling patients on physical activity in general practice: cluster randomised controlled trial. *BMJ.* 2003;326(7393):793.

68. Orrow G, Kinmonth AL, Sanderson S, Sutton S. Effectiveness of physical activity promotion based in primary care: systematic review and meta-analysis of randomised controlled trials. *BMJ.* 2012;344:e1389.

69. Bully P, Sanchez A, Zabaleta-del-Olmo E, Pombo H, Grandes G. Evidence from interventions based on theoretical models for lifestyle modification (physical activity, diet, alcohol and tobacco use) in primary care settings: a systematic review. *Prev Med.* 2015;76 Suppl:S76–93.

70. Northouse L, Williams AL, Given B, McCorkle R. Psychosocial care for family caregivers of patients with cancer. *J Clin Oncol.* 2012;30(11):1227–34.

71. Turner D, Adams E, Boulton M, Harrison S, Khan N, Rose P, et al. Partners and close family members of long-term cancer survivors: health status, psychosocial well-being and unmet supportive care needs. *Psychooncology.* 2013;22(1):12–9.

72. Geller AC, Keske RR, Haneuse S, Davine JA, Emmons KM, Daniel CL, et al. Skin cancer early detection practices among adult survivors of childhood cancer treated with radiation. *J Invest Dermatol.* 2019;139(9):1898–905e2.

73. Henderson TO, Amsterdam A, Bhatia S, Hudson MM, Meadows AT, Neglia JP, et al. Systematic review: surveillance for breast cancer in women treated with chest radiation for childhood, adolescent, or young adult cancer. *Ann Intern Med.* 2010;152(7):444–55; W144–54.

74. Children's Oncology Group. Long-Term Follow-Up Guidelines for Survivors of Childhood, Adolescent, and Young Adult Cancers. Version 5.0 – October 2018.

75. Loprinzi CL, Lacchetti C, Bleeker J, Cavaletti G, Chauhan C, Hertz DL, et al. Prevention and management of chemotherapy-induced peripheral neuropathy in survivors of adult cancers: ASCO guideline update. *J Clin Oncol.* 2020;38(28):3325–48.

76. Smith EM, Pang H, Cirrincione C, Fleishman S, Paskett ED, Ahles T, et al. Effect of duloxetine on pain, function, and quality of life among patients with chemotherapy-induced painful peripheral neuropathy: a randomized clinical trial. *JAMA.* 2013;309(13):1359–67.

77. Denlinger CS, Sanft T, Baker KS, Broderick G, Demark-Wahnefried W, Friedman DL, et al. Survivorship, version 2.2018, NCCN Clinical Practice Guidelines in Oncology. *J Natl Compr Cancer Netw.* 2018;16(10):1216–47.

78. Oktay K, Harvey BE, Partridge AH, Quinn GP, Reinecke J, Taylor HS, et al. Fertility preservation in patients with cancer: ASCO clinical practice guideline update. *J Clin Oncol.* 2018;36(19):1994–2001.

79. Carter J, Lacchetti C, Andersen BL, Barton DL, Bolte S, Damast S, et al. Interventions to address sexual problems in people with cancer: American Society of Clinical Oncology Clinical Practice Guideline Adaptation of Cancer Care Ontario Guideline. *J Clin Oncol.* 2018;36(5):492–511.

80. Simard S, Thewes B, Humphris G, Dixon M, Hayden C, Mireskandari S, et al. Fear of cancer recurrence in adult cancer survivors: a systematic review of quantitative studies. *J Cancer Surviv.* 2013;7(3):300–22.

81. Moore CW, Rauch PK, Baer L, Pirl WF, Muriel AC. Parenting changes in adults with cancer. *Cancer.* 2015;121(19):3551–7.

82. Zafar SY, Abernethy AP. Financial toxicity, Part I: a new name for a growing problem. *Oncology (Williston Park).* 2013;27(2):80–1, 149.

83. Zafar SY, Peppercorn JM, Schrag D, Taylor DH, Goetzinger AM, Zhong X, et al. The financial toxicity of cancer treatment: a pilot study assessing out-of-pocket expenses and the insured cancer patient's experience. *Oncologist.* 2013;18(4):381–90.

84. The USA Today/Kaiser Family Foundation/Harvard School of Public Health. National Survey of Households Affected by Cancer. 2006.

85. Denlinger CS, Sanft T, Moslehi JJ, Overholser L, Armenian S, Baker KS, et al. NCCN Guidelines insights: survivorship, version 2.2020. *J Natl Compr Cancer Netw.* 2020;18(8):1016–23.

86. Alfano CM, Mayer DK, Bhatia S, Maher J, Scott JM, Nekhlyudov L, et al. Implementing personalized pathways for cancer follow-up care in the United States: proceedings from an American Cancer Society-American Society of Clinical Oncology summit. *CA Cancer J Clin.* 2019;69(3):234–47.

87. Cancer Australia. Shared cancer follow-up and survivorship care: early breast cancer. Available from: https://www.canceraustralia.gov.au/clinical-best-practice/shared-follow-care/early-breast-cancer.

88. Cancer Australia. Shared cancer follow-up and survivorship care: low-risk endometrial cancer. Available from: https://www.canceraustralia.gov.au/clinical-best-practice/shared-follow-care/low-risk-endometrial-cancer.

89. Earle CC, Neville BA. Under use of necessary care among cancer survivors. *Cancer.* 2004;101(8):1712–9.

90. Snyder CF, Earle CC, Herbert RJ, Neville BA, Blackford AL, Frick KD. Trends in follow-up and preventive care for colorectal cancer survivors. *J Gen Intern Med.* 2008;23(3):254–9.

91. Snyder CF, Earle CC, Herbert RJ, Neville BA, Blackford AL, Frick KD. Preventive care for colorectal cancer survivors: a 5-year longitudinal study. *J Clin Oncol.* 2008;26(7):1073–9.

92. Snyder CF, Frick KD, Herbert RJ, Blackford AL, Neville BA, Lemke KW, et al. Comorbid condition care quality in cancer survivors: role of primary care and specialty providers and care coordination. *J Cancer Surviv.* 2015;9(4):641–9.

93. Snyder CF, Frick KD, Herbert RJ, Blackford AL, Neville BA, Wolff AC, et al. Quality of care for comorbid conditions during the transition to survivorship: differences between cancer survivors and noncancer controls. *J Clin Oncol.* 2013;31(9):1140–8.

94. Snyder CF, Frick KD, Kantsiper ME, Peairs KS, Herbert RJ, Blackford AL, et al. Prevention, screening, and surveillance care for breast cancer survivors compared with controls: changes from 1998 to 2002. *J Clin Oncol.* 2009;27(7):1054–61.

95. Garwood V, Lisy K, Jefford M. Survivorship in colorectal cancer: a cohort study of the patterns and documented content of follow-up visits. *J Clin Med.* 2020;9(9).

96. Snyder CF, Frick KD, Herbert RJ, Blackford AL, Neville BA, Carducci MA, et al. Preventive care in prostate cancer patients: following diagnosis and for five-year survivors. *J Cancer Surviv.* 2011;5(3):283–91.

97. Steele CB, Townsend JS, Tai E, Thomas CC. Physician visits and preventive care among Asian American and Pacific Islander long-term survivors of colorectal cancer, USA, 1996–2006. *J Cancer Surviv.* 2014;8(1):70–9.

98. Grunfeld E, Mant D, Vessey MP, Yudkin P. Evaluating primary care follow-up of breast cancer: methods and preliminary results of three studies. *Ann Oncol.* 1995;6 Suppl 2:47–52.

99. Grunfeld E, Levine MN, Julian JA, Coyle D, Szechtman B, Mirsky D, et al. Randomized trial of long-term follow-up for early-stage breast cancer: a comparison of family physician versus specialist care. *J Clin Oncol.* 2006;24(6):848–55.

100. Grunfeld E, Gray A, Mant D, Yudkin P, Adewuyi-Dalton R, Coyle D, et al. Follow-up of breast cancer in primary care vs specialist care: results of an economic evaluation. *Br J Cancer.* 1999;79(7–8):1227–33.

101. Augestad KM, Norum J, Dehof S, Aspevik R, Ringberg U, Nestvold T, et al. Cost-effectiveness and quality of life in surgeon versus general practitioner-organised colon cancer surveillance: a randomised controlled trial. *BMJ Open.* 2013;3(4).

102. Wattchow DA, Weller DP, Esterman A, Pilotto LS, McGorm K, Hammett Z, et al. General practice vs surgical-based follow-up for patients with colon cancer: randomised controlled trial. *Br J Cancer.* 2006;94(8):1116–21.

103. Murchie P, Nicolson MC, Hannaford PC, Raja EA, Lee AJ, Campbell NC. Patient satisfaction with GP-led melanoma follow-up: a randomised controlled trial. *Br J Cancer.* 2010;102(10):1447–55.

104. Vos JAM, Wieldraaijer T, van Weert H, van Asselt KM. Survivorship care for cancer patients in primary versus secondary care: a systematic review. *J Cancer Surviv.* 2020.

105. Railton C, Lupichuk S, McCormick J, Zhong L, Ko JJ, Walley B, et al. Discharge to primary care for survivorship follow-up: how are patients with early-stage breast cancer faring? *J Natl Compr Cancer Netw.* 2015;13(6):762–71.

106. Jefford M, Emery J, Grunfeld E, Martin A, Rodger P, Murray AM, et al. SCORE: shared care of Colorectal cancer survivors: protocol for a randomised controlled trial. *Trials [Electronic Resource].* 2017;18(1):506.

107. Zhao Y, Brettle A, Qiu L. The effectiveness of shared care in cancer survivors—a systematic review. *Int J Integr Care.* 2018;18(4):2.

108. Cheung WY, Neville BA, Cameron DB, Cook EF, Earle CC. Comparisons of patient and physician expectations for cancer survivorship care. *J Clin Oncol.* 2009;27(15):2489–95.

109. Lewis R, Neal RD, Williams NH, France B, Wilkinson C, Hendry M, et al. Nurse-led vs. conventional physician-led follow-up for patients with cancer: systematic review. *J Adv Nurs.* 2009;65(4):706–23.

110. Lisy K, Kent J, Dumbrell J, Kelly H, Piper A, Jefford M. Sharing cancer survivorship care between oncology and primary care providers: a qualitative study of health care professionals' experiences. *J Clin Med.* 2020;9(9).

111. Lisy K, Kent J, Piper A, Jefford M. Facilitators and barriers to shared primary and specialist cancer care: a systematic review. *Support Care Cancer*. 2020.
112. American Cancer Society. American Cancer Society Survivorship Care Guidelines. Available from: https://www.cancer.org/health-care-professionals/american-cancer-society-survivorship-guidelines.html.
113. American Society of Clinical Oncology. Available from: https://www.asco.org/practice-policy/cancer-care-initiatives/prevention-survivorship/survivorship-compendium-0.
114. Thompson CA, Ghesquieres H, Maurer MJ, Cerhan JR, Biron P, Ansell SM, et al. Utility of routine post-therapy surveillance imaging in diffuse large B-cell lymphoma. *J Clin Oncol*. 2014;32(31):3506–12.
115. Rustin GJ, van der Burg ME, Griffin CL, Guthrie D, Lamont A, Jayson GC, et al. Early versus delayed treatment of relapsed ovarian cancer (MRC OV05/EORTC 55955): a randomised trial. *Lancet*. 2010;376(9747):1155–63.
116. Jochelson M, Hayes DF, Ganz PA. Surveillance and monitoring in breast cancer survivors: maximizing benefit and minimizing harm. *American Society of Clinical Oncology educational book American Society of Clinical Oncology Annual Meeting*. 2013.
117. Snyder RA, Hu CY, Cuddy A, Francescatti AB, Schumacher JR, Van Loon K, et al. Association between intensity of post-treatment surveillance testing and detection of recurrence in patients with colorectal cancer. *JAMA*. 2018;319(20):2104–15.
118. Hiramanek N. Breast cancer recurrence: follow up after treatment for primary breast cancer. *Postgrad Med J*. 2004;80(941):172–6.
119. Australian Cancer Survivorship Centre. Recommendations for implementing and delivering shared survivorship care: full version. Melbourne, Australia; 2020.
120. Nekhlyudov L, Aziz NM, Lerro C, Virgo KS. Oncologists' and primary care physicians' awareness of late and long-term effects of chemotherapy: implications for care of the growing population of survivors. *J Oncol Pract*. 2014;10(2):e29–36.
121. Potosky AL, Han PK, Rowland J, Klabunde CN, Smith T, Aziz N, et al. Differences between primary care physicians' and oncologists' knowledge, attitudes and practices regarding the care of cancer survivors. *J Gen Intern Med*. 2011;26(12):1403–10.
122. Evans J, Nolte L, Piper A, Simkiss L, Whitfield K, Jefford M. A clinical placement program for primary care professionals at a comprehensive cancer centre. *Aust Fam Physician*. 2016;45(8):606–10.
123. Piper A, Leon L, Kelly H, Bailey A, Wiley G, Lisy K, et al. Clinical placement program in cancer survivorship for primary care providers 2017–2019. *J Cancer Surviv*. 2020;14(1):14–18.

Index

Note: Locators in *italics* represent figures and **bold** indicate tables in the text.

Printed and bound by CPI Group (UK) Ltd, Croydon, CR0 4YY

24/10/2024

01778288-0007